black skin

THE DEFINITIVE
SKINCARE GUIDE

DIJA AYODELE

DEDICATION

For my dearest angels Ōlùwàpāmìlérìn and Ōlùwàtāmìlòrē, the sun and the moon shine for you and I pray you stay true to yourselves and own your beauty. Head up, always!

HQ
An imprint of HarperCollinsPublishers Ltd

1 London Bridge Street
London SE1 9GF

www.harpercollins.co.uk

HarperCollins Publishers
Macken House, 39/40 Mayor Street Upper, Dublin 1, Ireland

First published in Great Britain by
HQ, an imprint of HarperCollinsPublishers Ltd 2021

A catalogue record for this book is available from the British Library.

ISBN: 978-0-00-863981-5

This book contains FSC™ certified paper and other controlled sources to ensure responsible forest management.

For more information visit:
www.harpercollins.co.uk/green

Editor: Nira Begum

Page design and typesetting: Emily Voller Design

Photography: Alamy / Bianca Lawrence / Charisse Kenion / Getty Images / John Godwin / Mackoy Family Collection / Nateisha Scott / Paula's Choice / Pexel / Ruvimbo Kuuzabuwe / Shutterstock / Sophie Harris Taylor / The Hot Mess Photography / Unsplash

Printed and bound in Malaysia by Papercraft

contents

foreword by Caroline Hirons

IN the modern arena where mediocrity is not only endorsed but encouraged, Dija Ayodele personifies the word 'excellence.'

Never settling, always challenging both herself and her peers, to be in the presence of Dija is to fully experience what it looks like when passion comes to life.

To say that the beauty industry has ignored Black women since its inception is an understatement. We all know the names Helena Rubinstein, Elizabeth Arden and Estée Lauder, but not many people have been told the stories of Annie Malone or Madam C.J. Walker.

At a time when all SPF protocols are still written for Caucasian people, and most of the products released by multi-nationals are only trialled on white skins in global territories, the wilful ignorance shown to the Black community by the powers that be in the beauty industry is as shameful as it is unforgiveable.

In 2017, Dija majestically stepped into the skin arena and said, 'if you won't represent us, and you don't talk to us or let us sit at the table, not only will we make our own table, but we'll put it in our own house.' Spotting the huge gap in the provision for Black women across not only professional services, but general skincare information, Dija utilised her professional expertise to the maximum and launched The Black Skin Directory, connecting consumers with highly-qualified and experienced professionals and further connecting those professionals with access to deeper education and information specifically tailored to support the needs of Black skin.

> **We all know the names Helena Rubinstein, Elizabeth Arden and Estée Lauder, but not many people have been told the stories of Annie Malone or Madam C.J. Walker.**

Whether you have purchased this book for personal use, or to support your own professional learning, you will not be disappointed. It is a manual that not only should and will be integrated into professional curriculums, but passed onto friends and family far and wide.

Dija is not only a cheerleader for her community, she's an ally. She is a true visionary and leader in our field, an absolute expert and an exemplary human being that I am privileged to call my friend.

This book is as exceptional as the very fine woman that wrote it.

Caroline Hirons

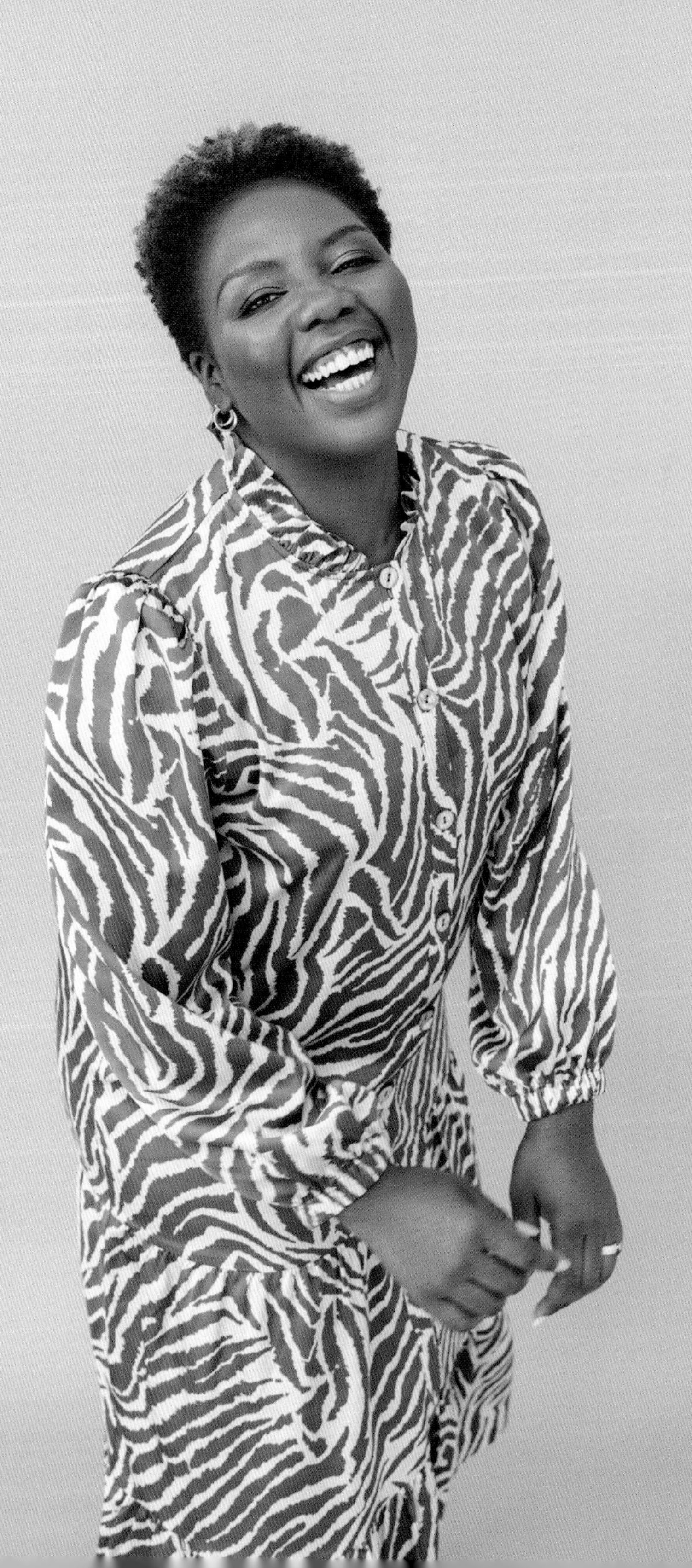

introduction

HELLO, I'm Dija Ayodele (#AuntieDija to some), an aesthetician who specialises in Black skin. I want everyone to have healthy skin, especially Black women and girls. Too often when it comes to beauty, and by extension skincare, we're the last to be considered, so I'm going to flip this around and place you front and centre within these pages.

Healthy skin is happy skin, and I know that both these two things together mean increased self-esteem and confidence. The link between these concepts is very clear and well researched. I see this link play out in my clinic, West Room Aesthetics, in London, every day when I consult with women and they tell me how much make-up they have to apply to cover up the dark marks left from breakouts and acne. Or when they ask – with pleading eyes – if there's a way I can just peel back layers of their skin to make it flawless again.

The bulk of my clinic work is focused on hyperpigmentation concerns and general skin discolouration – key complaints on Black skin – and this has left me with a profound understanding of how confidence is related to the appearance of our skin.

You've heard the phrases 'good skin day' and 'bad skin day' – three little words that can put a pep in your step or trample your self-esteem, because, for many of us, how we feel about our skin impacts our quality of life, our mindset and how we choose to show up in the world. As an aesthetician, I know that, even though I have the best products and tools at my disposal, if I'm not happy about my skin it can dent my confidence and the activities I engage in. I may find myself applying more make-up, or even turning my camera off on a video call. Whilst skin is personal to each of us, it has a social element too, because how we think our skin is perceived by others can take a toll on our mental well-being. Skin is as much a social construct as it is an individual one. One of my favourite books, *The Remarkable Life of the Skin* by Monty Lyman, describes skin as a 'book in which scars, wrinkles and tattoos tell our story and can be read by others.'

A study by Benjamin Barankin and Joel DeKoven in 2002[1] concluded that skin diseases such as acne and dermatitis seriously affect our psychosocial well-being, and that most people under-appreciate this connection. Anxiety and depression are common amongst sufferers, occurring in similar levels seen in patients who have arthritis or other disabling illnesses. Very visible skin disease can lead to societal exclusion and stigmatisation with a massive detrimental effect on quality of life. On top of that, when age and race are factored in, the mental impact of skin disease on Black women at any age is even greater, and I also know this from my own experience.

I've spent enough time speaking to women in my clinic to know that our pursuit of happy skin is an ongoing one. For some it feels like they've been on a desperate journey forever, throwing money and hope into a skincare abyss. By the time they get to me some women are so despondent they are simply looking for someone who looks like them to cut through the noise and bullshit and reassure them of what they should be doing to have healthy skin.

This book is me, on paper. I've over a decade's worth of advanced practical experience caring for skin, mainly Black skin at that. Aside from my CIBTAC (Confederation of International Beauty Therapy and Cosmetology) Level 4 qualification in skincare, I have pursued knowledge about Black skin to the highest level, often working with medical doctors and dermatologists to keep my skills and understanding sharp and relevant. Likewise, my heritage affords me first-hand knowledge of the concerns, the physical legwork and emotional labour that Black women, and other darker skin tones, face in the pursuit to access beauty on equal terms as white women.

Note that when I speak about wanting everyone to have happy skin, I don't say I want everyone to have flawless skin. Before you go any further, I'll just tell you now: flawless skin is for babies. For you and me, adulting in this thing we call life, the flawless skin boat has sailed. There are kinks in everyone's skin; what this book will do is help you iron them out so you can have your *best* skin,

skin that is supple, clear and healthy. Skin is dynamic and my favourite way to describe it is that it's always on the move, changing day to day and month to month. If we want to have our best skin, it's important we move with it, both in our thoughts about our skin and the actions we take to look after it.

For as long as I have been in the skincare business, I have stood on the platform that Black women should have access to the relevant information they need to care for their skin, and without breaking the bank. I've always been about access, availability and affordability, and I shall continue to champion these three tenets, especially for brown-skinned girls who have always been on the back foot when it comes to skincare products and also to information about skincare itself.

Prioritising Black skin

The beauty industry – and, by extension, the skincare world – mainly caters for white skin. There is little or no information specifically focused on Black skin, so with a lot of what we read, we have to infer its relevance to us. Things are changing slowly, but I believe a book dedicated to darker skin tones' skincare is much needed. The excuses that Black women aren't engaged, or only want 'natural skincare', or don't have money to spend on their beauty and skincare needs are complete tosh. Historical data has often pointed to the fact that Black women tend to outspend white women in certain beauty categories, such as

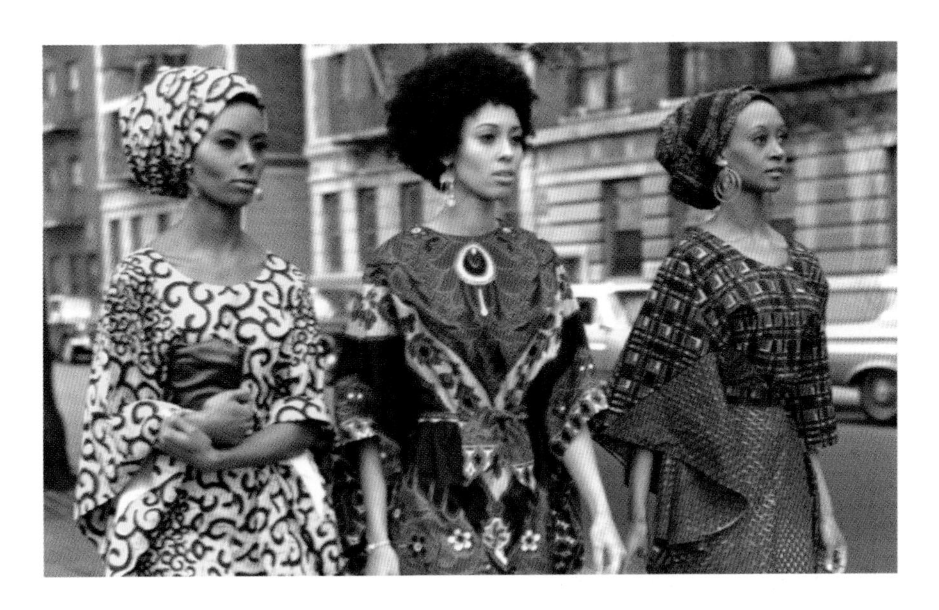

hair and make-up. The 2016 Shades of Beauty Report by Superdrug, which surveyed 559 women, found that 70 per cent of Black and Asian women feel left out of high-street offerings, and 36 per cent felt beauty advice for their skin tones and concerns was lacking. This is backed up by a 2023 Black Skin Directory Report in which, of the 300 women surveyed, only 8 per cent felt that mainstream skincare brands understood or acknowledged their needs. There's clearly a lot of work still to be done.

I always say that Black women come from a lower base when it comes to beauty. What I mean by that is that the beauty ideal that has been celebrated since time immemorial has always been that of the western white woman. The only way for us to gain acceptance was to try to emulate white and European standards of beauty: straighten our hair, lighten our skin, and contort our facial structures with make-up. It's only been since the mid-twentieth century that the narrative around Black beauty started to change because of the will and courage of the Black community to carve out spaces for itself, such as Naturally '62, a community-focused fashion show by Harlem-based Grandassa Group, which showcased models with rich Black skin, sporting full lips, proudly African noses and natural hair with kinky textures. Magazines like *Ebony* also supported this by feeding out images that honoured the uniqueness of Black skin. This progress and fight for mainstream acceptance was hard won, and, despite the problems that still exist today, we have come on in leaps and bounds!

Changing the narrative

For centuries we were actively told that Black is not beautiful. Black skin was derided, our features were denigrated, and we were told we were beastly and put on show as spectacles to be gawped at and ogled. In the 1800s, Saartje Baartman, an enslaved African from where we now know as South Africa, was held in a cage and put on display as a biological curiosity in both London and Paris. Ota Benga, a Congolese Pygmy, was captured in Africa and in 1906 he was exhibited next to apes as part of the Monkey House exhibit at Brooklyn Zoo. Sadly, he subsequently committed suicide in 1916.

I receive hundreds of messages a month on social media, mainly from Black women, in different parts of the world, asking for skin advice. From Lagos and Dubai to Tokyo and Los Angeles, Black women worldwide are craving skincare advice that is tailored them. I get all sorts of queries: 'Are chemical peels OK for

Black skin?' 'How do I get my top lip and bottom lip the same colour?' 'How do I get rid of dark marks?' 'Any tips on how I can safely lighten my skin?' (I only have one: don't!) It breaks my heart because, as a rule, I don't give personalised advice on social media. Without taking into account your current skin condition, general health, lifestyle, products and routines it is improper – not to mention nigh impossible in the majority of cases – for me to give any tangible, useful advice. I am limited to being very general in my comments and, trust me, I hate having to generalise as much as you dislike having to read it. I always imagine you screwing your face up and saying, 'She hasn't really told me anything!'

Additionally, there is so much information on the internet it can make your head spin. From bloggers and influencers to brands and professionals, everyone and their mama is giving advice. We are awash with plenty of pseudo skincare experts who lack the experience and qualifications on which to base their 'advice'. I know that some of this information can appear well put-together, but be careful. It can also be sometimes downright confusing or extremely technical; many a time I've consulted with a client who has been the victim of a dodgy blog post or spent their rent money on products that sadly haven't delivered.

The number of products, and the sheer amount of advice, out there is humungous – even I sometimes get fed up. But I'm driven by the same passion that used to get me up early, aged 6, to sit in my mama's dressing room to watch her meticulous grooming ritual. The standout parts of this routine were Oil of Ulay (I am old enough to remember when it was Ulay, not Olay as we know it now) delicately massaged into her skin, a deliberate dusting of Fashion Fair face powder, a maroon lipstick that oozed Madame-like power, a spritz of something expensive (YSL Paris or Opium) always behind ears and on the wrists, and she was ready to sashay into the day. My 8-year-old now watches me get ready, and I want to make sure that as she grows up her Blackness is celebrated and reflected back at her in what she reads and consumes about her beauty, that she is armed with the tools and knowledge to navigate the skincare world, and to know that she isn't anyone's afterthought. I have this same desire for every Black woman, regardless of age.

The only book you need

So, I'm putting some of my skin health knowledge together in one place for you to access. I've cut through the noise to bring you the real deal of what you *actually* need to know and what you *actually* need to be doing for healthy skin. I admit now that some of the ritualist romance of skincare has been cut out in some places, because, fundamentally, a lot of what we're sold sits in the 'nice to have' category rather than being absolutely fundamental to good skin health. I'm proud to carry on my tradition of writing in simple English, because you shouldn't need a science degree to know how to care for your skin.

This book is my way of making the latest skin health advice available to all Black women in a way that is quick and easy to digest. A sassy tour in skin health, if you like – from the function of skin, the difference between Black and white skin, why hyperpigmentation is such a pain, what treatments are safe for Black skin, whether Black people need sunscreen (spoiler: yes!), and whether there is any truth in the statement 'Black don't crack.'

Myths and misconceptions are plentiful in the Black community, as is the reliance on heritage skincare items like shea butter and coconut oil. I will start by examining this reliance from a historical, cultural and race-relations perspective, because to understand our present relationship with skincare we must understand our past interactions.

That said, whilst my writing centres on Black and melanin-rich skin, this book is also for everyone and anyone interested in skin, whether you're in the wider beauty industry as a student, a therapist or in management, or you may be mum to a mixed-race child or your partner is Black, this book will widen and sharpen your understanding of what it means to have Black skin and how to care for it.

The skincare and beauty industry has long failed to consider and reflect the needs of Black skin. Awareness of physiological differences is lacking, such as why melanin is more impactful on Black skin, and cultural sensitivities such as colourism and the effects of slavery and racism often fail to be considered or engaged with empathetically. For this to change, we have to look at history and understand how it has shaped and contributed to our experiences in beauty today: a process that is both poignant and empowering.

This book will unpack it all. It is the book I wish I had all those years ago when I fell in love with beauty and aesthetics. The information is timeless and will never be out of step in how you care for your skin at any age, so I hope you will treat this guide as a close companion and refer to it frequently.

black skin

a history

It's a cliché but beauty has always been more than skin deep. The ability of Black women to enjoy and partake in the rituals of beauty today is rooted in our historical experiences. It is so important for us to be included in and to lead beauty and skincare conversations, and to claim our identities by owning our beauty, our skin colours and our heritage.

It is my hope that this chapter will galvanise you as much as it strengthened me to take back control of my image and to take even more concerted pride in my ethnic and cultural heritage. We cannot understand the underlying significance of this book if we are unable to find, place and appreciate Black beauty in a historical context. This is the only way we can create equitable concepts of beauty for *all* women.

Beauty and skincare are close bedfellows; to understand the attitude of Black women towards skincare, we first have to examine and answer the question, 'What is the relationship between Black women and beauty?' Likewise, we must also understand the impact of perceptions of beauty, especially perceptions of Black beauty, and which must extend also to understanding the hierarchy and guardianship of the concept of beauty.

> 'You can't really know where you are going,
> until you know where you've been.'
>
> Maya Angelou

African Beauty

The concepts of beauty and beautification have been expressed in different ways across the continent of Africa. The Pharaohs of Egypt bathed in milk and honey to keep their skin smooth and soft and drew attention to their eyes with the use of kohl, whilst the rituals of communities in sub-Saharan Africa demonstrate more physical expressions of beauty: the Makonde people in Mozambique practise facial cutting; the Yoruba people in Nigeria inscribe tribal markings; and there's scarification in Benin and Togo. In the Democratic Republic of Togo, the Barega tribe performs both facial cutting and scarification, whilst the Wanyabungo tribe consider trimmed teeth a mark of beauty. In Kenya, the Maasai tribe pierce and stretch the earlobe as a sign of beauty and strength.

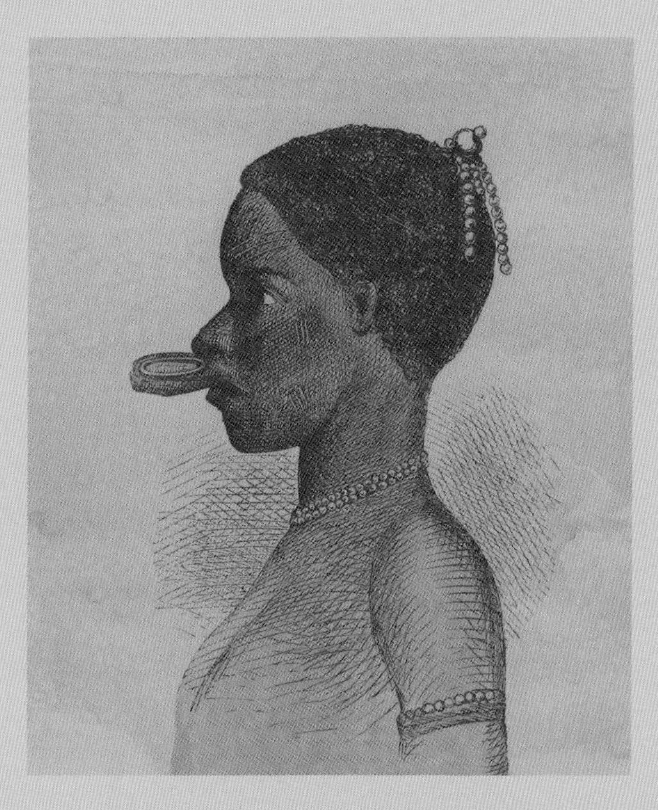

Lip-plate of an African woman, probably a Makonde native in east Africa, mid-1800s. © Alamy

Within the tribes of Southern Nations, Nationalities, and People's Region in Ethiopia, the women are known for their clay lip plates (sometimes up to 16cm in size), which stretch their lips. The bigger the stretch the more beauty is bestowed. Additionally, the tribes are famous for adorning their bodies with paints and flowers to draw attention to their beauty. In South Africa, the Khoikhoi community removed their front teeth in a practice that is now largely attributed to beauty and fashion but has its origins in the concept of owning their beauty during slavery. Teeth were used a barometer of health by slave merchants and their removal made sales more challenging.

For generations, the Himba women of Northern Namibia have considered their hair and skin as a mark of their power and beauty. They are known to spend a considerable amount of time on their appearance, rubbing their skin with Otjize – a special mixture made from tree resin, animal fat, soil, and a milled red-pigmented stone. They use this paste not only to cleanse their skin and hair but also as a form of sunscreen, and to look good too. The paste gives their skin a glowing red look, which symbolises blood as the essence of life and earth.

Africans have always taken time, care, and pride in their beauty. The desire to be and feel beautiful is omnipresent. The richness of Black skin was admired and preserved. As was Afro hair, which was a tool for expressing status, rank, and power. All these practices served a dual purpose – beautification, but also to identify and define belonging to particular families, groupings and communities.

> The concepts of beauty and beautification have been expressed in different ways across the continent of Africa.

The Concepts of Light and Dark, Good and Evil, White and Black

The idea of light and dark standing for good and evil can be traced back to teachings of the early Christian Coptic church. Many credit the scholar Origen as the first to explore these dualities in the third century AD. Yes, that's right, I'm taking you to way back when because, believe me, when I say that our twenty-first-century understandings have to be grounded, they *have* to be grounded. As we like to say, how can you know where you are going if you don't know where you are coming from.

In many of Origen's works, he refers to Jesus Christ as being the 'light': 'The word of Christ opens the soul and we see differences between light and darkness, and choose in everyday to stand in the light.' The act of choosing to stand in the light is a rejection of the dark, therefore implying 'something bad' or not worthy of being chosen.

Overlay the conceptual teachings of good and evil on to light and dark and we can see how the physical colours of white and black come to take on a new meaning: white used to imply lightness, divine intelligence, purity and innocence; black being associated with absence of life, ugliness, evil and fear. Within religious iconography and art it was common for devils and demons to be depicted as black or in black clothing. Blackness had come to represent something that was against good, and these ancient doctrines give us the first insights into colourism.

Though unclear (and subject to much interpretation by scholars and religious leaders) the Jewish Talmudic texts refer to Black skin being a consequence of the curse of Canaan. The Book of Genesis tells us that Noah cursed his grandson Canaan, for the sins of his father Ham. The curse was to blacken the skin of Ham's descendants and subject them to slavery. This curse has even been used as a justification for slavery. Records show that in 1578, English sea captain George Best was one of the first to start a narrative of Africans being Black and loathsome on account of them being descendants of Ham's offspring.[2]

Black Riches and Fertility

All this said, there was a time when Black people were powerful and our skin colour was celebrated. In ancient Egyptian texts, the colour black was aligned with nature and represented fertility. It was seen as the colour of the earth, and the black silt of the river Nile provided rich soil for crops to grow.

The wealthy Malian Empire, which covered huge swathes of West Africa from c. 1235 to 1670, and, even before that, the Ghanaian Empire, which existed from c. 300 to 1100, were ruled by dynamic Black kings. Their heirs, such as Dinga Cisse in Ghana and Sundiata Keita in Mali, developed their territories' education, language, laws, customs and trade in salt, gold, iron ore and – sadly – humans.

The Moors of Spain and Portugal came from Black Islamic North Africa. They were a prosperous and enlightened people who cultivated cultural, educational and economic excellence in their territory for over eight hundred years, from c. 711.

Another exultation of Blackness is the reverence of the Black Madonna within Christianity, and Catholicism specifically, who at various times in history has been named Mother of the Universe, hailing from Africa. There are thousands of paintings and statues of her likeness all over Europe and the Americas and her devotees associate her Blackness with love, fertility and transformation.

It is clear to see that over the course of history Black skin has been both celebrated and dehumanised by various powers, including Africans.

There was a time when Black people were powerful and our skin colour was celebrated.

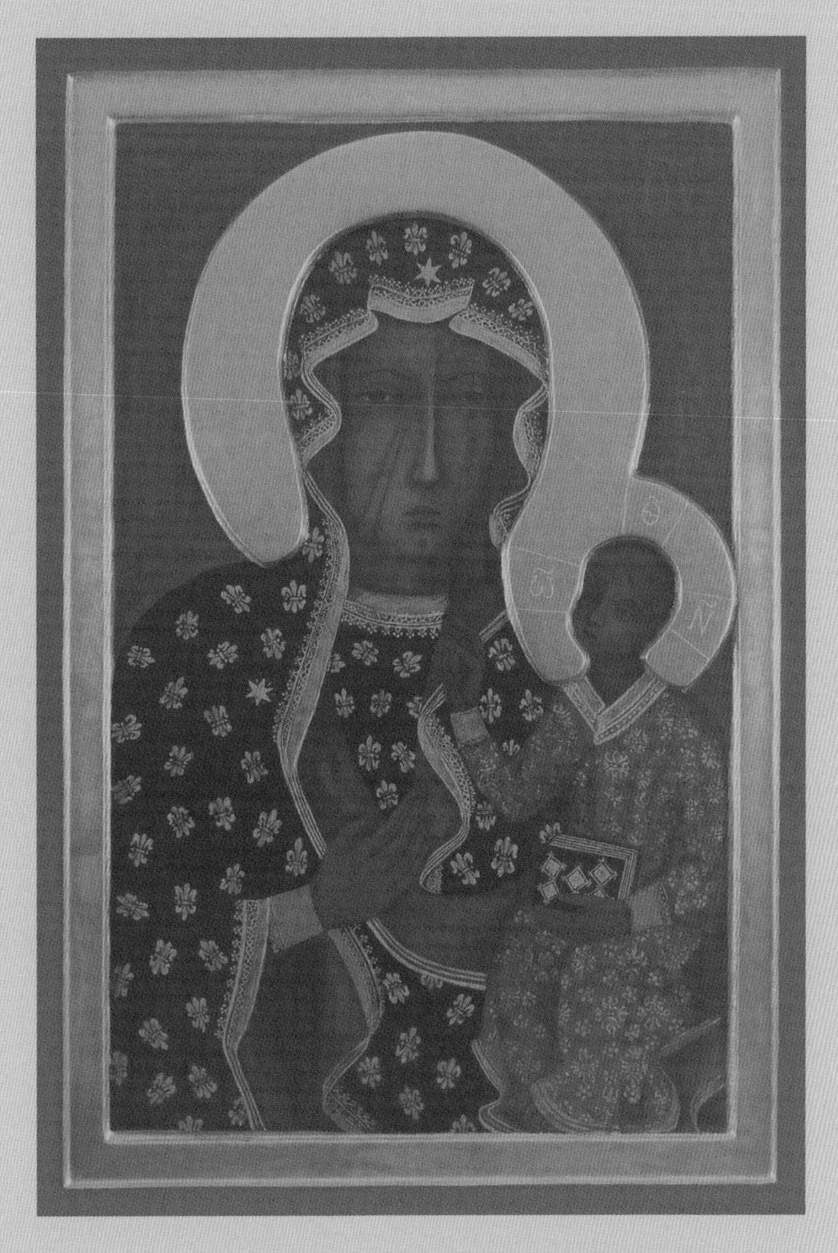

The Black Madonna of Czestochowa (Copy). Museum:
Jasna Gora, Czestochowa. © Alamy

Seize, Season and Strip

White enslavement of African people was premeditated and systematic, and it dehumanised the whole race. Africans played a role in this process, but the vast expanse of this crime against humanity was controlled and orchestrated by whites.

Enslaved Africans were groomed to make them compliant. They went through a process of 'seasoning', the removal of any sense of their own identity and, therefore, self-worth. Young and old people, who were considered of no value, were murdered in front of their captured relatives in a power display designed to shock captives into submission. Many historians have taught that the effects of this practice would have induced post traumatic stress disorder (PTSD) as, when captives arrived at sale locations dotted along the west coast of Africa, they were described as being in a form of stupor and lethargy.[3]

Men, women and children would be separated, and women often subjected to the torment and anguish of rape by white slave traders and agents. On Bunce Island, off the coast of what is now Sierra Leone, which was notorious for the British slave trade, there was a grim outhouse called the 'rape house'. Although in ruins, the main structure still stands today. Before captives left African soil to become slaves in the Americas, they were branded with the insignia of their traders using a hot iron, marking them out as property, not people with free will. Additionally, their feet and ankles were forced into shackles, all under the shadow of a giant cannon designed to instil fear and compliance.

The journey to America across the Atlantic Ocean was called the Middle Passage; it was treacherous, and many did not survive. Abolitionists wrote of men, women and children being packed like sardines in the boat hulls, meaning sickness and disease were rampant. Often captives who fell ill were thrown overboard to prevent the spread of sickness, or even if the ships were too laden. This further jaded the captives and emphasised that they were subhuman and deemed worthless.

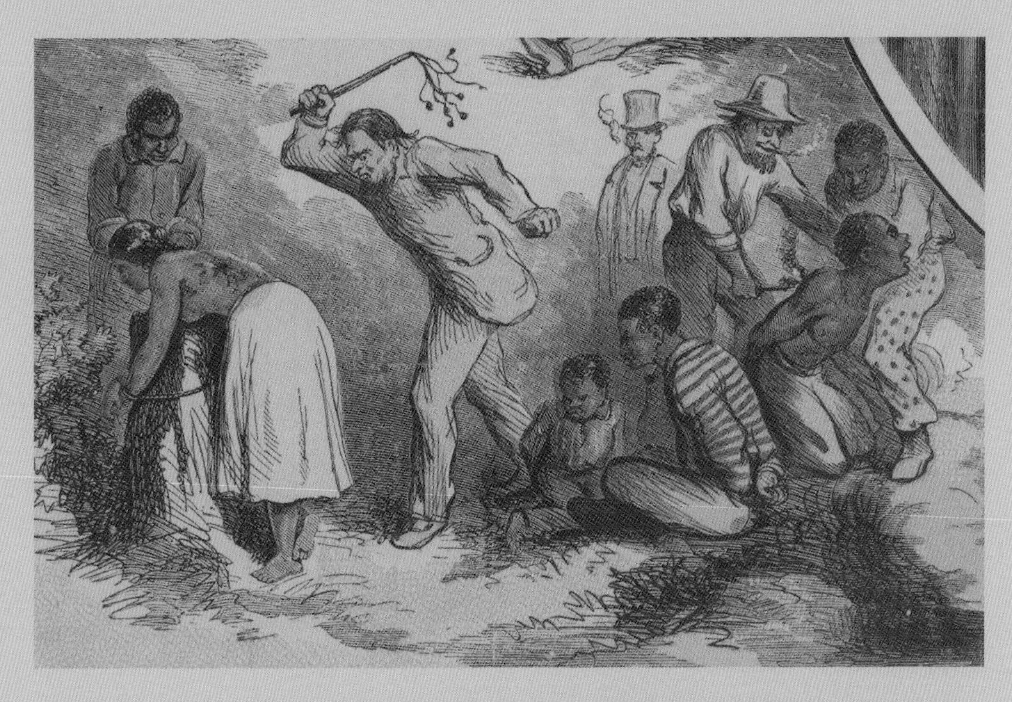

A female slave is whipped and a male slave branded. Detail from the Emancipation, end of the slave trade print by Thomas Nast (artist) & King & Baird (engraver), 1865. © Alamy

On arrival in the Americas, and after further degrading inspections, sales and transactions in the open-air markets of Alabama and South Carolina (amongst other places), captives would be taken to plantations to start their lives as slaves. There they would undergo further 'seasoning' – beatings, rapes, harsh punishments including public hanging, cultural deracination, humiliations and orders designed to break the spirit, to imbue both helplessness and hopelessness – to instil resignation to this new life.

It is of no doubt that the overall intention of these practices was to strip Africans of their identity, beauty, heritage, pride and any feelings of worth and agency. Africans were treated no better than beasts from the jungles of Africa. The seismic effects of four hundred years of slavery cannot be ignored. If we are to ever understand the relationship that Black men and women have with beauty today, we have to delve into and accept the mental effects of slavery and its impact on the perception of beauty and worth, both for whites and Blacks.

Slavery created a hierarchy of Black skin and, in so doing, created a grading for beauty and skin tone. At the bottom of the pile were those who looked most African: darker skin, Afro hair and the classic features of a broader nose and full lips. They had a very low beauty rating in comparison to lighter-skinned slaves who had features, hair and skin tone of closer resemblance to whites and Europeans. It was a system of 'Pigmentocracy', as defined by Kobena Mercer,[4] in which slaves with a white bias had more upward social mobility because in some circumstances they could pass as white. This meant these slaves stood more of a chance of working inside, as opposed to darker-skinned slaves who had to toil the fields.

One of the Founding Fathers of the American Constitution, Thomas Jefferson, who hypocritically declared that 'All men are created equal' in the US Declaration of Independence in 1776, went on to coin the classifications of 'mulatto' – half mixed race; 'quadroon' – quarter mixed race; and 'octoroon' – eighth mixed race, further propagating the image of Africans being subhuman and unequal. In a society where Black people simply wanted the right to stay alive and survive, these sorts of categorisations promoted a tonal hierarchy and, though demeaning, became a form a social currency. Black people wanted to marry 'light' in order to increase their life's lot. These phrases brought about reductive descriptions such as 'blue-Black' and 'high yellow' as a means of rating Black people within a system and allocating them a beauty score. Being lighter skinned afforded some Black women a higher status as it was a more palatable form of Blackness, one that in certain circumstances white people would accept as beautiful. The messaging is significant, and we see it play out in arguments about colourism today.

'Race science' took hold in the eighteenth and nineteenth centuries, and European scientists and artists such as Cuvier, Blumenbach and Schopenhauer took to strengthening their unfounded and racist stereotypes by depicting Black people as inferior, criminal, sexually deformed and related to animals. In his 1774 book, *The History of Jamaica*, the once-dubbed 'father of English racism', Edward Long, depicted Africans as inferior and a different species to white people. He described Africa as the parent of 'everything that is monstrous in nature', Black people as having 'tumid nostrils', and Afro hair was described as a 'bestial fleece'. The dissemination of the ugliness and inferiority of Blacks was, sadly, so brilliantly executed that both whites and Blacks believed it.

Where race science left off, a crude entertainment industry took over, building on the notions of race science to further degrade the Black experience. Minstrel shows became a grotesque entertainment form around America that perpetuated the 'ugliness' of Blacks.

SLAVES!

LONG CREDIT SALE

OF

PLANTATION HANDS

FROM ALABAMA, WITHOUT RESERVE.

BY N. VIGNIÉ, AUCTIONEER,

Office----No. 8 Banks' Arcade Passage, and corner of Conti street and Exchange Alley.

THURSDAY, MARCH 25, 1858,

AT 12 O'CLOCK, M.

Will be sold in the Rotunda of the ST. LOUIS HOTEL,

No. 1. **ABSALOM**, aged 28 years, Plantation hand, fully guaranteed.
No. 2. **NED**, aged 45 years, Plantation hand, fully guaranteed.
No. 3. **TOM**, aged about 46 years, Plantation hand, fully guaranteed, except having a defect in the right knee.
No. 4. **BILL**, aged about 23 years, Plantation hand, fully guaranteed, except a slight defect in one finger.
No. 5. **FRANK**, aged about 25 years, a plantation hand, fully guaranteed, except a burn on his back and right side.
No. 6. **ALFRED**, aged 35 years, plantation hand, a good subject, has worked in a Blacksmith shop; powerful built man.
No. 7. **POLLY**, Negress, aged 23 years, No. 1 plantation hand and fair Cook, Washer and Ironer, fully guaranteed.
No. 8. **GEORGE**, Griff, aged about 23 years, good plantation hand and carriage driver, very likely and intelligent. MARTHA, his wife, aged about 30 years, Cook, Washer and Ironer, with her four children: NED, aged 7 years; NANCY, aged 6 years; HORACE, 4 years, and MARY, aged 1 1-2 years.

☞ All of the above Slaves are from the State of Alabama, and sold under a full guarantee, except the defects above stated.

ALSO, at the same time and place the following

LIST OF ACCLIMATED SLAVES.

No. 9. **DAN**, Black, aged about 23 years, a good Cooper, acclimated.
No. 10. **LEWIS**, aged about 35 years, general laborer, and accustomed to work in a brick yard.
No. 11. **FIRMAN**, aged about 40 years, general laborer, and accustomed to work in a brick yard.
No. 12. **MARY**, Griff, aged about 27 years, a good house servant and child's nurse, and No. 1 washer, and ironer, having absented herself once from her former owner.
No. 13. **JIM**, Black, aged about 26, a general laborer, and good subject.

☞ All the above Slaves are fully guaranteed against the vices and diseases prescribed by law, except the defects made known.

Terms---9 months for approved city acceptances, bearing 6 per ct. interest

US Slave Market Auction: Poster advertising a New Orleans slave auction of 18 enslaved persons ('Plantation Hands') from Alabama, USA, 1858 © Alamy

part one

know your skin

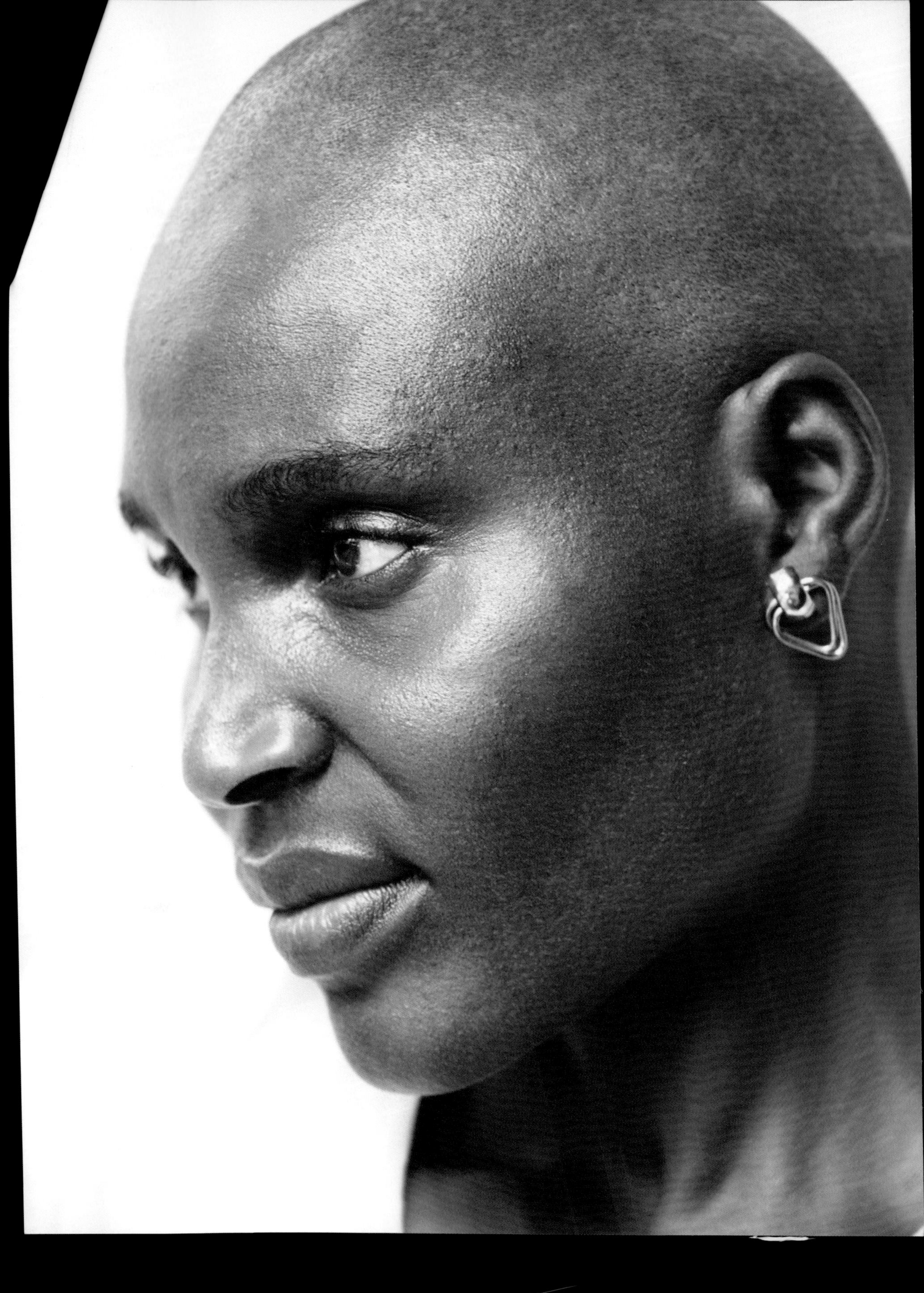

01.

skin 101 – the basics

skin 101 – the basics

'The wrapping that contains the substance of life.'

Angelo P. Thrower, MD

YOUR skin is the largest organ in your body, did you know that? Not many appreciate this fact, and that's because most people consider important organs to be the heart, lungs, liver...the things they see as vital to keep us moving and breathing. Skin is always the last to be considered, but I can guarantee you that you wouldn't last long if you didn't have your skin. Try getting around in just raw flesh. I'll leave you with that image! Skin is the most taken-for-granted part of our body, poked at, scratched at, rubbed and experimented with, never really being given the true respect it deserves – until, of course, there is a problem and your skin doesn't behave or look the way you want it to.

Your skin is so important; I can't stress enough how crucial it is to your health and happiness, but all so often I see it treated like an afterthought. Experience tells me most people just aren't clued up enough about the work their skin does for them, and whilst I don't believe you need a doctorate in biology to have healthy skin, you must have an understanding and appreciation of the fundamentals, so this is where we'll begin – let's call it Skin 101 – to save you a lot of confusion and heart ache.

The fundamentals

Your skin is a complex structure doing many things and carrying out different functions, but fundamentally it is a barrier; a multilayered, semi-permeable waterproof fence that keeps bacteria and germs from entering your body and causing infection and inflammation. But it also prevents you from losing moisture and drying out like a withered prune.

Its jobs are plentiful. Your skin:

- secretes oils and fats to keep you supple and comfortably lubricated,
- controls your temperature by encouraging you to sweat to release heat. Likewise, you get goosebumps to trap heat when you're cold,
- helps the absorption of lotions and creams including medication,
- physically protects you from the elements, such as rain, and from germs in the outside world,
- produces melanin to protect us from the sun,
- excretes waste products such as sweat, sebum and toxins,
- helps you to feel touch, pain and pressure sensations,
- converts UV rays from the sun into vitamin D for strong bones, and
- provides an immediate healing response to injury and infection.

So you see, your skin is just the ultimate multitasking machine, tough and durable but, in the most fascinating way, super soft, flexible and elastic all at the same time. It is your most visible organ, hence why we have such a complex relationship with it and why it can easily influence our moods and how we perceive ourselves in relation to others. You will never hear someone say, did you see how spotty her lungs were? But it's not uncommon for us to use such language to describe our skin.

I also like to think of skin as a communicative organ that can easily tell the world what you're going through. Skin shows up poor lifestyle habits, such as a diet lacking fresh food, recreational choices such as smoking, drugs, drinking, partying too hard and sleep deprivation. These will all make your skin appear dull, grey and tired. Likewise, if you're bossing it in those departments, your skin will tell all too – 'Oh my, you're looking well!' – with increased radiance, glow and vitality.

Your skin is strong and firm enough to give your body shape and structure, yet due to its suppleness you can move around easily with no rigidity. Your skin continues to grow even after muscle, fat and skeletal structures start deteriorating. Skin is simply the work of a higher power and I bow down to its intelligence.

> Your skin is so important; I can't stress enough how crucial it is to your health and happiness

FACT

Every square inch of skin has:

- 6 metres of blood vessels
- 100 oil glands
- 659 sweat glands
- 65 hair follicles
- 3,000,000 cells
- 60,000 melanocyte cells
- 1,000 nerve endings
- 78 sensory heat apparatus
- 70 metres of nerves
- 160 pressure apparatus for tactile stimuli
- 19,500 sensory cells at the end of nerve fibres
- 13 sensory apparatus for cold

basic building blocks of skin

The skin is a team player, made up of three distinct layers all performing unique but complementary roles: the epidermis; the dermis; and the hypodermis (also known as the subcutaneous layer). It is your first line of defence against the outside world.

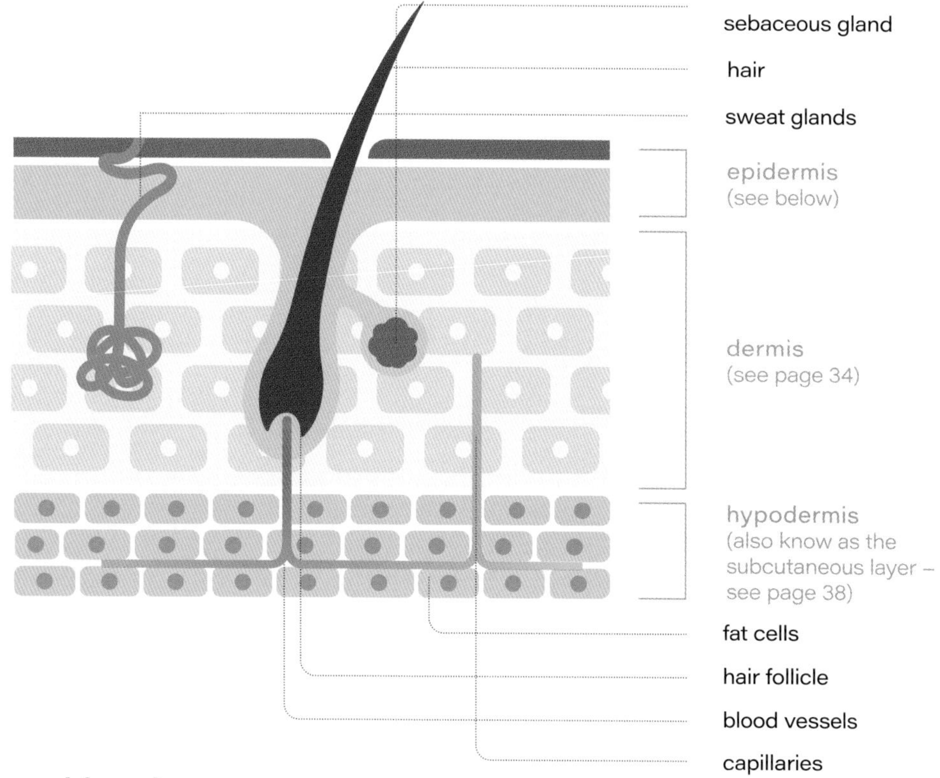

the epidermis

The all-important epidermis is not much thicker than this page. Depending on where it is in the body, it is made up of 4 or 5 distinct layers of protein cells, called *keratinocytes*, that sit on top of a thin membrane. They start off round, plump and squidgy in the first layer – called the *stratum basale* – and become progressively flatter, drier and skinny as they reach the fifth and uppermost layer, the *stratum corneum*. This is the layer that we see and touch. It blows my mind because although this visible layer is thin, it's still made up of 20 layers of skin cells.

The entire epidermis is thin but, my goodness, it is tough and resilient! It's also as active as a game of musical chairs, because skin cells are constantly moving and replacing each other as old cells expire. This cycle can take anything from 21 days, for young skin, up to 60 days for mature skin. It's important to know that even though the juice has been sucked out of our skin cells by the time they get to the upper layer, they're not completely dead: they are still doing a really important job of signalling to the cells below to keep reproducing. This is why I always refer to 'old cells' and not 'dead cells' in the hope that we will be less aggressive with our skin. We're kinder to things that are still living.

As you can see, these cells are arranged in a neat brick-like pattern forming a type of defensive wall. The glue (technically called the *natural moisturising factor*) that holds the cells together is made up of a cocktail of fats, amino acids, salt, sugar, urea and lactic acid. Together the cells and the glue form a strong waterproof barrier that we in the business like to call the *lipid bilayer structure*. Think of it like a waterproof waxed Barbour jacket!

Layers in the epidermis

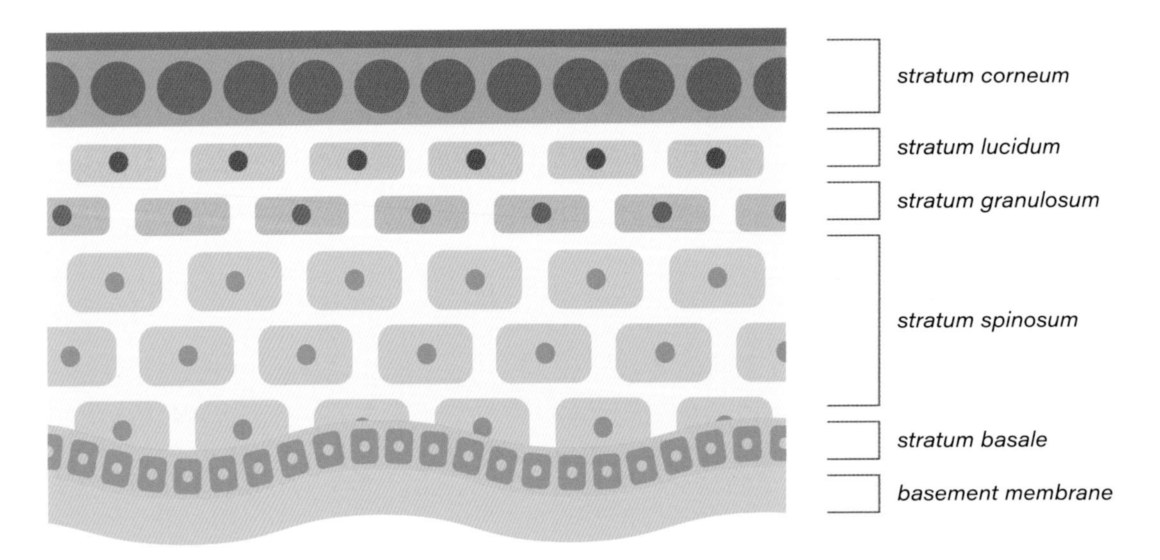

FACT The thickness of the epidermis varies from 0.4mm to 1.5mm. On the eyelids the thickness is less than 0.1mm. Only the palms and soles of the feet have a stratum lucidum, a thin, clear, fatty layer to protect against friction.

Are you still with me? On we go!

Sitting right on top of the stratum corneum, you have the invisible *acid mantle*, which is also made up of fats, water, sugar, amino acids and non-pathogenic bacteria. The pH of the acid mantle is 5.5–5.6 and (when balanced) its job is to act like a protective big brother, maintaining the integrity of your skin and protecting it from harmful bacteria.

FACT You may hear the stratum corneum also called the horny layer (stop sniggering!), because the cells are compact and strong like an animal's horn.

Together these two elements (the lipid bilayer structure and acid mantle) form the *natural barrier function*, acting as your first line of defence, protecting your skin from outside influences, and also preventing moisture and water loss, something that Black skin is prone to doing at higher rates than white skin. If too much water escapes from your skin it becomes a hot, dry and flaky mess. You've heard of Black skin being described as 'ashy' before, right? This is what it refers to, but we'll cover this when we talk more specifically about skin types in Chapter 3.

If we were going to war, your natural barrier function would form the infantry soldiers at the front.

Also within the epidermis are the *melanocyte cells*, spread out in the bottom layer. These cells are responsible for producing melanin pigment, thus giving them a very important role in determining our skin colour. Each melanocyte cell feeds melanin to between 35 and 40 skin cells for distribution throughout the upper layers of our skin.

If we were going to war, your natural barrier function would form the infantry soldiers at the front.

Other residents of the epidermis include the *Langerhans* and *Merkel cells*, which form part of the body's immune and sensory systems.

the dermis

Commonly referred to as the 'living tissue', the dermis is the thickest of the three layers of skin, housing collagen and elastin fibres all suspended in a gel-like 'skin soup' made of proteins, water and hyaluronic acid, known scientifically as the *extracellular matrix* (ECM). Together they all exist in tandem to give shape and resilience to the skin.

Collagen and elastin are types of strong connective protein tissue found throughout the body and are like scaffolding. Their bouncy elastic fibres provide cushioning and shape to the epidermis layer that sits directly on top. Collagen is super important for our skin health and makes up about 70 per cent of the dermis – it's that important. Its job is to provide strength and plumpness to the skin. It is also directly affected by UV rays, which penetrate the skin and attack

FACT Hyaluronic acid is a very large sugar molecule and each one can hold 1,000 times its own weight in water or, to look at it another way, a single gram of hyaluronic acid can hold up to 6 litres of water. It's a super-smart ingredient, helping to keep skin soft, plump, balanced, hydrated and moisturised. It even works within your skin cells to regulate the moisture levels and you will find it in a lot of skincare products; it features heavily in injectable products such as dermal fillers.

it, leaving the skin with fine lines and wrinkles. Additionally, sugar is its enemy; eating too much sugar will harden your collagen and, over time, it will become stiff and brittle to the point where the fibres break. When this happens, again, you get lines and wrinkles.

Remember – Black will crack if you're slack!

When we talk about 'Black don't crack' we're really referring to the ability of Black skin to hold off showing lines and wrinkles as early as white skin. This is because Black skin has a thicker dermis with tightly packed bundles of collagen.[5] One of the advantages of our abundant melanin is that the skin has a high degree of inbuilt protection from the sun's UV rays, so our precious collagen is somewhat protected from the damage that leads to premature ageing.

Collagen and elastin are types of strong connective protein tissue found throughout the body and are like scaffolding.

Elastin fibres make up a very small amount of the dermis, about 2.5 per cent, and they are what gives your skin its bounce and allows it to return to its original form after you stretch or pull it. From the age of 20, collagen and elastin start to degrade, and as you advance in years, your skin gradually loses its plumpness and elasticity; that's when droopy and sagging skin texture starts to show. Granted this is much later than white skin, but it's only a matter of time, which is why you must start looking after your skin as early as possible.

When we talk about 'Black don't crack' we're really referring to the ability of Black skin to hold off showing lines and wrinkles.

What else is in the dermis?

Cells, cells, and more cells! That's what!

Sweat glands

Up to 4 million sweat glands live in our skin and are connected to the brain. They help keep us safe and healthy by regulating our temperature through our skin.

There are two types of sweat glands. First, eccrine glands, which we have all over our bodies, but especially in our palms and the soles of our feet. Do you get clammy palms when you're nervous? That's the eccrine glands at work. Then there are the apocrine glands, producing a more oily type of sweat. These are located specifically in the armpits, groin, and around the nipples. This is the type of sweat that produces body odour, as it interacts with the bacteria on our skin and gives us our individually distinctive scent.

FACT Heat and emotional stress will kick the eccrine glands into action. Apocrine glands are only stimulated by emotional stress.

Fibroblasts

Hardworking cells that secrete pro collagen, a protein necessary for the production of collagen.

Immune cells

Mast cells, T cells, B cells, macrophage cells all form the skin's defence force. Following signals from Langerhans cells stationed above in the epidermis, they sprint into action whenever we experience trauma, damage or foreign invaders.

Nerve endings

Be it pain, pressure or temperature, your ability to touch and feel starts in the dermis, as nerve endings live here too, providing various degrees of sensitivities.

Hair follicles

They enclose, protect and hold in place individual hairs from deep in the dermis to their protrusion at the epidermis.

Hair

Hair is made from the same protein as the skin, keratin, and grows in columns through the dermis to the epidermis. Afro hair has a distinct thick and coily pattern, which makes it quite fragile and prone to curling back into the skin, causing painful in-growing hair.

Sebaceous glands (aka oil glands)

The skin's very own personal oil well, the sebaceous glands are also located in the dermis, as a sac attached to the side of the hair follicles. Their job is to secrete an oily, waxy and fatty substance called sebum, which provides lubrication to keep skin supple, contributes to the overall 'waterproofness' of the skin and keeps the skin within the necessary acidic limits of pH 4.5 to 6.

These glands are directly affected by fluctuations in our sex hormones, especially testosterone, which can cause an increase in oil production, causing spots and breakouts.

FACT Sebaceous glands are found all over the body, except on your palms and the soles of your feet. You have loads on your face, chest, back and scalp though.

Blood vessels

Transport blood vessels also live in the dermis to supply oxygen and nutrients, whilst also removing waste products. They also play an important role in regulating our temperature.

FACT The blood vessels in the skin trump other blood vessels in the body because they have a greater ability to contract and dilate in order to regulate the body's temperature.

It's clear to see that the dermis is a very busy intersection of the skin. If it was part of the UK road network, the dermis would be the equivalent of Spaghetti Junction in Birmingham.

the hypodermis (also known as the subcutaneous layer)

Sitting underneath the weighty dermis is this third, fatty layer. A much-needed fatty layer, I might add, because one cannot underestimate its important job in providing cushioning for the body and protecting us from daily knocks and bumps – especially if, like me, you err on the side of clumsy. The amount of subcutaneous fat you have is dependent on the body area.

FACT The hypodermis is also responsible for the appearance of cellulite in different parts of the body.

The reason why you don't just sit on bones when you flop into your favourite chair? The subcutaneous layer of fat in your bottom. The reason why chubby faces look more youthful? Yep, fat! Why your palms are so fleshy and soft? Yes, you guessed it, fat! Respect the subcutaneous layer.

Bar its ability to cushion, prevent injury and, in some cases, cleverly mask our government age, with the help of other connective structures the subcutaneous layer is also the connecting link between the dermis and our muscles and bones. It provides a support function to the blood and lymphatic vessels, nerves and glands that pass through it on their way to other parts of the body, such as the dermis.

As we age, we tend to lose the subcutaneous layer as it naturally thins. This leaves our skin looking roughened and veiny.

what else is on the skin?

You may have heard of the gut microbiome...well, your skin has a microbiome too and it's totally unique to you, influenced by your genetics, lifestyle, diet and environment. It's a flourishing safari of millions of bacteria, fungi, viruses and even mites that, on the whole, live happily on the skin everywhere from in between our toes to inside the oil glands on our face. They play an important role in keeping the skin balanced and functioning healthily.

FACT The most studied microbiome infection is *Acne vulgaris*, caused by the newly categorised *Cutibacterium acnes* (formerly known as *Propionibacterium acnes* – you may recognise it as its shortened form: *P. acnes*).

Most of the time, your skin microbiome causes no harm, but if it is disrupted it can contribute to all manner of issues, such as acne and eczema.

the difference between male and female skin

It's important to give a shout-out to the men in our lives, because no doubt they have skin issues, too. So, the important things you should know:

- Men have more androgen hormones, so their skin is 25 per cent thicker than female skin.
- They have even more compact collagen bundles, so they will age even more slowly than women. Men define the 'ageing like fine wine' phrase. Cases in point: Idris Elba, Denzel Washington, Will Smith – I could go on, but you get the picture.
- Male skin produces more sebum so tends to be oilier. Oily skin ages better. See point above.
- The stratum corneum (the uppermost layer of skin) is thicker and with a rougher texture.
- Male skin has an increased tendency for acne-type conditions but, conversely, tends to be better hydrated than female skin due to differences in pH levels.

FACT Androgens are hormones that are commonly, incorrectly, classified as male hormones, but they are present in both men and women. The most noted androgen is testosterone.

So, there you have it, a crash course in the fundamentals we should know in order to understand how our skin lives and works. This is key to unlocking how best to look after it.

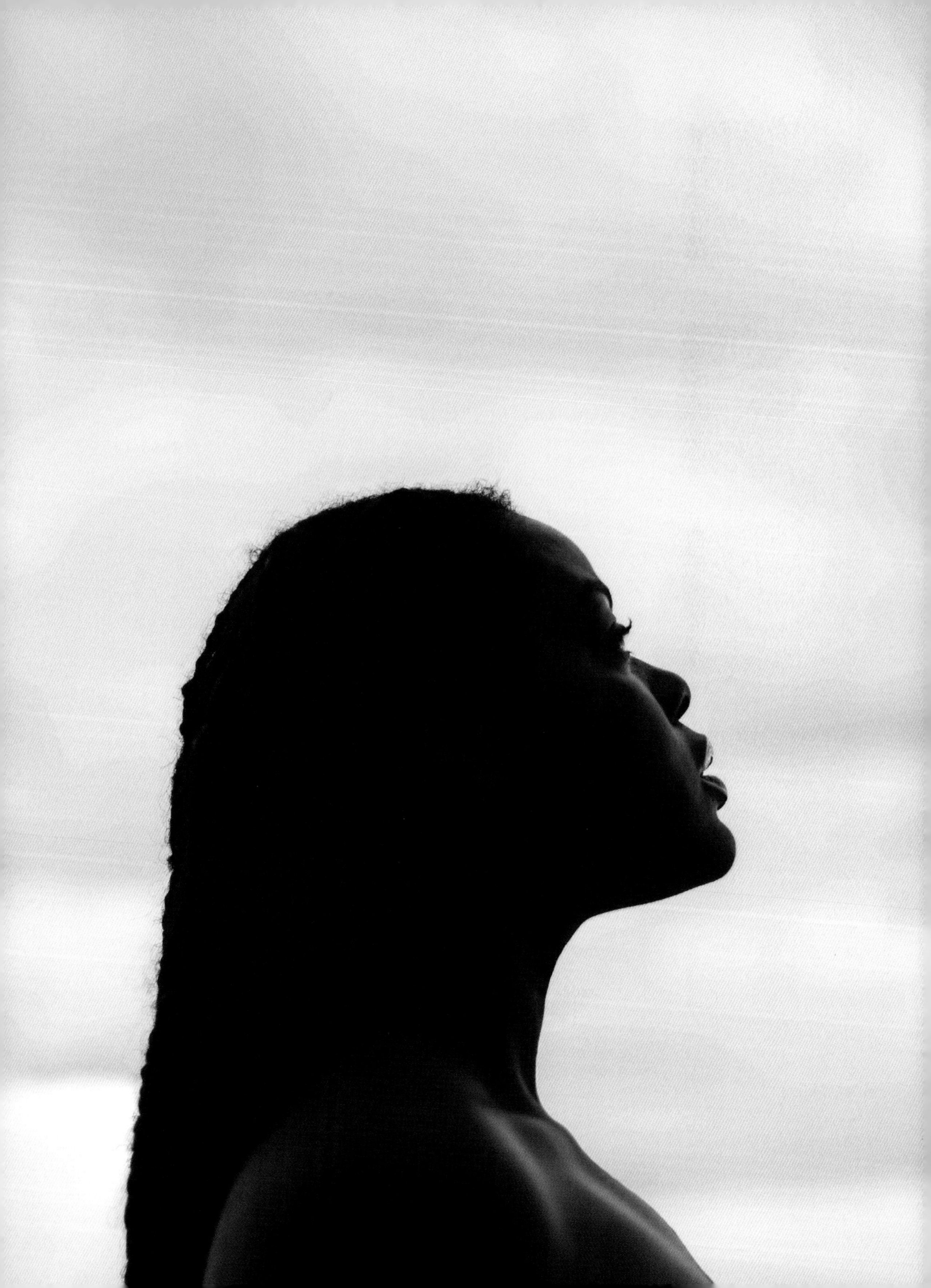

02.

the uniqueness of black skin

the uniqueness of black skin

ONE of the most popular questions I get asked is, 'Is skin not just skin? Bar colour is it that different? Really? Really, really?'

Yes really, really. There are similarities, but Black skin is physiologically different to white skin in a few ways. There are also cultural differences in the way we treat the skin.

How melanin is distributed in the skin

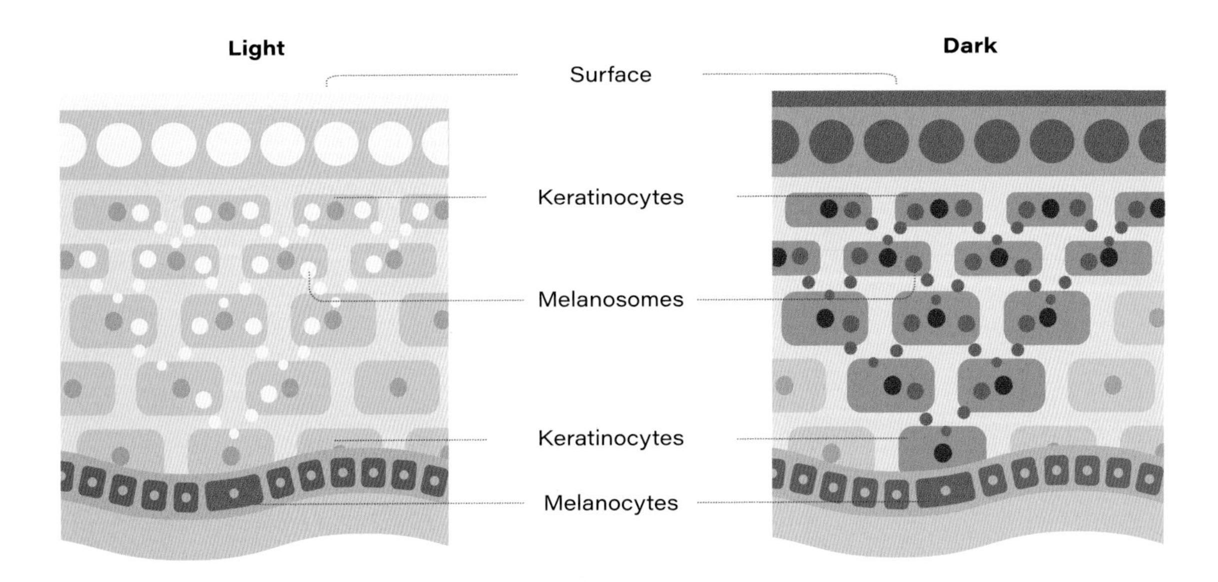

> There are similarities, but Black skin is physiologically different to white skin in a few ways. There are also cultural differences in the way we treat the skin.

melanin

The differences in our skin colours are down to our genetic backgrounds, location, and our individual environmental exposure to the sun. Those closer to the Equator generally have Black or darker skin tones to protect against the high UV exposure that comes from the sun. White skin is predominantly found in the northern latitudes and tends to be lighter to enable it to absorb vitamin D from the sun. However, global travel has moved us all over the world, so these are not hard and fast rules.

Everyone – be you of Black, white or mixed-race heritage – has melanocyte cells, living in the very bottom layer of your epidermis, the stratum basale. Within these melanocyte cells are the melanosomes, granules that contain the pigment called melanin. At this very early stage, the granules are actually transparent with no colour at all. As they migrate through the layers of skin, they then take on their distinctive colour.

FACT Eumelanin and pheomelanin can co-exist in the same human cell, but not within the same melanosome.

There are two different types of melanin pigment produced by the melanocytes: eumelanin – a dark brown pigment, and pheomelanin – a red or yellow tint. Black people and those with darker skin tones have more eumelanin, hence our different shades of brown skin colour, whereas white and lighter skin tones have pheomelanin.

The melanocyte cells have tentacles, just like an octopus, that extend to our many keratinocyte cells to help distribute the melanin pigment throughout our epidermis, giving us all our unique individual skin colours. The key factor when it comes to skin colour is the size and the amount of melanocytes and melanosomes. Black and darker skin tones have larger individual melanosomes that are evenly distributed through the epidermis. The melanosomes in Black skin are also more active and produce more melanin. In fact, some studies have shown that Black skin produces twice as much melanin as white skin. It is noted that melanosomes also age more slowly in darker skin tones.

FACT A tan is *not* a sign of healthy skin. It is evidence of the skin protecting itself from sun damage by producing more melanin.

White and lighter skin tones, conversely, have smaller melanosomes, which are clustered together and rarely found in the upper layers of the epidermis. The melanosomes in white skin are stimulated by UV radiation from the sun, hence why white skin goes brown in the sun. In the middle sit those of Asian descent, who also have large melanosomes that are found individually as well as grouped together.

Together, the combination of increased melanin and its distribution in the skin gives Black skin some protection from premature ageing caused by UV radiation from the sun. On average, research points to Black skin having an approximate natural sun protection factor (SPF) of 13.4. White skin sits somewhere around 3.3.[6]

But before you run amok with no sunscreen, remember that the increased melanin levels in Black skin also make it more vulnerable to discolouration, be it loss of colour (hypopigmentation) or patchy, uneven deposits of colour (hyperpigmentation).

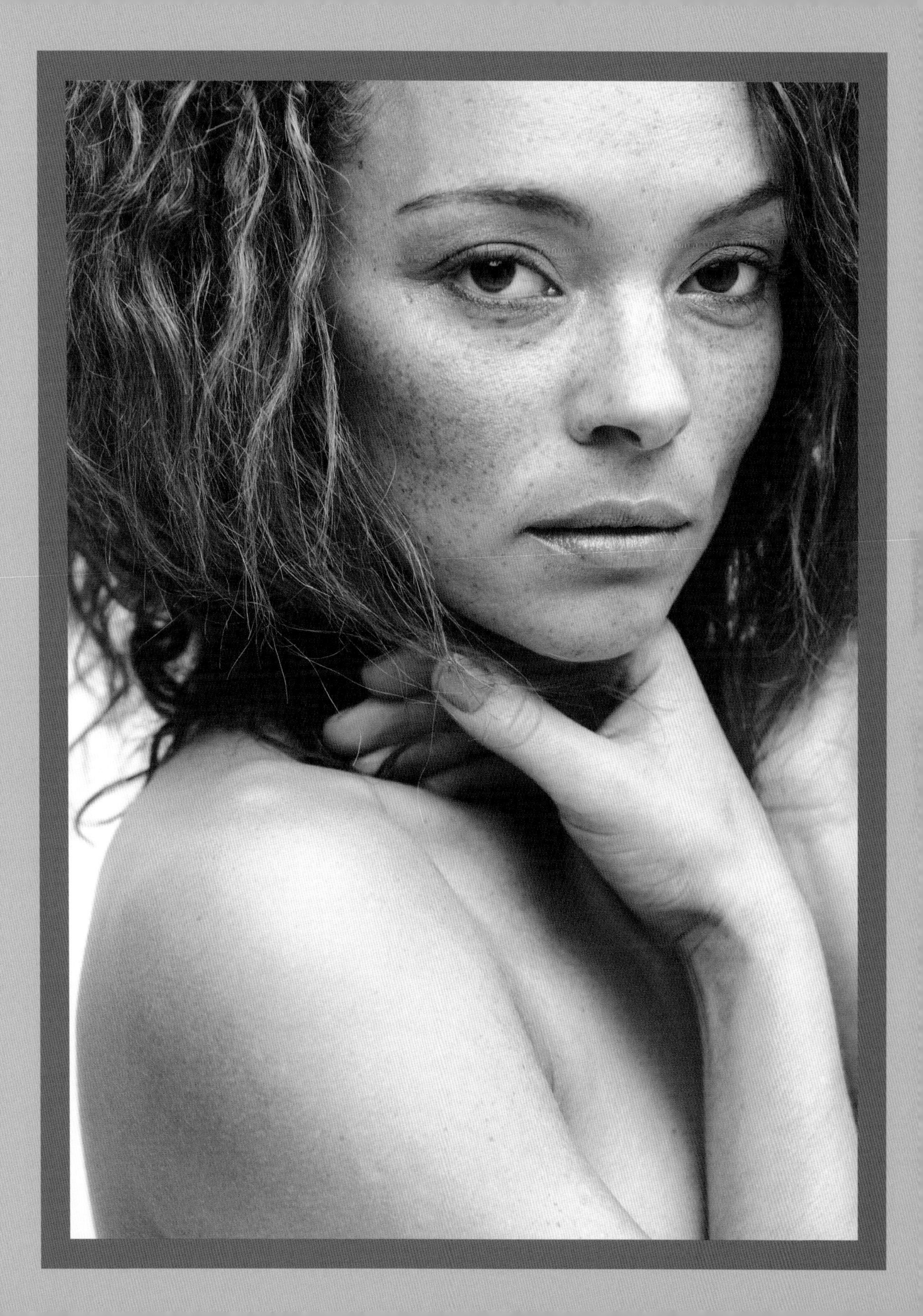

water retention

Another point of difference between Black and white skin is the rate at which water is lost through the skin. One of the functions of the skin is to provide a barrier against water loss and to help the skin stay hydrated. Anything that disrupts the skin's delicate barrier can cause increased water loss, which we in the business refer to as TEWL: 'transepidermal water loss'. A significant number of studies show that whilst Black skin has on average a higher sebum content and a more compact stratum corneum than white skin,[7] it also has lower ceramide levels, so it is prone to increased water loss.[8] This contributes to increased dryness of the skin and the increased likelihood of us experiencing dry, flaky and ashy skin conditions.

I tend to find most women, even if they usually have an oily skin type, will complain of drier skin in the winter months. This is because cold weather and winter wind whips moisture away from the skin and, combined with warm homes, your skin will feel parched and dehydrated, easily losing its glow and vitality.

FACT Ceramides are a type of waxy fatty acid that help form a waterproof barrier on the skin.

Ever get that dry, itchy feeling on your pins after removing your tights? That is TEWL in action.

scarring

They say too much of a good thing isn't good for you, and that can be the case with collagen. Black skin is more prone to what's known as 'hypertrophic' and 'keloid' scarring, both caused by the overproduction of collagen after injury. White skin can also get keloid scarring, but it has been noted to be more common in Black skin.[9]

A regular scar will heal at the site of the injury; these scars will not be elevated or abnormal. Hypertrophic scars will heal at the site of the injury but may be raised, although there is a chance that they could spontaneously turn back into a normal scar. Keloid scars, on the other hand, are larger than the point of the original injury. They can be hard, raised, shiny, hairless and smooth; they are also often uncomfortable, unsightly, itchy and painful, depending on their location.

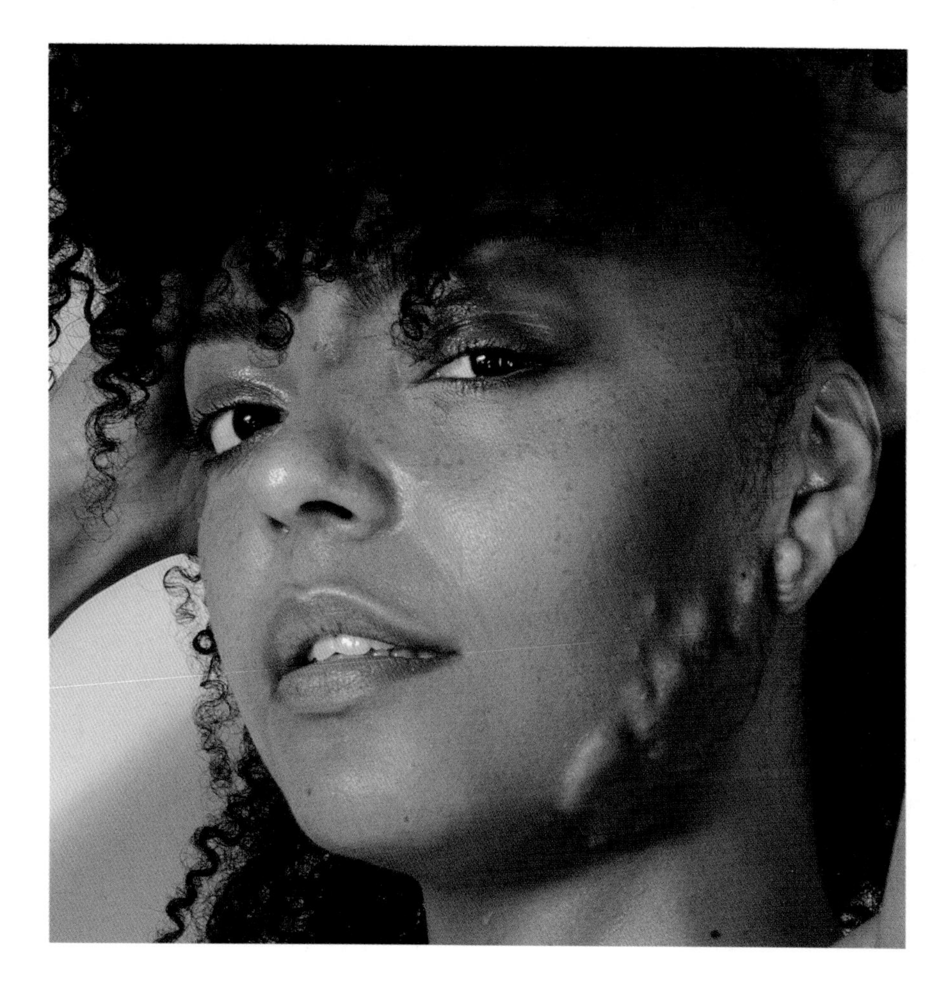

FACT You can't get a keloid scar on your eyelids, palms of the hands or soles of your feet.

A keloid forms when an injury penetrates the epidermis through to the upper portion of the dermis, stimulating collagen production. If the collagen doesn't receive a signal to stop regenerating, it continues to be produced at a higher rate and this accumulates as keloid scar tissue into the surrounding skin. Some people can be so prone that even a pimple can cause a keloid scar and they have to be especially vigilant about treatments and products that work on the basis of controlled injury (e.g. micro-needling) to the skin as it is difficult to predict how their skin will react.

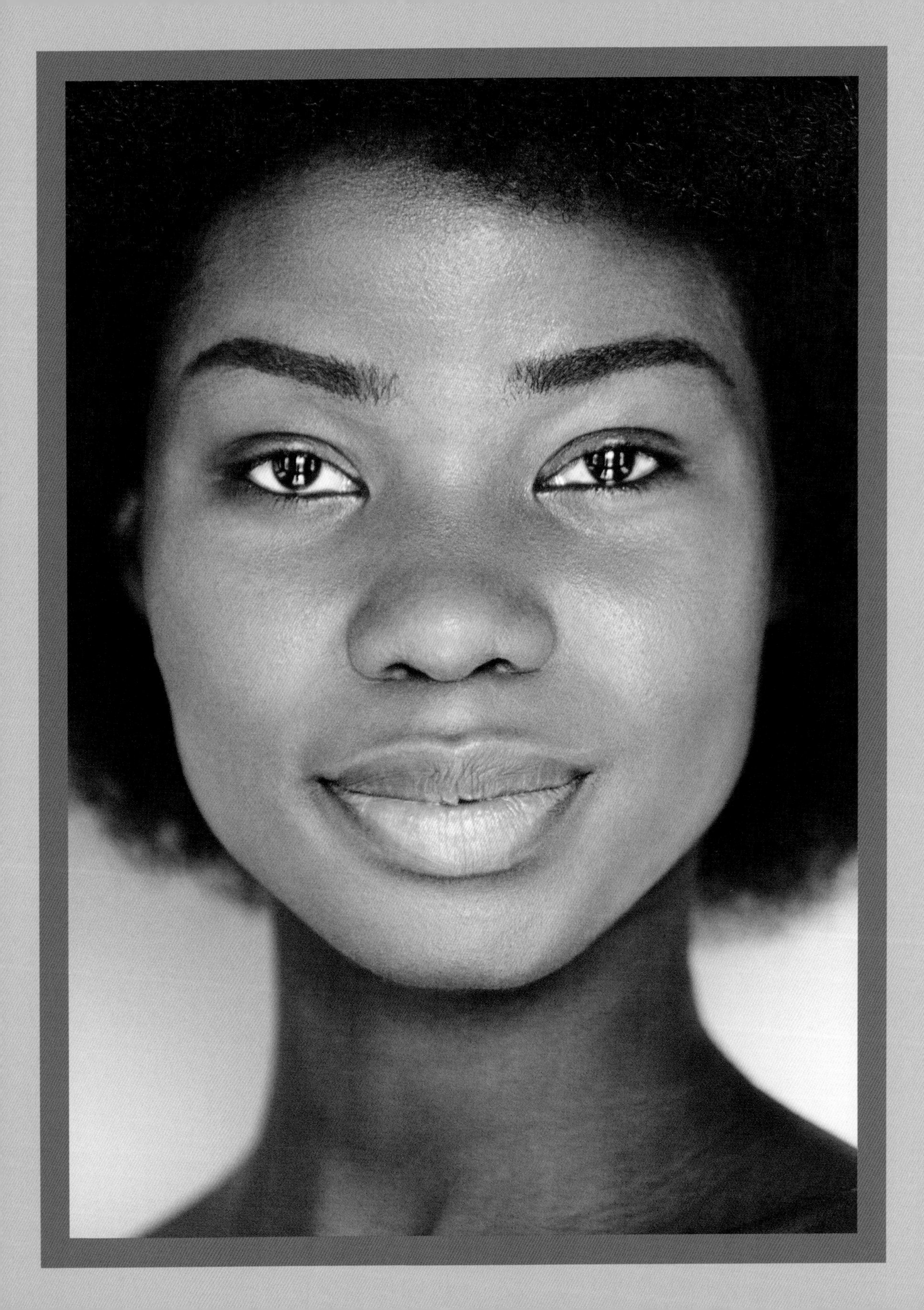

It would be great if there was more research into keloid scarring, not so much so that we can understand the causes, but so that we can find more successful treatment options. Currently treatment options are basic, ineffective, and produce inconsistent results. They vary from topical and injectable steroids to hydrogel compression sheeting, all designed to stunt the overdevelopment of collagen. Surgery is also an option, but there is always the risk that the keloid will return bigger and badder than before. See why there needs to be more research?!

differences in collagen

The statement 'Black don't crack' is often used as a compliment because Black women tend to have a later onset of fine lines and wrinkles compared to white women of a comparable age. There is a reason for this and it's all to do with collagen and the effect of UVA rays on the skin. Black skin has thicker, tighter and smaller collagen fibres, formed into bundles, and melanin acts like an overcoat protecting these bundles from the damage that UV causes when it penetrates the skin. So they stay intact for longer, firmly propping up skin. In comparison, collagen in white skin is much more susceptible to UV damage due to the lack of readily available protective melanin. The collagen construction in white skin is under much more stress and strain from extrinsic ageing factors because it is not as robust.

Whilst skin may be 'just skin', understanding the differences between Black and white skin is crucial in knowing how best to look after yours, as we'll explore further in the book.

> The differences in our skin colours are down to our genetic backgrounds, location, and our individual environmental exposure to the sun.

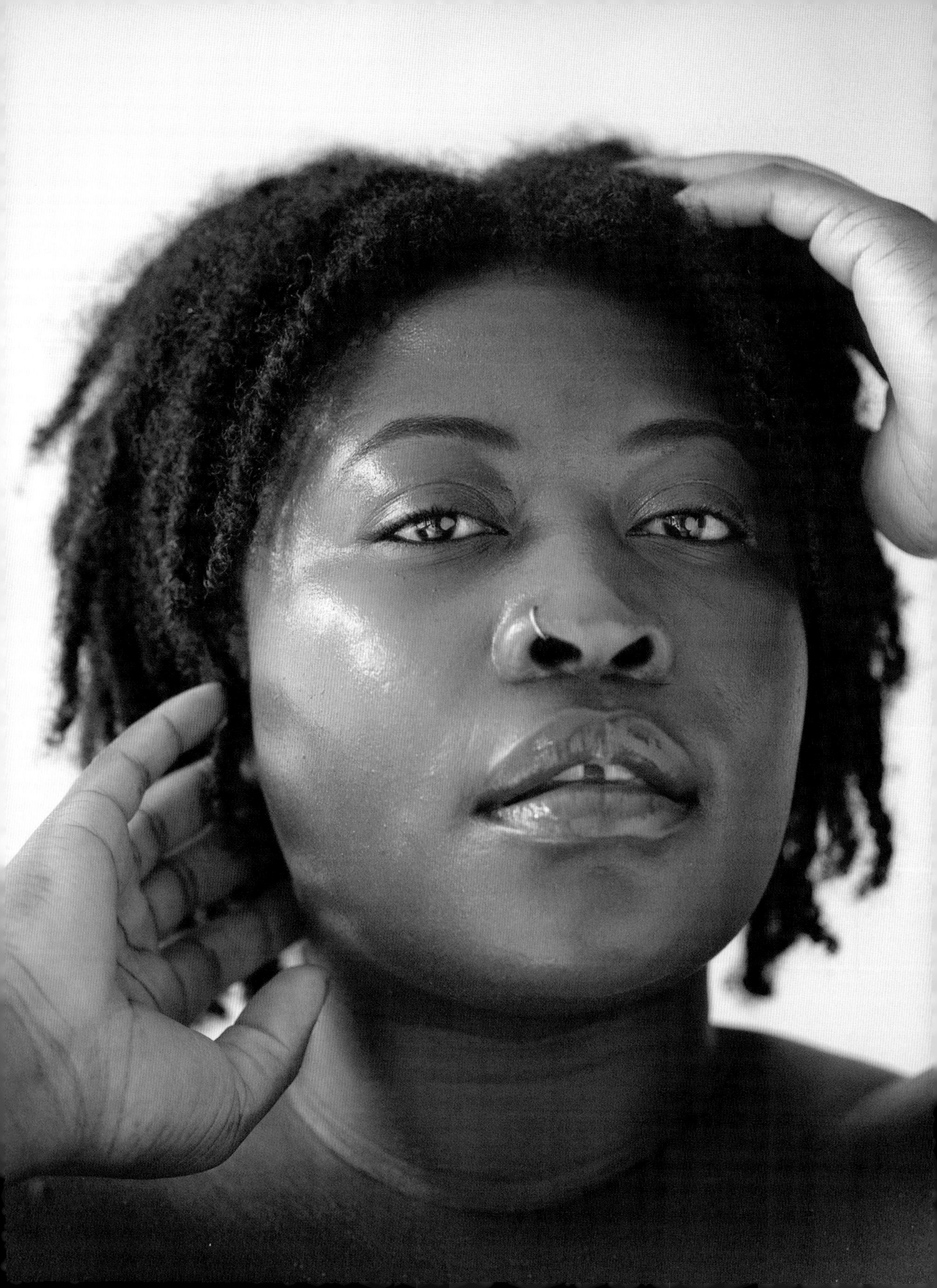

03.

what's your skin type?

what's your skin type?

UNDERSTANDING your skin is essential and one of the single best things you will do for its health. Period. We call this 'skin typing'. Is your skin dry? Do you think your skin is sensitive? Are you oily 'ish' or 'oil slick'? Does your make-up slide off by lunchtime and do you, like me, constantly find foundation fingerprints on your papers? Is your skin dehydrated? Do you experience summer skin or is it winter skin that bothers you the most? Are you hankering after the smooth skin you had as a child?

Seeing all the questions thrown up about skin types, I hope you can see how important it is to know where your skin sits and what sort of condition it is in.

Skin type and skin condition are two different things, but I often hear people using them interchangeably and it can create a lot of confusion, so let's clear it up once and for all:

Your **Skin Type** is what you were blessed with at birth.
It's a genetic present from your mum and dad.

Your **Skin Condition** is the state that your skin is currently in.
This 'state' is a result of your lifestyle, habits,
and can be a result of your skin type.

A good level of understanding will form the basis of all the decisions you make about your skin, from what cleanser to use to whether you could get away with skipping moisturiser before sunscreen. It will inform your make-up choices, so this is definitely a chapter to play close attention to. From a professional point of view, understanding your skin type helps us to place your current skin condition in context, and then to guide you to the most suitable treatments that will deliver the best results for your skin goals. It's one of the first things I do during your skin health consultation: establish your 'current' skin type, alongside looking at your skin's current condition.

I say 'current' because skin types change throughout life. I've never met anyone who has the same skin they had 10 years ago. Yet, so many people will sit on my very bougie velvet hot-pink chair and start their skin health consultation by saying, 'My skin never used to cause me any problems, I just want to have that skin back.' The skin from way back when. Or they say, 'I've never had any problems with my skin, my skin has always been good.' And it can happen this way; you feel that one day you woke up and your skin started being problematic. But I can assure you that the problems started a lot earlier and have slowly crept up on you over time; it's just that, unfortunately, life doesn't always allow you to pay as close attention as you would like.

I'm not a fan of assigning 'good' and 'bad' titles to skin. People always seem to be more aggressive with skin they deem 'bad', which invariably throws their skin into more of a funk. Whereas, when I come across clients who say they have good skin, they have a false sense of security that it will always remain so, regardless of how much (or how little) effort they spend looking after it.

Skin is such a dynamic and reactive force, so I encourage you to think about what your life was like during the time you thought you had 'good' skin. For most people it's their early teens, but it's more than likely life has taken several twists and turns since then, so your skin has gone on a journey, too. Skin will always reflect its present intrinsic and extrinsic environment.

Generally, we use 4 different classifications to categorise your skin type, looking mainly at the appearance of your skin, its oiliness, texture and pore size.

Dry skin can be one of two things: first, oil dry, meaning that the skin doesn't produce enough (or sometimes any) oil to naturally lubricate itself. Secondly, it can also be water dry, i.e., dehydrated, meaning there is insufficient moisture in the uppermost layer. This is a very common issue for Black skin as research shows that our skin is less able to hold water.[10] Although the pore size will be small, the dry skin will indeed feel dry, tight and rough, perhaps even with some flaking. Make-up doesn't sit well on dry skin and constantly looks patchy. Or your skin literally drinks your foundation because it's so parched.

Oily skin produces more oil than is needed for the skin to function normally. It will have a rough and thickened texture, tending to be greasy and look shiny. The pores are quite visible, and this skin can easily suffer from congestion and blackheads. Having oily skin does not necessarily mean you have strong, resilient skin that can take everything and the kitchen sink thrown at it. Whilst this skin type can be less reactive, it is not a licence to saturate it in harsh ingredients and products – its bite back isn't pretty!

Normal skin is one that is balanced, with the right amount of sweat and sebum that delicately lubricates and moisturises the skin. The texture is smooth and the pores are not overly noticeable on the skin. This is an ideal skin type but very few people will have it. If they do, they probably also have a sixth toe!

Combination skin is where most women sit as it is rare to be just one skin type. You will find yourself oily in some areas and dry in others. The most common combination skin I see is an oily t-zone (nose and forehead) with dry cheeks and temples. The degree of oiliness and dryness will always fluctuate and vary. Additionally, don't forget that Black skin is much more efficient at reflecting light, so don't confuse surface shine with oiliness.

FACT Skin typing was developed by Helena Rubinstein in 1910 as a way of classifying skin according to its nature and its needs. Cleverly, this also made it easier to sell skincare products in specific categories.

Your skin type is what you were blessed with at birth. Your skin condition is the state your skin is currently in.

As skin changes and matures as the body ages, you can easily move through different skin types. You can be in your 40s and suddenly start experiencing acne breakouts that you may associate with teenagers. Likewise, all of a sudden you could start experiencing facial hair in your 50s and 60s as androgen (mainly testosterone) levels rise and oestrogen levels fall during the menopause. Skin responds to both its internal and external environments. If you get a stressful job that has you reaching for sweet treats to fend off the three o'clock slump, and then follow it up with a bevvy or two when you get home, you may find once unproblematic skin becomes quite sluggish, grey-looking, oilier and more spot prone as sugar and alcohol cause a trail of inflammation in the body, making you more susceptible to breakouts or worsening dermatitis-type conditions such as eczema and psoriasis.

FACT The other pores that we have are sweat glands and they are also openings in the skin, but these rarely become clogged and act as a personal air conditioner to keep the body cool. Sweat glands are found all over the body but are concentrated in the underarm and groin areas, as well as the hands and feet.

I hate to be the bearer of bad news, but understanding your skin type will involve paying attention to everything else that's going on in your life. Skin typing is always a work in progress that takes time and patience; it may even be helpful to keep a diary. You need to search for clues. I always ask in consultations, 'What was going on in your life at the time?' What kind of transitions were happening? A new job, marriage, children, divorce, house move, illness, death?

Sometimes there are no hard and fast answers; it's a case of working through things to arrive at probable answers and probable solutions.

finding your skin type

A common question I get asked all the time is *'Dij, how do I find out my skin type?'* and you'd be surprised how many people don't quite know their skin type or understand that its condition can change through the seasons, or even through life events such as puberty, pregnancy, illness or menopause. Personally, it would make my skincare dreams come true if we just started including skincare classes in the National Curriculum. Let's start with working out our skin type, before we look at different skin conditions you may experience from time to time.

As skin changes and matures as the body ages, you can easily move through different skin types.

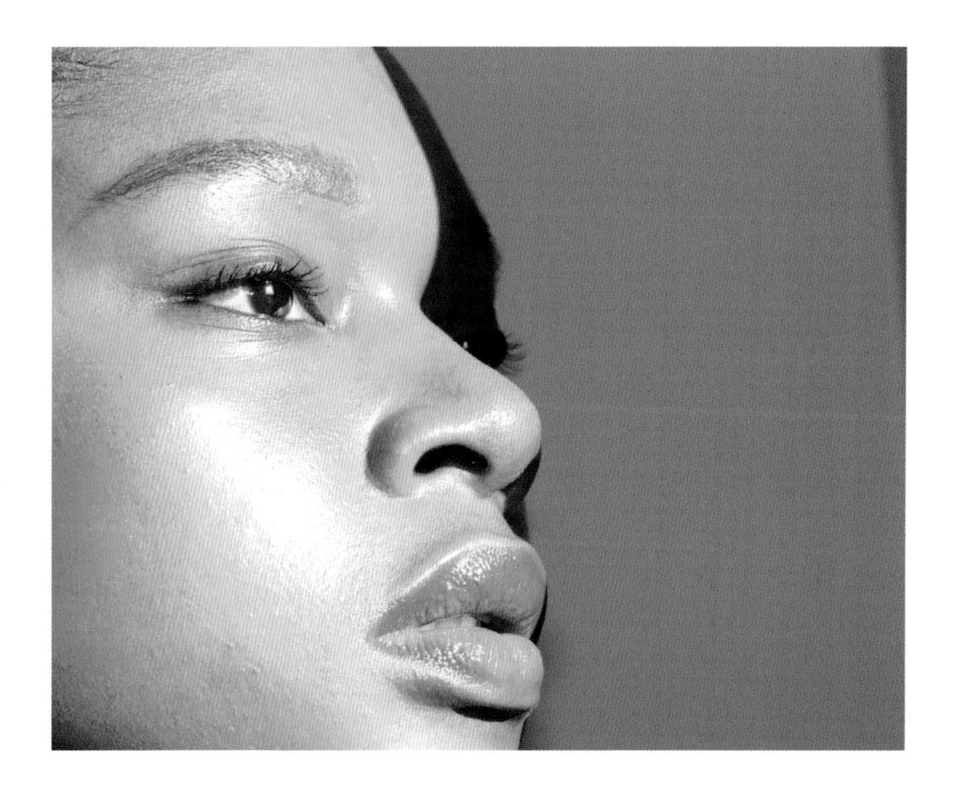

discover your skin type

How does your skin feel after washing, if you don't apply moisturiser or serums?

A. tight | B. comfortable | C. greasy

How would you describe your pores?

A. large and visible | B. visible only on t-zone | C. what pores?

On a normal day, without make-up, how does your skin tend to feel and look?

A. dry, screaming for moisture | B. greasy, like an oil slick | C. slight sheen

Do you ever have dry and flaky skin?

A. yes, story of my life | B. in some areas, e.g. cheeks | C. no flakes here!

If you wear make up, how quickly do you get shiny?

A. never, team matte | B. in a few hours | C. disco ball, within an hour

mostly As	mostly Bs	mostly Cs
dry	combination	oily

Psst...It's not that simple

It is possible for you to be a mix of two skin types or have a dominant skin type and still experience dehydration and/or be reactive to products.

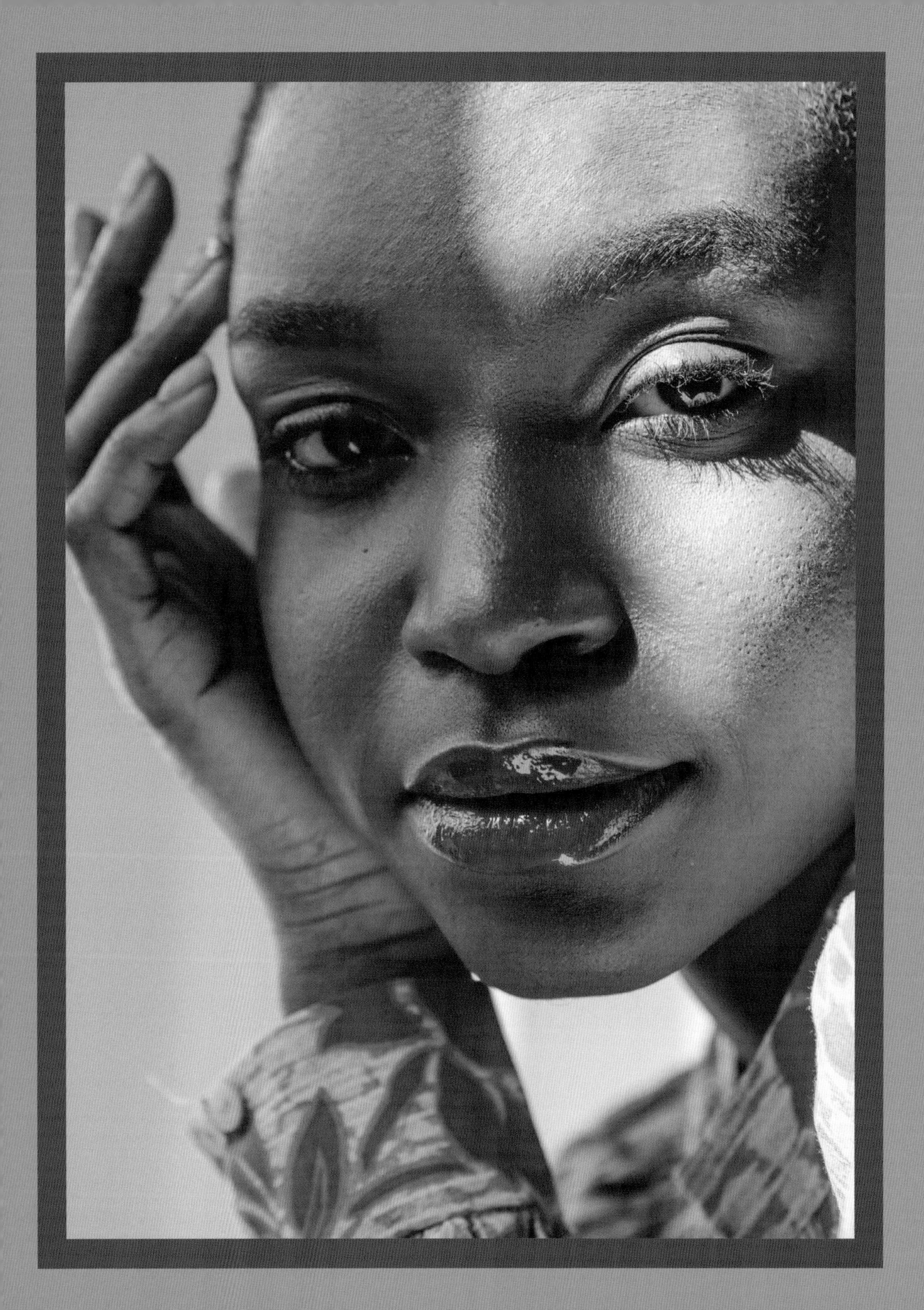

Pores

If I got a pound every time someone tells me they wished to close their pores, I'd be chilling in my pyjamas in the Bahamas by now. Firstly, we cannot close pores – they are not doors – and nor should we want to as they play a crucial role keeping our skin healthy and allowing it to fulfil its important roles of excretion and absorption.

There are two types of pores on the body but the one that we are mainly concerned with is actually a hair follicle that has a sebaceous gland attached. These glands secrete oil through the pore to the surface of the skin so that your skin stays lubricated and supple. Without this, your skin would dry up and shrivel like California raisins.

If this process of oil rising to the surface of the skin through the pores doesn't happen you end up with congestion and spots under the skin. Simples. Apart from the soles of your feet, your palms and lips, these pores are all over your body. A few things impact on the size of your pores. Firstly, genetics: the hand mum and dad gave you will have a major impact on the size of your pores. Pollution, excess oil, dirt, make-up and sunscreen also play a role. If you are prone to whiteheads and blackheads this will also create a larger pore size. This is why I labour the point of proper cleansing, because it's the first step in controlling the size of your pores. Age is a big factor as well. As the skin matures, collagen and elastin, which provide structural support to the pores like a scaffold, start to deteriorate. This causes the skin to stretch and sag, which ultimately makes pores appear more prominent on your close-ups.

minimising the appearance of pores

The same way a balloon swells when you fill it with air, pores will expand when filled with oil and gunk. When you let the air out of the balloon it shrinks; when you take oil out of the pores, they shrink too. This is my favourite pore-size explanation!

So, to control pore size and minimise their appearance, you have to regularly draw excess oil out of them.

- Use salicylic acid somewhere in your routine. This is an ingredient that loves oil and is able to penetrate your pores for a deep cleanse to dislodge any congestion. Cleansers and toners are good places to look for salicylic acid.
- Washing your face properly twice a day is key to sweeping away oil, dirt, make-up and sunscreen that contribute to large pores.
- Regular gentle exfoliation will help to remove the build-up of old skin cells that can lead to clogged pores. Look out for glycolic, lactic and mandelic acid in your skincare products because they are excellent exfoliators and perfectly safe for Black skin. (More about these key skincare ingredients in Chapter 11.) Additionally, they retexture your skin, so overall not only is pore size minimised, the feel and quality of your skin is improved. Bonus!
- Consider swapping your basic night moisturiser for a retinoid serum like retinol instead. This will make a massive difference in the long term because it improves your overall skin quality.
- Use a minimum SPF30 broad-spectrum sunscreen daily to prevent damage to collagen that can make pores appear more visible.
- If you are particularly oily and your pores are getting you down, a weekly clay-based face mask will help to draw out excess oil and instantly shrink your pore size.
- Use skincare labelled as 'non-comedogenic' as they are less likely to clog your pores. Non-comedogenic means that the product has been formulated with lightweight, pore-friendly ingredients that won't clog your pores. Many products in the oily-skin category are non-comedogenic and will be advertised as such, so it's easy to spot them. Whatever you do, avoid using heavy ingredients such as coconut oil or shea butter on your face because they can just sit in your pores, contributing to your unhappiness when you look in the mirror.
- Keep on top of your pores with professional in-clinic treatments. If large pores are becoming bothersome, then turbo-boosting rejuvenating treatments such as chemical peels will always help to deep-cleanse your skin to remove oil and debris.

The bottom line is that you need your pores, they are not your enemy and you don't have to be constantly fighting against them. Treat them nicely and they will fall in line and not be so in your face – pun intended.

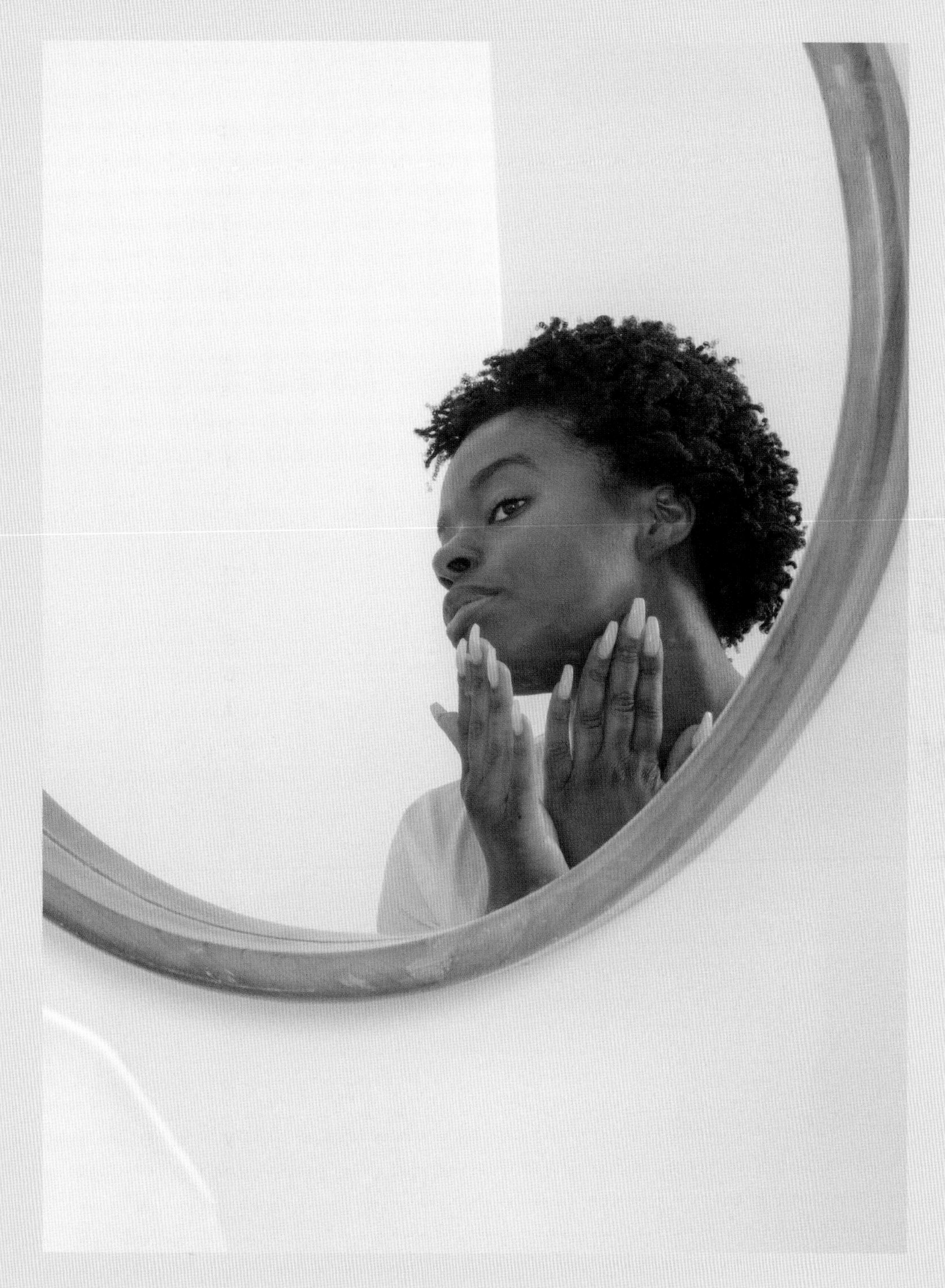

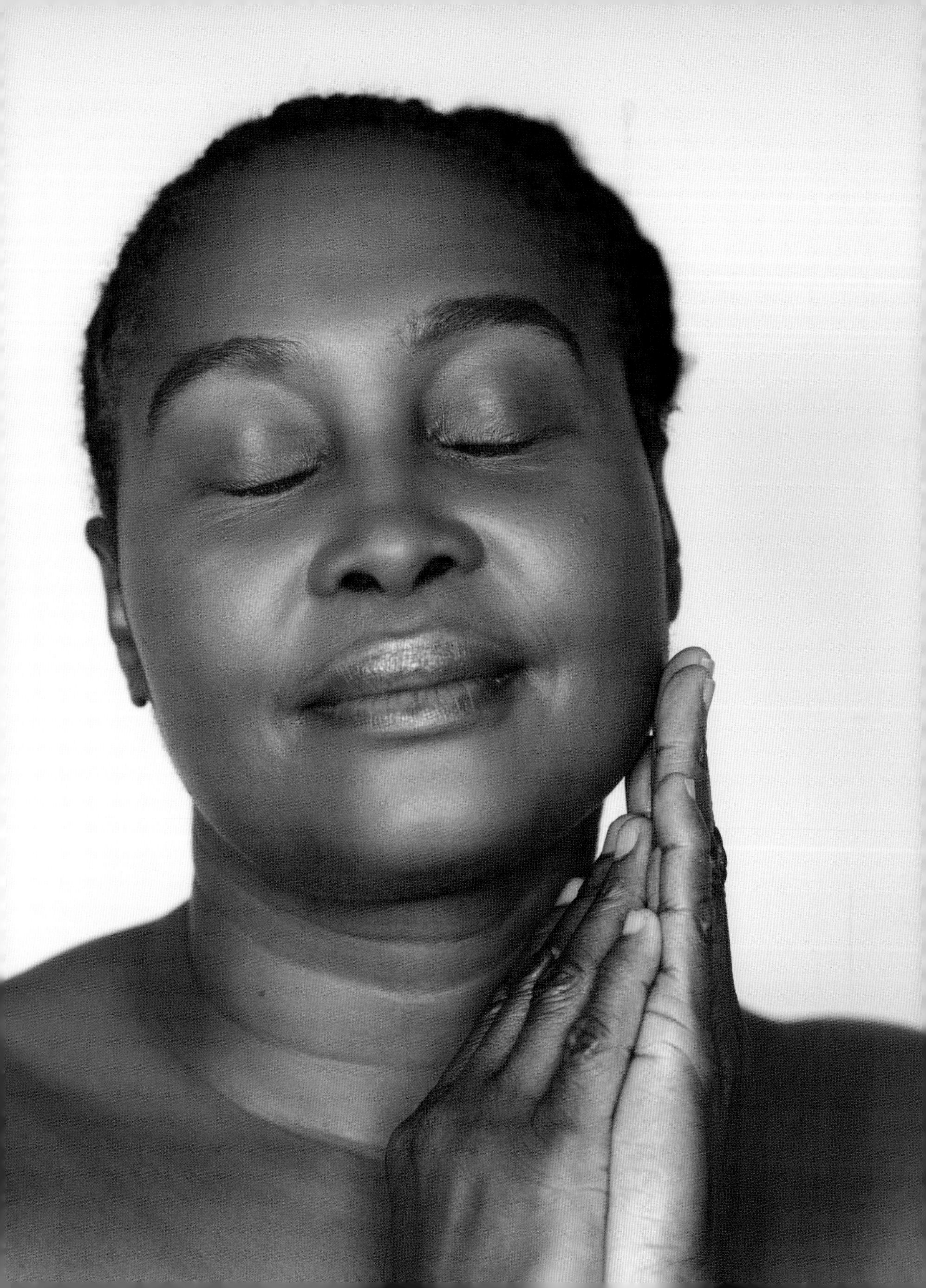

04.

skin across a lifetime

skin across a lifetime

THERE are times in your life when the quality of your skin is more noticeable. Most of the time, we're just ticking along then, woosh bang, our skin gives us a tap on the shoulder to say 'pay me some attention.' I'm not talking about a new spot here or there – those are easily dealt with. It's more things like how the texture of your skin has changed, how pores are more noticeable, how many more freckles you have, how dark marks seem to never fade, and how many more lines are framing your eyes.

Sadly, the body isn't designed to last forever, and skin cells are automatically programmed to be born and to die after a certain time. Obviously, our lifestyles can impact this process (more on that in the next chapter), so it's worth bearing in mind that the story your skin is telling right now is based on how you've looked after it as well as how your genetic clock is set.

After doing my job for over a decade, it's clear there is a pattern that defines skin at different ages. I love doing the 'life vs skin' analysis with clients, where we plot changes in their skin against milestones in life. This helps us clarify what we should be thinking and doing for our skin at certain milestones.

puberty

Skin shifts can start to happen from age 8 upwards and continue well into teenage years. My transition from girlhood to adolescent is immortalised in a particular grainy picture of me, aged 14, in the backyard of the house I grew up in in North London. I'm stood by the washing-line, a vision in unimaginative brown leggings and brown top, and there is a very visible spot on my chin. One of those spots that can't help but call your attention. 'Yoohoo!' (Frantic wave.) 'Look at me, I'm over here!' Large and bulging with a white top and virtually ready to pop. I didn't really suffer from acne or breakouts as a young girl, but from time to time I did have these mahoosive whoppers on my face.

Androgen hormones pick up during puberty, giving the sebaceous glands a kick to start producing more oil – hence those pesky breakouts. Both boys and girls will produce more testosterone and, along with rises in oestrogen and progesterone, this will result in some degree of acne. For some, like me, it will be one or two spots; for others it may be full-face acne that will wreak havoc on self-esteem and self-confidence. As if teenage life isn't difficult enough!

Teenage skin has the advantage of 'bouncebackability' because it is young and able to regenerate quickly, and pretty successfully, so the main thing to concentrate on is taking control to put solutions into place quickly. See Chapter 9 for more on teenage skincare.

> The story your skin is telling right now is based on how you've looked after it as well as how your genetic clock is set.

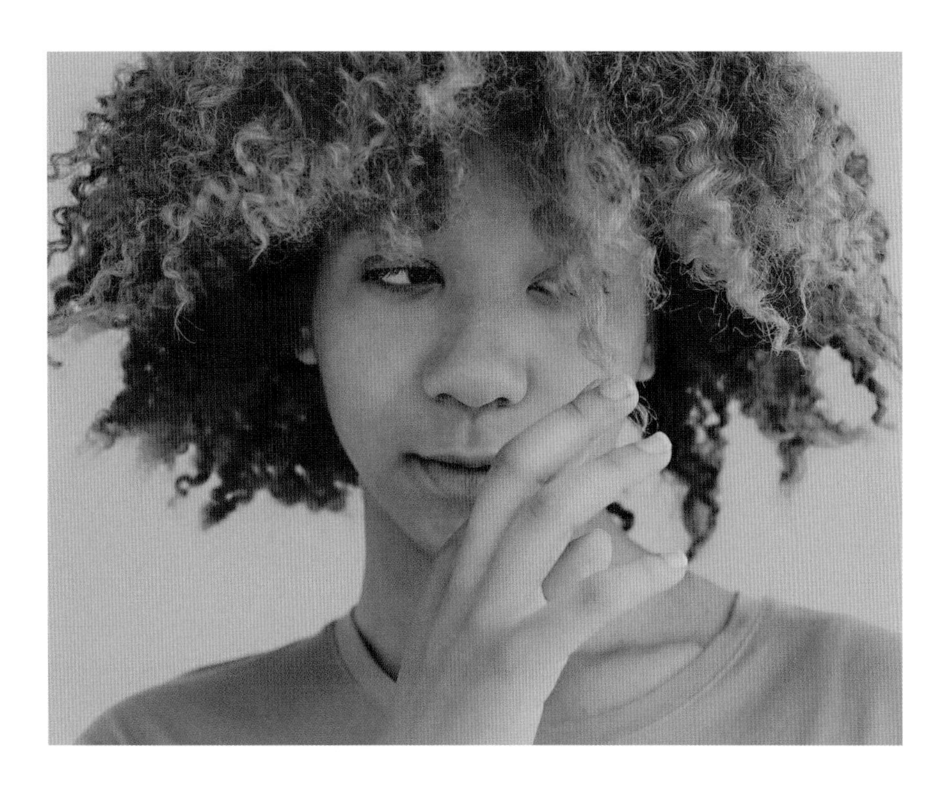

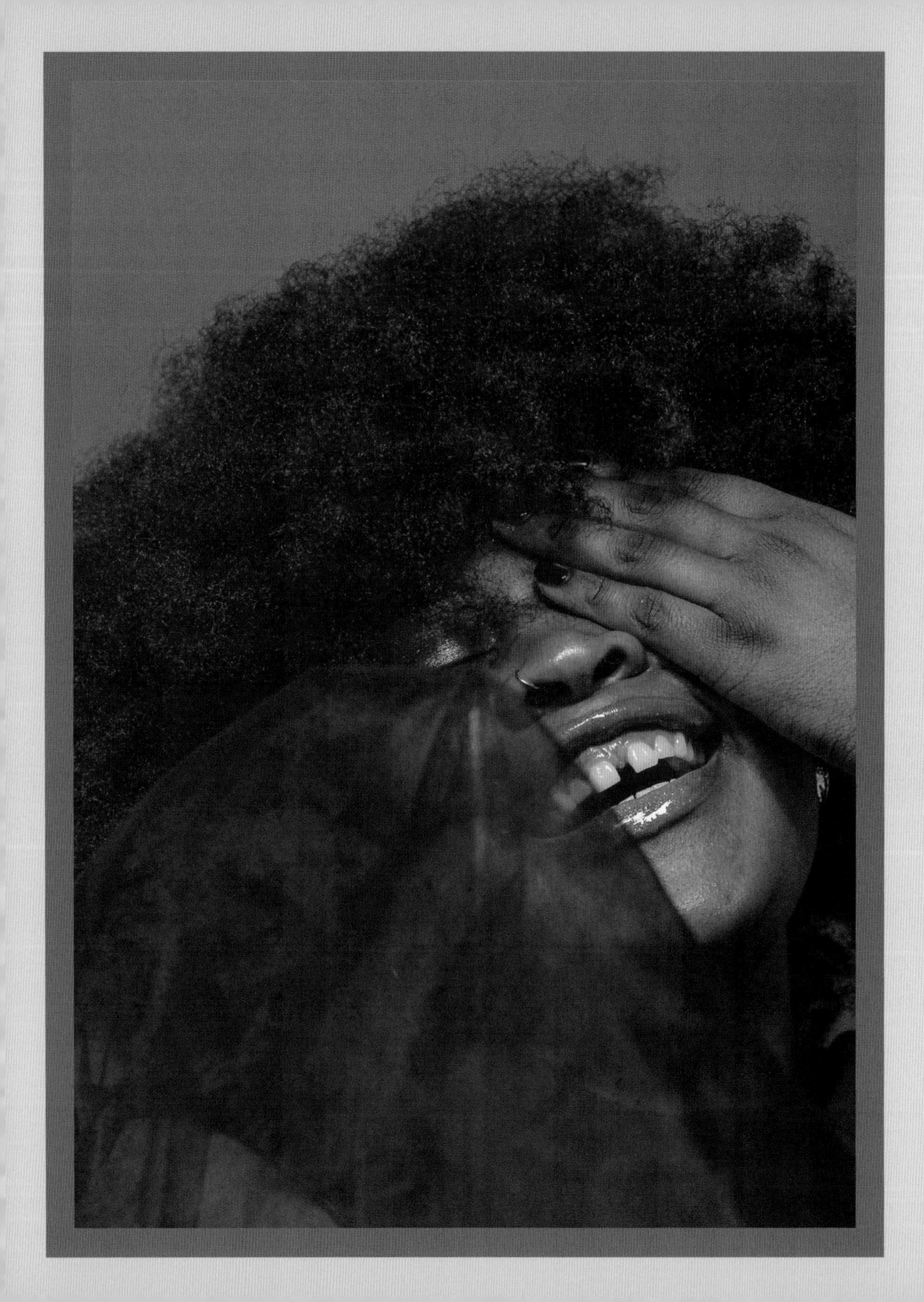

20s–30s

Even though you're just starting out, this is when you really start setting the foundation for the skin you will enjoy in later life. So if there is any time you want to pay close attention to your skin, it's now. This is when your skin starts losing its ability of near-perfect youthful regeneration. Your lifestyle will have the most impact now, and, if my 20s were anything to go by, you're working hard (late nights, stress, poor diet, smoking) and you're playing hard (clubbing, drinking, flying, beach holidays). So my advice is to look after your skin as much as you can. Believe me when I say prevention is better than cure.

I'll get the downsides out of the way first: collagen starts depleting in your skin from age 25 onwards, albeit more slowly than your white counterparts. But it does start to deplete nevertheless, along with elastin, which – sadly – doesn't regenerate once it's lost.

Childhood sun damage also starts to show, and you start noticing the dark marks left over from spots more. It's not that you didn't get them before, it's just that they faded much quicker, so you didn't really notice them that much. If you are on the oily-skin spectrum, pore size and texture may become more noticeable because the skin cell turnover cycle starts to slow down, leaving the surface of your skin feeling rough. Lines and dark circles may also start creeping around the eyes.

This is the time when skin can become sensitised, due to overuse of products and ingredients because you are more willing to, and can afford to, experiment – much to the chagrin of your skin and the disappointment of skin practitioners everywhere as we really need you to practise patience, commitment and consistency at this point.

It's not all bad though, because if you seriously treat your skin with a good and consistent routine, using decent products and skin-type appropriate ingredients, you can make it play the game you want.

> When it comes to skin, practise patience, commitment and consistency.

Weddings

The pressure to look your very best can be very real. From the dress, show hair style, make-up and skin. Having been a bride with both a UK and destination wedding, I appreciate just how much focus is on perfection, skin included.

If you're not used to looking after your skin in any significant way but you'd like to do so on account of your upcoming wedding, I gotchu!

Start with booking a skin and lifestyle consultation as soon as you're engaged. Do this a minimum of 6 months ahead of the date – and it's even more important if you have active concerns such as acne and hyperpigmentation. It's also a good time to consider your body skincare: hands, arms, lips, back and shoulders. This is especially important if you are wanting to stun in a backless, sleeveless, low-neckline number.

The consultation will get you using the right types of products for your skin concerns. But also, you'll learn about the things you have to watch out for, like, perversely, how your skin will break out more leading up to the big day because you're under so much stress.

You can start treatments at the 6-months-to-go mark as well. This is enough time to see some decent results from mainly rejuvenating programmes that stimulate your skin with hyaluronic acid, help to fade discolouration, increase clarity and glow. Black skin needs to focus on brightening, so tyrosinase inhibitors (see Chapter 11) should play a big role in your skincare. You want the battery packs in your skin cells to be fully charged and operating at full power.

Ideally, you don't want to be starting any new stimulating treatments 3 months before the day. In my experience, that's when the stress starts ramping up and it will show on your skin, so combining that with new skincare can be a recipe for disaster, *especially* if your skin goes through a purge. If time is not on your side but you want to have some treatments, consider LED light, micro-current and some lasers like the Byonik.

Destination brides, especially if in the tropics or somewhere mega warm – the best thing you can do is to arrive 5–7 days ahead of time to give your skin time to acclimatise to a drier or more humid climate. Don't be tempted to go for any new treatments on arrival either: don't tempt breakouts or worse! An emergency skincare kit will be handy, see Chapter 12. Make-up artists can work wonders with their brushes, and photographers can airbrush pictures to perfection; however, your guests and their mobile phones may not be so kind!

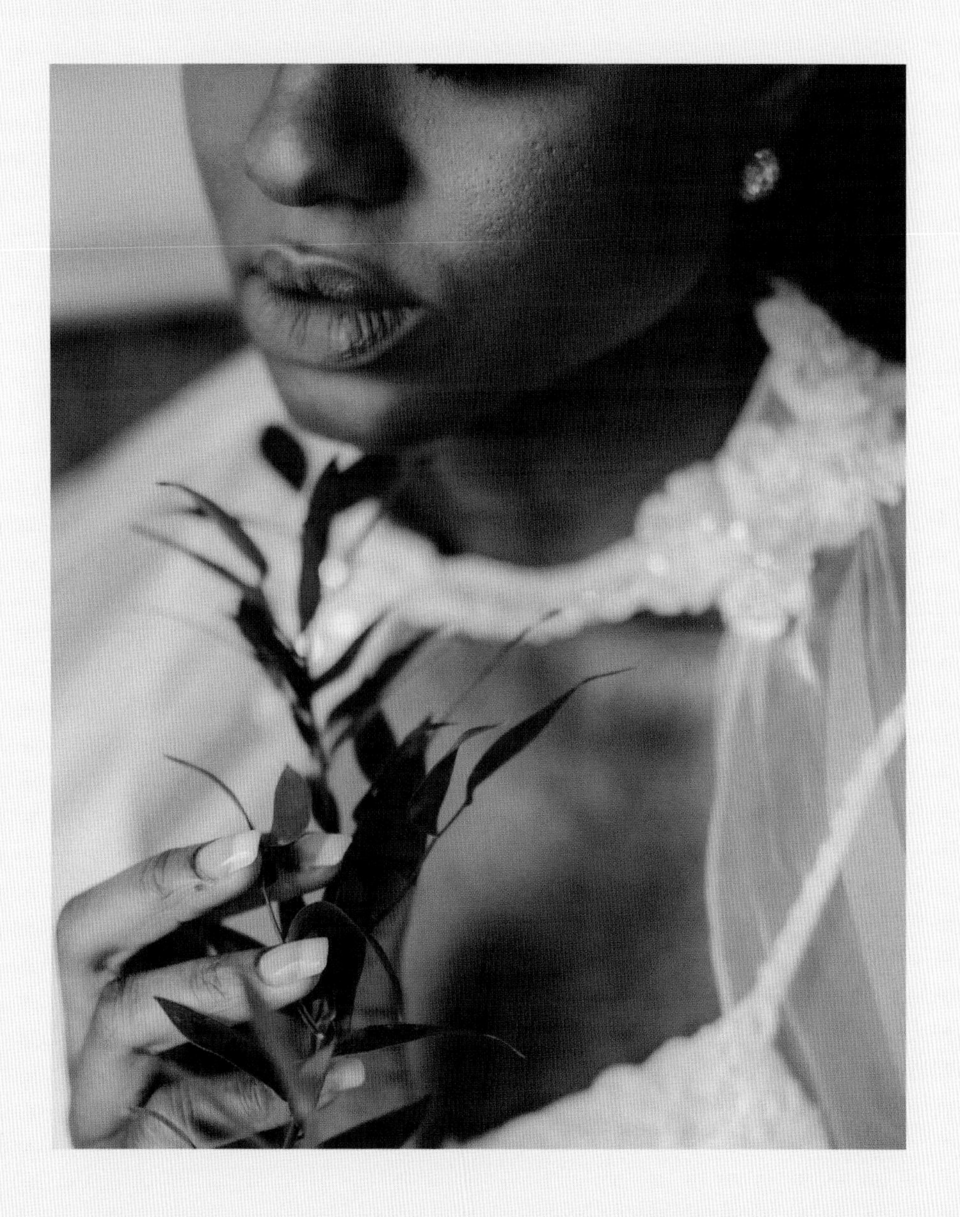

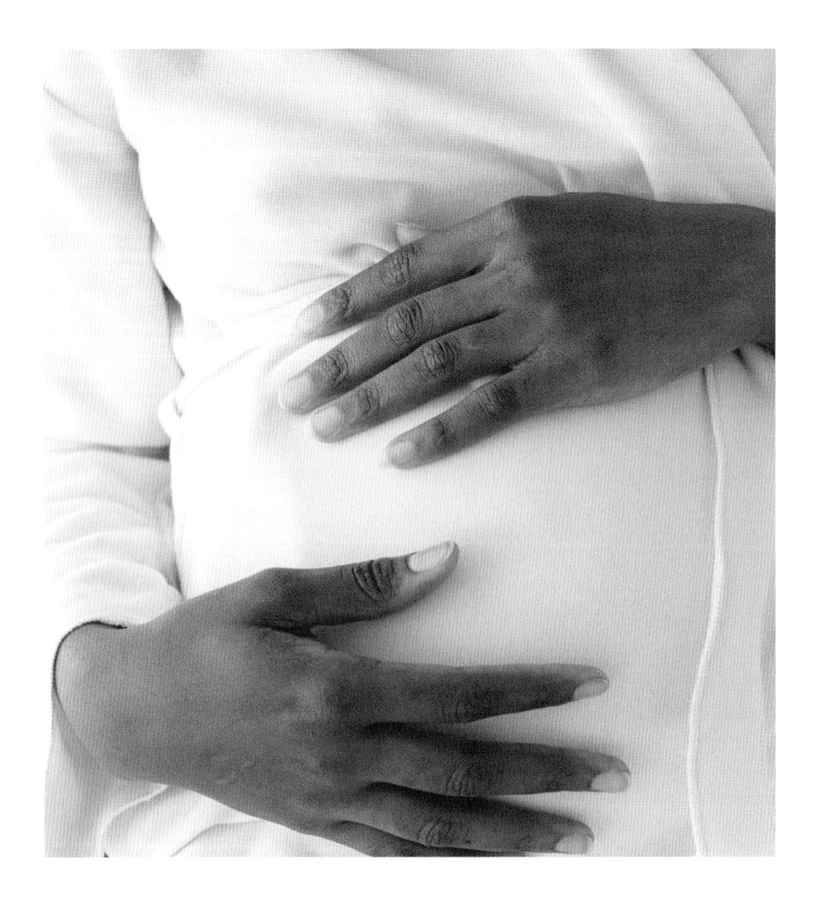

pregnancy

Pregnancy is a massive upheaval in all senses of the word. Black women are prone to increased darkening of the skin, notably on the face – foreheads and cheeks bearing the hallmark of what is often called the mask of pregnancy. With both my pregnancies, by the time I was 7 months gone, my face was at least three shades darker than the rest of my body. This did fade after I gave birth and for many women that will also be the case. There is a small number of women for whom the discolouration lasts a very long time though. It's simply the luck of the draw.

It's also a myth that pregnancy means radiant skin. This is not the case for everyone; acne and breakouts can set in, creating a lot of hyperpigmentation in their wake. Itchy skin irritations are more common, and these too can discolour the skin, causing hyperpigmentation. If you get severe itching all over your body, this is called obstetric cholestasis and you must seek medical advice from your doctor.

Stretch marks are very common because of the sudden increase in your size and how much your skin has to stretch to accommodate a growing bump. This expansion causes elastin to break, so applying deeply moisturising creams with ingredients such as plant oils – shea butter and jojoba oil, ceramides, glycerine and Vitamin E can protect the skin from their development and reduce the accompanying darkening and flushing. Stretch marks tend to fade after you've given birth.

It's a myth that pregnancy means radiant skin. This is not the case for everyone.

40s–50s

They say life starts at 40 and I would like to add that this is also the prime time to start earnestly supporting your skin, especially if you weren't doing so before.

Collagen and elastin are breaking down at a faster rate and, given the onset of peri-menopause, you will notice that your skin is drier and more rough textured as the natural exfoliation process of the skin slows down. Lines will arrive and stay like unwanted visitors; the ones around the eyes will become deeper; the lines running either side from the corners of your nose to the corners of your lips will become more prominent; and the middle of your face will start to lose its plumpness. Dark circles are also much more visible because the skin around the eyes is getting even thinner, making issues of poor circulation and even genetic darkness more apparent.

Black skin will look dull and lacklustre; I have had many a 40-something sit on the hot-pink velvet chair and say the words, 'My skin just looks so dull!' These are all signs that the skin's natural processes that would normally keep it vibrant are slowing down. Code for you have to take things up a notch to meet your skin where it currently is.

This is the age group that complains the most about pigmentation, especially melasma and pent-up sun damage (most Black women today in this age bracket would not have grown up wearing sunscreen simply because the messaging about its benefits would not have been communicated). It's a double whammy; not only does skin look dry and tired, it also looks patchy and discoloured. DPN (short for Dermatosis Papulosa Nigra, harmless but fleshy pigmented raised bumps often called skin tags) that were barely noticeable years before are now more bothersome, because you've amassed a few more lumps and bumps or the existing ones may have grown in size.

From a skincare point of view, include everything good you did in the previous decade, but include more moisture-boosting ingredients such as hyaluronic acid and ceramides to prevent excessive dryness. Now I'd definitely be encouraging you to consider supporting treatments such as chemical skin peels, micro-needling, laser and LED light to stimulate, improve hydration and rejuvenate your skin. At this point, creams alone are not going to cut it as the skin needs a boost in the deeper layers to preserve its health.

I know I sound like the harbinger of doom (imagine sitting in a face-to-face consultation and I'm coming at you with all this information! Consider yourself lucky that you can just turn the page if you want to shut me up.) Jest aside, even with all I have said, all is not lost as not everything here will happen to you all at once. It may be only one or two things, but the point is that if you don't want it to become three or four things, then now is the time to intervene.

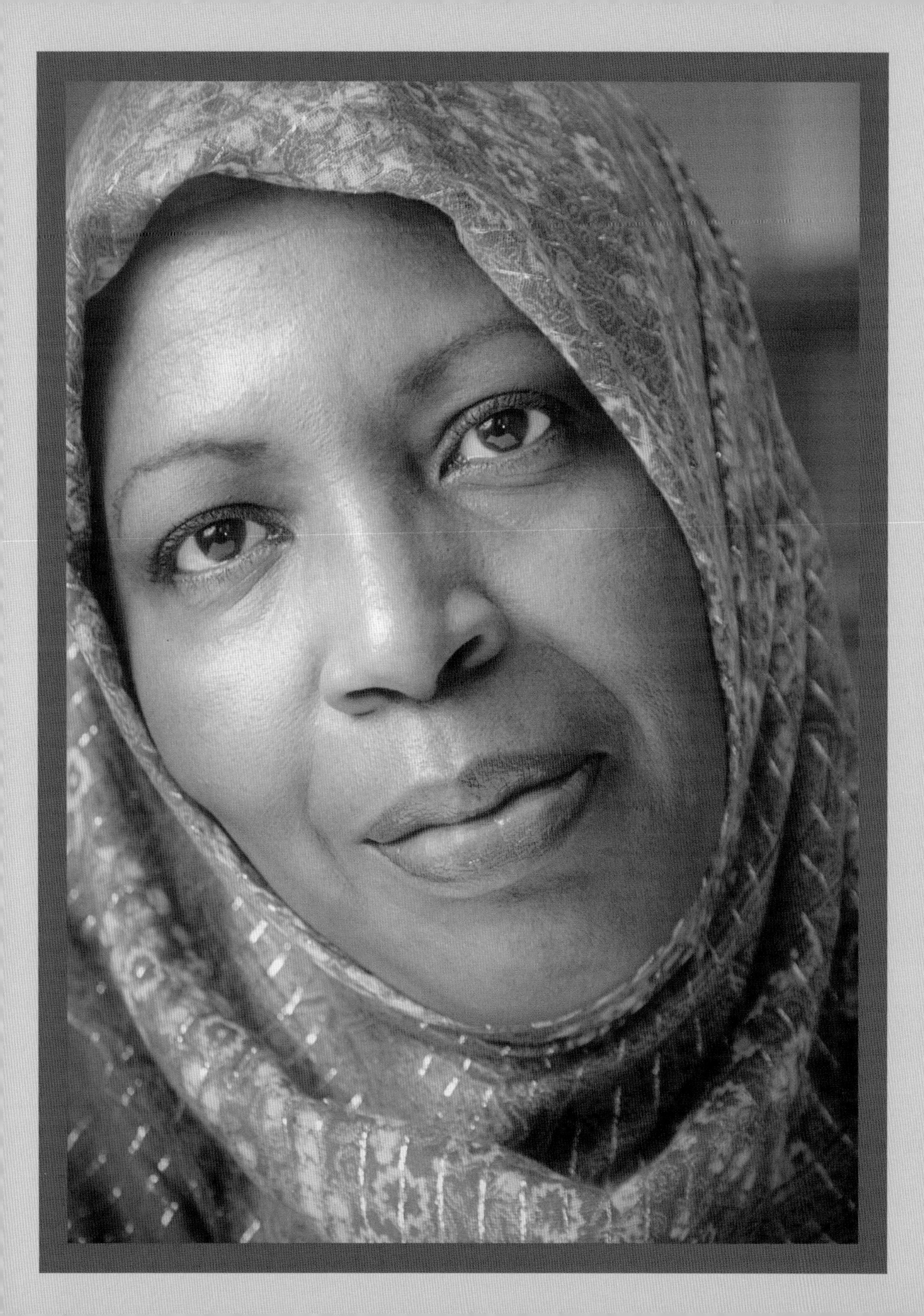

50+

This is the golden decade where you can reclaim your time and money and plough it into looking and feeling good; typically the kids have flown the nest and you've cut the purse strings. Realistically, you're in the throes of menopause. According to NHS statistics, the average age to reach the menopause is 51, so your skin will be experiencing the physical and physiological changes that the menopause brings with it.

The drop in oestrogen levels, along with other hormones, will impact the quality of your skin big time. Black skin is already prone to losing moisture and the menopause will worsen this. The turnover of your skin cells will slow down considerably, increasing the buildup of old and dull cells on the surface of the skin and you may find an increased need to exfoliate to improve the texture and restore your glow. Be careful not to use grainy scrubs, though, as their likelihood of scratching and damaging fragile skin will be higher. Enzyme or acid-based exfoliators are the best option to keep skin in smooth shape.

Furthermore, your skin will feel considerably parched and thirsty because it will start to struggle to hold on to water; the protective skin barrier will be weaker because the pH level of the skin changes, and this makes it easier to pick up rashes and irritations as the skin will be thinner. Pigmentation concerns – which Black skin is already prone to because of more active melanin cells – such as melasma and blemishes that were once masked by the thickness and suppleness of your skin, will be more apparent, especially around the eyes, where you will also be contending with more pronounced dark circles. If you spent lots of time in the sun without UV protection in your younger years, you are sure to see the effects now. It is also possible to develop acne and start sprouting facial hair because the body continues to produce testosterone, even whilst other hormones are decreasing, but in a cruel twist of fate you may start to lose hair on your head.

Your skin's ability to regenerate itself becomes much slower, so things like bruises (which you will be more prone to), cuts and wounds will take longer to heal. This means that if you're having professional skin treatments, the gap between appointments has to be longer. Instead of the usual 4 weeks, appointments may be 6 weeks apart so that your skin has as much time to heal and strengthen as possible.

The skincare focus here is on boosting collagen and stimulating the skin to produce as much hydration as possible, and then maintaining those gains. These will help the skin feel moisturised, plumped and comfortable, with a smoother and more radiant texture. Remember, it's never too late to start looking after your skin. Obviously, I wish you'd started in your youth (I would say that, wouldn't I?!), but the most important thing is that you start regardless of which age bracket you tick.

Alongside the chronological age-related changes that are happening to your skin, extrinsic factors are also taking their toll. Environmental damage in the form of pollution and UV radiation attacks skin from the outside in. At the same time adulting is also impacting on your skin. Modern stresses such as work deadlines, late nights, poor diets, sedentary days with long spells in front of screens, worries, all find a way to weave themselves into the fabric of your skin, not to talk of illnesses and drugs (prescribed or otherwise!), which can also impact the quality of your skin.

Over the course of our lives, skin can and will experience many changes. Accepting that some of these changes are inevitable is the first step in looking after your skin, and I want you to be assured that there's plenty available to help you manage your skin in good and in challenging times. And more often than not it starts with looking at our lifestyle.

The drop in oestrogen levels, along with other hormones, during menopause will impact the quality of your skin big time.

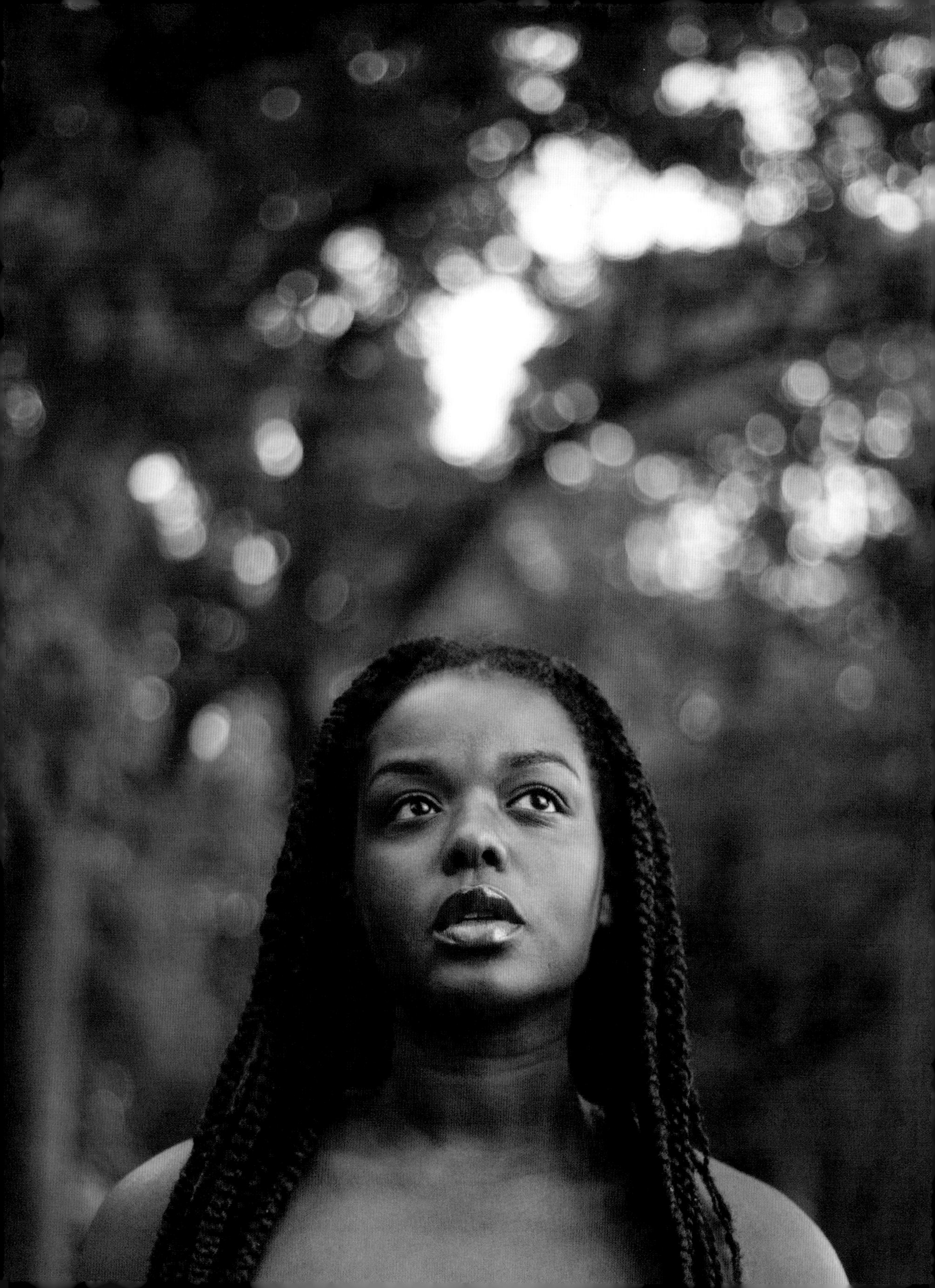

05.

lifestyle and skin

lifestyle and skin

HEALTHY skin is as much about how we live our lives as about the products we apply on top of it. Your skin is a flappy mouth snitch and will speak even when you are silent. When you've been in the skincare game as long as I have, you have a way of instantly assessing clients as soon as they walk through the door. It's not malicious, it's a very automatic 'what am I working with here today?' A quick visual assessment helps me to mentally tick off certain boxes and I can spot a poor sleeper, hay fever sufferer, too many sugars in the tea, stressed out, veg-phobic client even before they sit down. If you're sick, your skin will invariably look dull and washed out.

Likewise, if you're in good health, your skin will also reflect this, looking smooth and with a light radiance.

It's so important to listen to our skin cues. I once had a boss who broke out in multiple big red welts of hives on her face and neck in response to stress. I always knew when she was up against a deadline as her skin gave out all the signs. Eventually she changed roles because professionally she wasn't coping and, thanks to her skin, it was clear for the whole world to know.

My personal philosophy is to always approach skin health from a place of practicality, doing the best for your skin at any given time. Life is fluid, sh*t happens, and skin will follow the patterns of your lifestyle, but all too many times I find that we expect our skin to remain in a static condition and we give it (and ourselves) a hard time when it temporarily looks worse for wear.

That said, there are many aspects of our lives and lifestyles that we can and should keep in check so our skin can be the best it can be.

smoking

No. Just don't do it. Don't start and, if you are a smoker, figure out a way to stop. Having once been a smoker I do sympathise, but at the risk of teaching you how to suck an egg, smoking does your skin and health no favours.

Smoking speeds up the skin ageing, it worsens the impact on the skin of some diseases such as lupus and psoriasis as well as slowing down your skin's ability to heal after an injury, trauma or inflammation. Blood supply is reduced by smoking, and this starves the skin of oxygen; collagen and elastin are damaged so wrinkles set in earlier, the texture of the skin becomes dry and rough, and discolouration is more noticeable.

Stopping smoking will improve your skin health. Period. I've seen smokers go from looking a shadow of health to a picture of radiant vitality within a matter of weeks after giving up smoking.

> It's so important to listen to our skin cues.

diet

A colourful and nutritious plate full of healthy proteins, fats, vegetables and carbohydrates will do wonders for your body and, in turn, your skin. Over the years, diet has taken on a more prominent role in skincare and to a large extent I welcome this, as what you put into your body does need care and attention. But by the same token, I've seen clients get themselves into an agonising tizz over their plates, ending in varying degrees of stress and unhappiness (and hunger!).

I remember once consulting with a client who had been seeing a well-known naturopathic doctor who had advised what I can only call severe food restrictions, cutting out wine, cakes, wine, chocolate, butter, wine, cheese – did I say wine? My client fell off the programme because, in her words, 'I had the best skin I'd ever had, but I was miserable.' A very sociable person who suffered from occasional acne breakouts and enjoyed eating out with friends was now a very sad one with clear and smooth skin sitting indoors. I know who I'd rather be. Pass me the whole bottle of wine.

Restricting a particular food group without a sound basis given by a qualified medical professional, such as for allergies or intolerances, does more harm than good. So by all means, don't deny yourself anything, enjoy everything in moderation – sweet treats, coffee, alcohol, takeaways. An indulgence here or there will not derail any skin health improvements you're making.

Psst... A word about alcohol

Alcohol contains sugar and can do a double on your skin as it will dehydrate because it's a diuretic and the sugar will cause inflammation. If you're a big drinker, especially of cocktails, expect your skin to experience puffiness, broken capillaries and ruddiness/redness of the skin (though on very dark Black skin this is more a flushing as redness won't show).

sugar face

Yes, there is such a thing called sugar face and it happens when there is a lot of sugar in your diet, leading to a process called glycation.

This is when sugar attaches itself to the collagen in our skin and this makes it hard and brittle, leading to breakages which show up as fine lines and wrinkles. With collagen being the all-important scaffolding for the skin, once it breaks the skin starts to sag and droop and your pores become stretched and more noticeable. The problem is that glycation is a slow process and you often don't see it on Black skin until it's too late because we have tighter and more compact collagen bundles. Though when it starts to show, it's all at once, making the skin look dramatically aged.

As if that's not enough, sugar is also inflammatory and weakens the natural barrier function which protects and balances your skin. This makes any existing condition you are prone to, such as acne or eczema, worse.

And sorry, there's more: sugar influences the body's production of testosterone, eventually leading to more oil on the skin, which then makes your pores larger and more visible. As this increased oil mingles with bacteria on the surface of the skin, the likelihood of breakouts also increases.

One last point on sugar, it also slowly dehydrates your skin. It will look dull, lacklustre and sallow, meaning dark circles and discolouration are more noticeable. Black skin will have a shiny and grey undertone.

When we in the profession say 'sugar is the devil for skin,' this is what we mean. Avail yourself of the sweetie jar with caution.

> Skin will follow the patterns of your lifestyle.

dairy

We live in the time of milk, cheese and butter excess and, having a child who is allergic to dairy, I've come to understand just how much dairy we consume. It's in everything, and the confusing thing is that it is hidden behind so many names – whey, casein, caseinate, tagatose...the list is endless.

In the skincare world, there are some that believe there is a clear link between dairy, skin quality and inflammatory conditions such as acne. Official research is inconclusive, which leaves it up to us professionals to decide on our own personal approach in the absence of evidence. I have seen clients who cut dairy out of their diets and see their skin quality flourish, experiencing fewer breakouts and increased clarity. Likewise, I've seen clients who've done the same with little or no effect on their skin. So, when clients ask me about this, I always give both sides of the story and conclude with, 'It doesn't hurt for you to try giving up dairy for a few weeks to see what the effect would be.' And I'd say the same for you too, dear reader: if you think there's a link between your skin and your dairy intake, try eliminating dairy for two to three weeks, take pictures of your skin every couple of days and keep a daily diary to track your progress. At the end of the period, review your data to see whether there truly was an effect.

Because I don't believe you should just cut out a food group without professional oversight, I recommend you follow up with a nutritionist. They can provide appropriate advice if you do decide you want to cut out dairy based on its effects on your skin.

stress

I've come to accept that adulting will always mean we all live under some degree of stress. However, prolonged excessive stress puts a drain on our body by releasing the hormone cortisol into our system. This creates inflammation in the body and stimulates testosterone, which slowly increases oil production in the skin. Resulting in...you guessed it! A poorer skin condition and, worse still, dull skin, spots and breakouts.

sleep

Sleep is crucial for skin health and is a basic beauty directive so that your skin can rest and repair. Without it, your body is under more stress and your skin health suffers. It becomes dull and patchy and everything, including pigmentation and under-eye circles, worsens.

Skin cells follow your circadian rhythm, your body's internal clock system. In fact, research shows that the cells that make up the skin, such as the melanocytes and collagen-producing cells called fibroblasts, also have their own personal clock in addition to the master body clock that lives in the brain.[11] Both clocks work together for your body and skin health.

The quality of your sleep will impact your hydration and moisture levels, the strength and resiliency of your skin's natural barrier function, how much oil your skin secretes, how fast your skin ages, blood and oxygen flow to your skin, and how your natural exfoliation process functions. Research has also shown that at night and during sleep, the skin has the body's highest DNA repair capabilities, the highest cell division and highest absorption rates. This is key to why certain product ingredients like retinoids and alpha hydroxy acids have even more benefits when used at night.

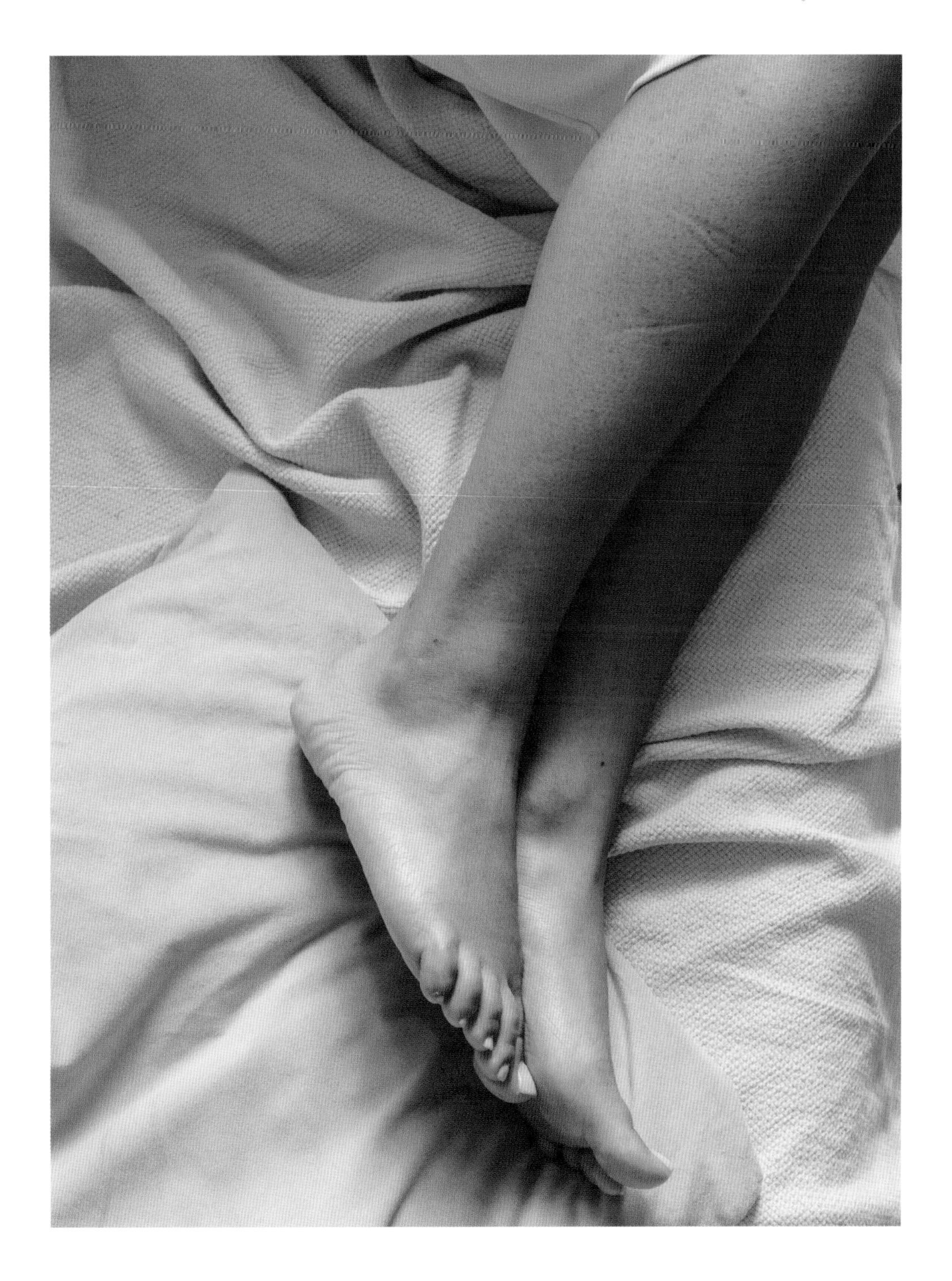

environment

Air pollution is a major problem around the world and according to the World Health Organization, it kills around 7 million people a year. We've known for decades that daily exposure to pollution has poor health outcomes, including leading to heart and lung problems – and especially for those who live in big cities like London, New York and Lagos. These air pollutants include (but are not limited to) polycyclic aromatic hydrocarbons, volatile organic compounds, oxides, particulate matter, ozone and cigarette smoke.

FACT A free radical is an unstable molecule that damages skin cells, DNA and collagen, eventually causing premature ageing.

With the skin being your first line of defence, prolonged exposure to pollution will affect it and increase flare-ups of inflammatory skin conditions like acne and eczema, not to mention speeding up premature ageing. People who live in big cities experience more skin dryness, hyperpigmentation and much earlier wrinkles because free radicals in the atmosphere attack and damage skin cell DNA.

Prolonged exposure to pollution will affect it and increase flare-ups of inflammatory skin conditions like acne and eczema.

It was only when I moved from London to the Kent countryside that I truly appreciated the environmental and pollution burden my skin was under. Within a few weeks I noticed my skin was clearer and calmer, and this was reinforced each time I spent a day in London and saw how quickly my skin quality would deteriorate. Granted, not everyone can up-sticks for a quieter life in the country, and you may not want to either. But including an antioxidant with vitamin C into your health regime, applying sunscreen and maintaining a consistent twice-daily skincare routine will make a big difference.

black skin

a history

The Long Fight for Freedom of Expression

It took nearly a hundred years to completely abolish slavery, from the first French decree in 1794 to the abolition of slavery in Brazil in 1888, but none of this brought about an up-valuation of Black people, our skin and our features. Lofty declarations of physical freedom and equality of all men did not take into account the psyches of individuals and identities that over the course of four hundred years had been savaged and dehumanised. Self-worth, esteem and value did not immediately come flooding back.

> Slavery may have been abolished, but it was replaced with a different kind of racism. A structural racism that kept (and in some regards continues to keep) Black people prisoners of their skin colour and excludes them from participating equally in beauty, skincare and self-care with their white counterparts.

In the southern US states, this was embodied in the 'Jim Crow' laws, the state-directed segregation of Blacks and whites that was only abolished in 1965. In South Africa it was Apartheid, which ended only as recently as 1994. Whilst no such segregation formally existed in the UK, up until the Race Relations Act was passed in 1968 it was common to see letting signs that read 'No Blacks [or Coloured], no dogs, no Irish', which served to informally segregate society.

> The legacy of the organised and systematic stripping and brutalising of the Black and African identity is still with us. A legacy that for the best part of five hundred years has said that Black is not beautiful, Black features are similar to those of baboons, Black characteristics are animalistic and Black skin is ugly and fearsome. When we look at the concept of beauty, white people got a head start with no challenges, and Blacks are still playing catch-up.

We are only just starting to dismantle this mental trauma as we reclaim and rebuild our identities and seize ownership of our beauty. White people have to understand their part within a societal system and beauty industry that often fails to acknowledge its complicity in this deep history.

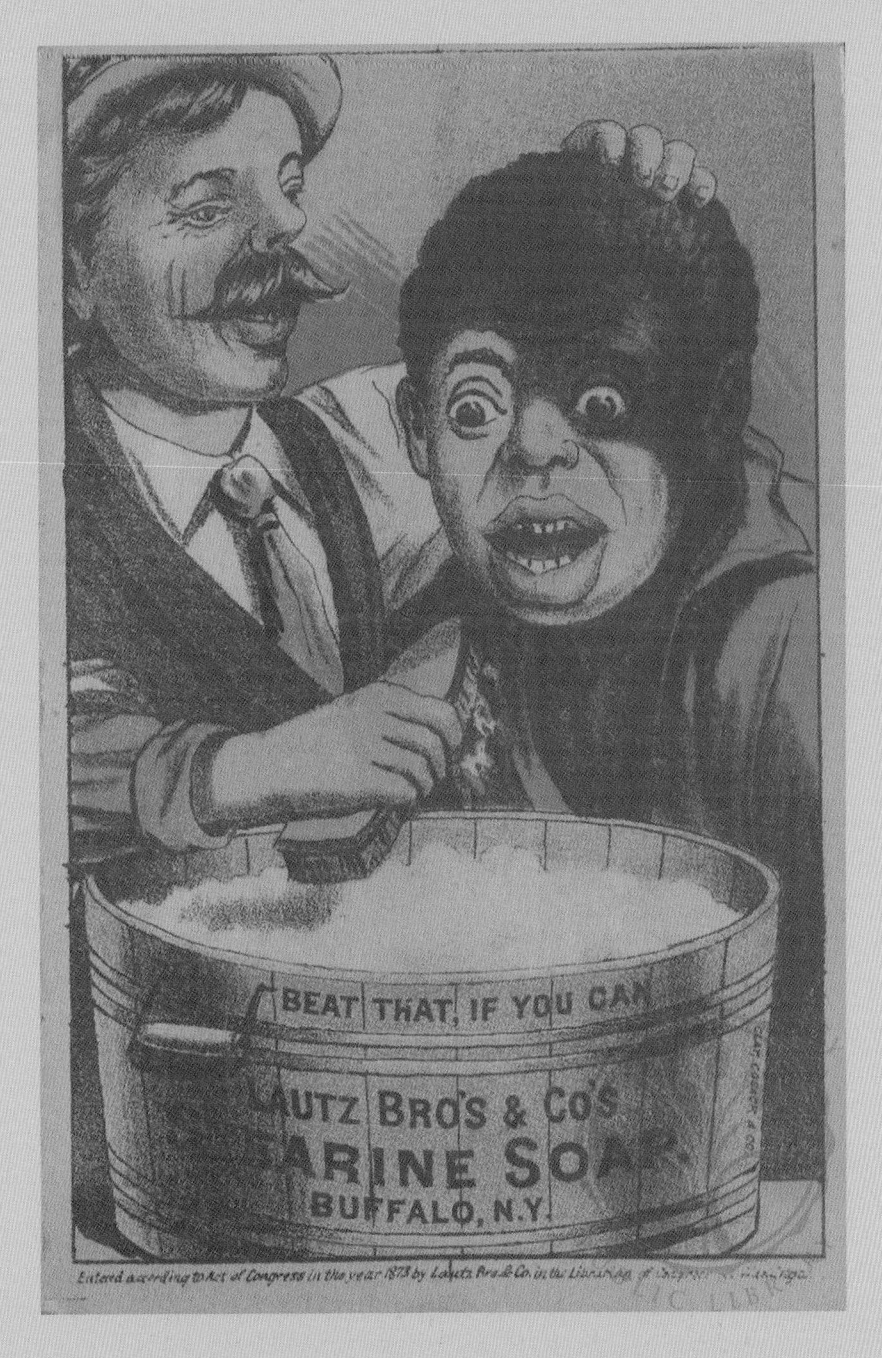

Lautz Brothers and Co. Stearine Soap Advertisment. Buffalo N.Y.
© MacKoy Family Collection donated by Betsy Schram

Black Freedom Under a White Gaze

> 'No more yallah gals for me!' Max announced with finality, sipping his drink. 'I'll grab a Black gal first.'
>
> 'Say not so!' exclaimed Bunny, strengthening his drink from his huge silver flask. 'You ain't thinkin' o' dealin' in coal, are you?'
>
> *Black No More*, George Schuyler

As we slipped into the first half of the twentieth century, three things were clear. Black people have been freed from physical slavery, they have agency of their beauty and identity, but they are still slaves to the white aesthetic.

> Freedom gave Black people the right to control how they show up in the world and control their identity, but after centuries of being brainwashed into a subhuman portrayal, that Blackness – Black skin, Afro hair and facial features – made them as ugly as animals, it's no surprise that even in freedom Black people still looked to whites as the benchmark of beauty. There was no guidebook or role models to emulate; Black people were culturally homeless. So in a new world at the turn of the century, under the gaze of a society and media that celebrated whiteness as the symbol of beauty, they had to forge new identities to ease painful memories of toil and abuse by rejecting Blackness.

Where there is demand, a supply will always spring up, and it wasn't long into the 1900s that the practice of ethnic alteration started to occur. Crude skin-lightening products that carried blatant anti-Black messages such as 'Black no More', 'Fair-Plex', 'Lucky Brown Bleaching Cream' and 'Cocotone Skin Whitener' started to appear on the market to enable Black people to deal with the problem of being Black.

Wigs and hair-straightening products to mimic European hair also came on the scene. Much-lauded African American beauty entrepreneurs, such as Annie Turnbo Malone, with her 'Poro Preparations' for skin and hair, and the world's first female self-made millionaire, Madam C. J. Walker, are credited for giving Black women hair that moved and met the preferred white aesthetic. In the 1940 Walker School of Beauty Culture textbook, hot combs and hair straightening is described as being 'in vogue now and when given correctly, will produce a decided improvement in the appearance of hair that is inclined to be very curly'.[12] Black women now had the option to meet a standard of beauty that excluded the natural appearance of most African Americans.

Madam C. J. Walker also sold skin-bleaching creams, further commoditising whiteness for Black people looking to develop a new identity. Her 'Tan-Off' cream was sold to Black women for 'brightening sallow or dark skin...and for clearing the complexion'.

Effectively, these skin-lightening and hair-altering products sold the hope of acceptance, the hope of being considered beautiful, the hope of a better life for Black people at a time of great identity and cultural insecurity in the shadows of slavery and outright racism, which reinforced a message that to be white is beautiful and to be Black is ugly.

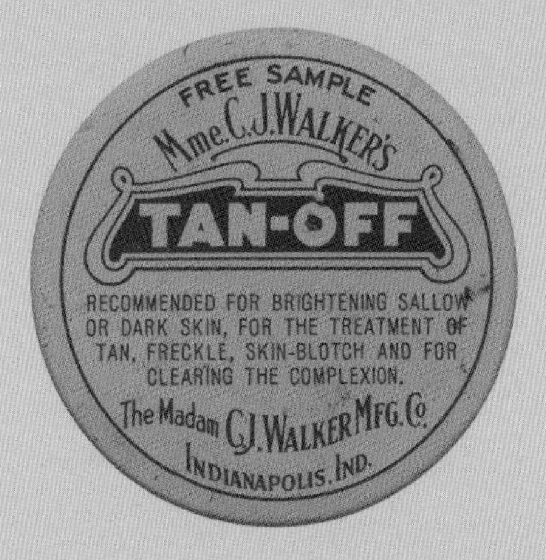

A free sample tin of whitening cream made by the Madam C.J. Walker Manufacturing Company. Contributor: SBS Eclectic Images. ©Alamy

The Impact of Music and Hollywood

Like today, Hollywood in the 1900s played a pivotal role in perpetuating images of beauty. Whilst Black women were taken on for films, it was mainly to fulfil the role of house servants, and their Blackness and size were specifically chosen to be the mirror opposite of the slim, white leading actress with perfectly coiffured hair. Black men played one of three types of role: inoffensive clowns; submissive and dependable servants; or hyper-sexual beasts. They were all united in being very dark skinned with noticeably more African features, to emphasise the 'Black is ugly and fearsome' narrative. In the 1920s, Hollywood still used white actors in Blackface to ensure they could present the most grotesque caricatures of Black people.

A legacy of early Hollywood which still exists today is that super dark Black skin is regarded as too Black to be beautiful, and these actresses are always made to feel second class. Multiple-award-winning actress Viola Davis has been at the front end of this discrimination:

> 'When you do see a woman of colour onscreen, the paper-bag test is still very much alive and kicking. If you are darker than a paper bag, then you are not sexy, you are not a woman, you shouldn't be in the realm of anything that men should desire.'
>
> Viola Davis, *The Wrap* magazine, 2015

Depictions of beauty on stage

The 1920s and '30s Jazz music scene provided an increased freedom of expression for Black people, but on stage it was still popular to portray Black people as animalistic, sexualised and exotic, sometimes even sharing the stage with performance animals such as leopards and lions, harking back to the descriptions of slave traders, plantation masters, and white scholars who painted Africa as a dark and uncivilised place where Black savages roamed like animals in an untamed jungle.

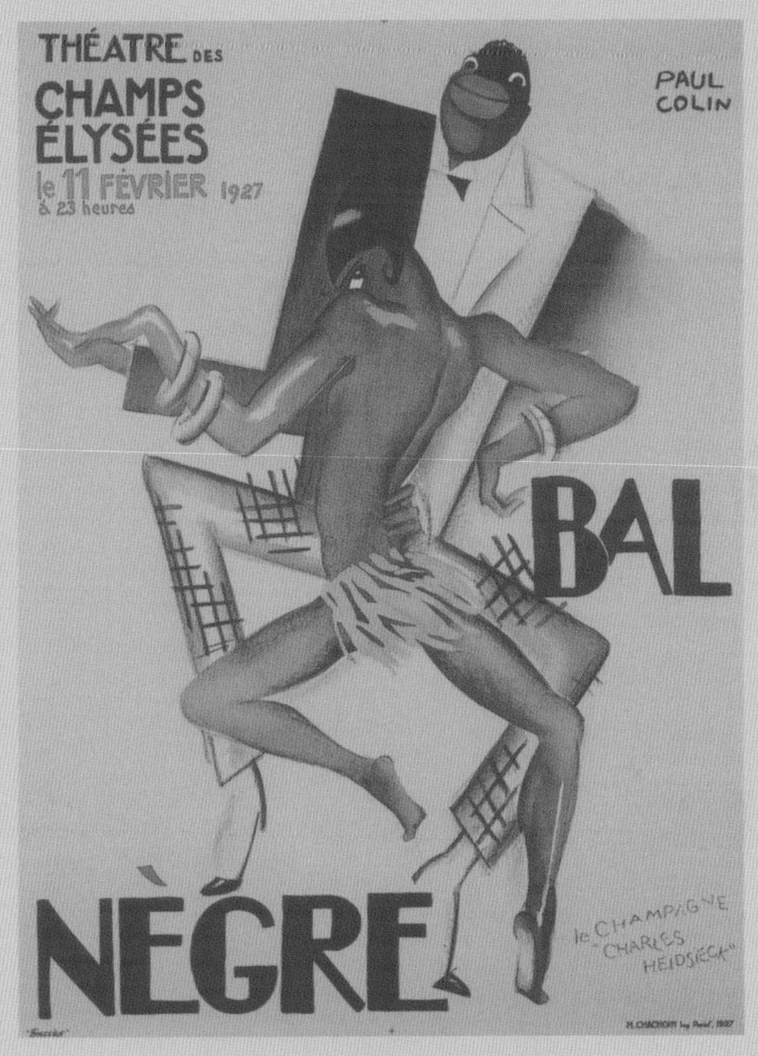

1920s France 'Bal Nègre' Poster. ©Alamy

When Josephine Baker opened La Rèvue Negre in Paris in October 1925, her lauded performance was reduced to commentary about her physical attributes. Newspaper *Candide* described it as 'apelike...with wild and superb bestiality'. The *New Yorker*'s correspondent Janet Flanner, said: 'Two specific elements had been established and were unforgettable – her magnificent dark body, a new model that to the French proved for the first time that Black was beautiful, and the acute response of the white masculine public in the capital of hedonism of all Europe – Paris.'[13]

Being crowned the sexiest Black woman on the planet did not free Baker from the clutches of the white beauty aesthetics. She was well aware that her success still depended on the lightness of her skin tone, as described in the 1993 book *Josephine Baker: The Hungry Heart* by Jean-Claude Baker and Chris Chase: 'I had to succeed, that's why I spent thirty minutes each morning rubbing my body with half a lemon to lighten my skin...I couldn't afford to take any chances.'

Depictions of beauty in film

In the white Hollywood and music scene, Blackness was controlled. There were times when lighter-skinned Black singers and actresses were deemed problematic if they appeared too white for their patrons. Billie Holiday was told to 'blacken up', Josephine Baker was passed over because she was deemed too light to play a harem girl, and Fredi Washington had her skin darkened so that she could feature alongside darker-skinned actors to avoid accusations that Black men were fraternising with white women at a time when mixing was prohibited.

During this time independent Black filmmakers rebelled against some of the constraints of Hollywood and society by casting and promoting their own Black superstars, especially in more diverse and less stereotypical roles where characters had more personality. However, centuries of conditioning meant that for these movies to appeal to a Black audience that subscribed to the dominant white aesthetic, many of the Black actresses were cast according to their resemblance to white Hollywood actresses. Ethel Moses was likened to Jean Harlow and Bee Freeman to Mae West.

Whilst society kept a tight lid on the acceptability of Black features, white women could borrow aesthetically from Black women and be seen as beautiful. Much like today when 'bee-stung' lips on white women were celebrated for shape and fullness, whereas the same on Black women were derided as thick and ugly.

Fashion designer Coco Chanel loved a tan, and for those who couldn't holiday on the French coast, Jean Patou launched the first suntan oil in 1927. Having brown skin became a marker of health and vitality for white women, when traditionally it had been a symbol of the toil and poverty of outdoor workers in the fields. Whilst Black women tried everything they could to rid themselves of the stain of having Black skin, white women treated dark skin as a fashion concept. If ever there was a paradigm shift, this was it. The sad reality for Black women is that they didn't have the option of washing their skin colour down the drain whenever they felt like it.

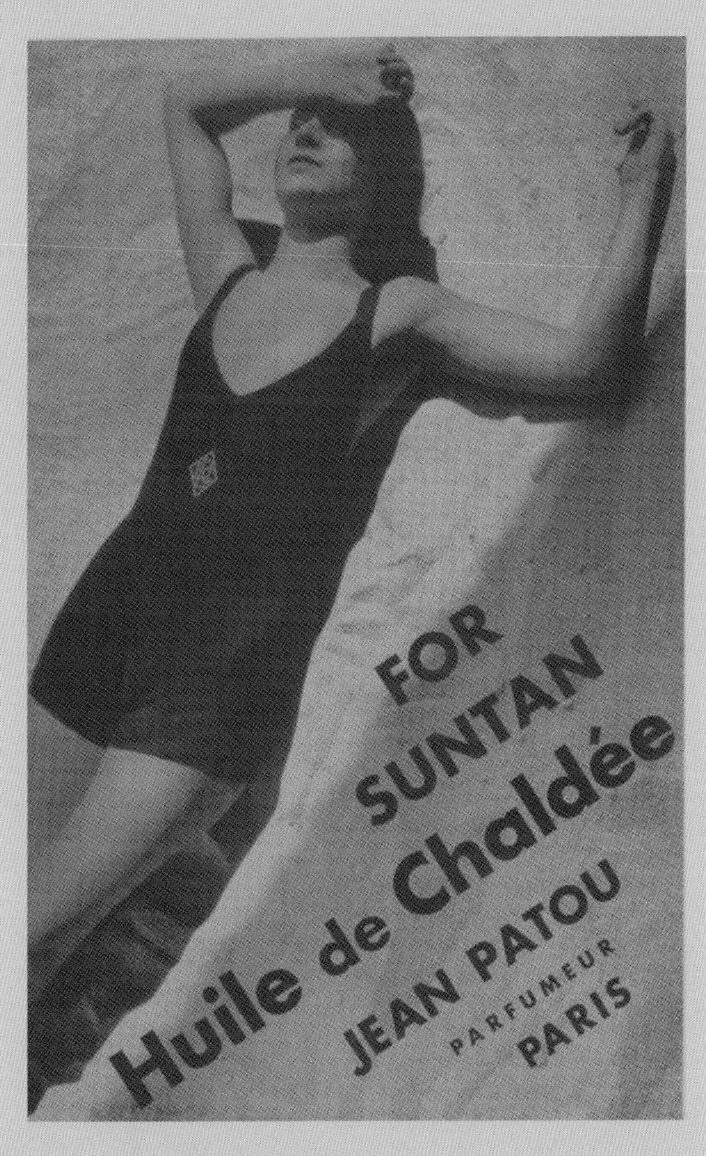

Photographic Print of Advert for suntan cream from Jean Patou, Paris 1930. © Mary Evans Library

War – Two Steps Forward, One Step Back

The frills and fripperies of the 1920s and '30s were replaced with the seriousness of war in the early 1940s. The war effort signalled the beginning of the end of the 'Jim Crow' laws and encouraged desegregation. There was a noticeable increase in Black people in formal employment, and higher incidences of civil unrest when Black people demanded their constitutional rights. Nineteen fifty-five saw the American Supreme Court declare segregated schooling unlawful and 6-year-old Ruby Bridges became the first Black pupil in a white school in America; a tired Rosa Parks refuses to give up her seat on the bus; and 14-year-old Emmett Till is slaughtered in Mississippi for allegedly cat-calling a white woman. There was a second wave of Black migration to northern states and again there was a palpable makeover of Blackness.

> Television had spread across American homes and *Ebony* magazine was founded in November 1945 as the first Black-owned beauty and lifestyle magazine. Sadly, in its first decade the magazine did not champion Black women, and reliance on advertising spend meant it focused on Eurocentric approximations of beauty for Black skin: light- and fairer-skinned cover girls and adverts for skin-bleaching and hair-straightening products.

The post-war economic boom saw Black people having more disposable income, and after five hundred years of vilification and institutionalised aesthetic shame, they were able – and could afford – to remodel their beauty based on a European standard. White women had been doing this remodelling for a long time, though without the emotional baggage and trauma. So again, when I say Black women are playing catch-up, this is a perfect illustration.

> Skin care and beauty had become heavily commoditised but the narrative was still centred around whiteness.

1945 was also the year that Afro hair stylist Rose Morgan built a beauty salon that set new standards for Black women. She wanted to provide Black women with access to a way of life and respect not typically afforded them at the time. Her salon, the Harlem-based Rose Meta House of Beauty, grossed $3 million in sales in the first few years. It provided treatments, beauty products, fashion, lessons in charm and etiquette as well as make-up to suit Black skin. She did for Black women what Estée Lauder was doing for white women in New York City, and only a year after launching, *Ebony* magazine dubbed the venture 'the biggest Negro beauty parlour in the world.'

The number of skin-bleaching companies marketing their wares in the new Black lifestyle press increased. Popular brand Nadinola touted that 'Few men can resist the charm of a honey light complexion' and 'Lighter skin leads to brighter evenings'. Bleaching creams often contained high levels of hydroquinone and/or mercury to stop the production of melanin, thus creating a lighter skin tone whilst slowly poisoning you.

Skincare and beauty had become heavily commoditised but the narrative was still centred around whiteness. It appeared that Black women had more choices, but there still was only one option: choose whiteness to succeed economically, politically and socially because Black just isn't beautiful enough.

FACT Barbie dolls were created by Mattel in 1945, but the first Black Barbie doll only hit the scene thirty-five years later, in 1980.

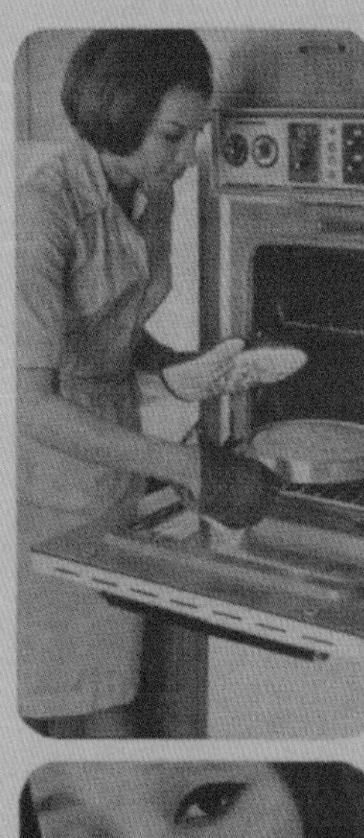

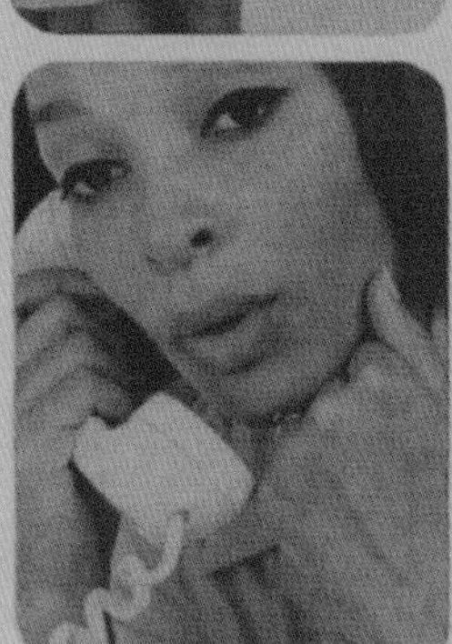

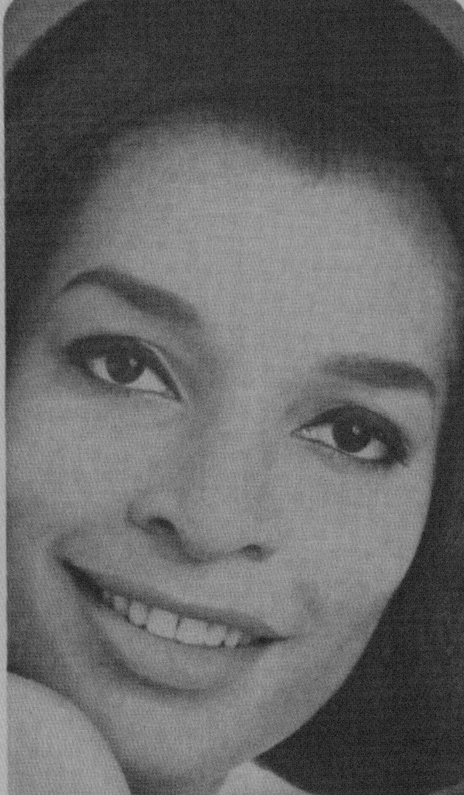

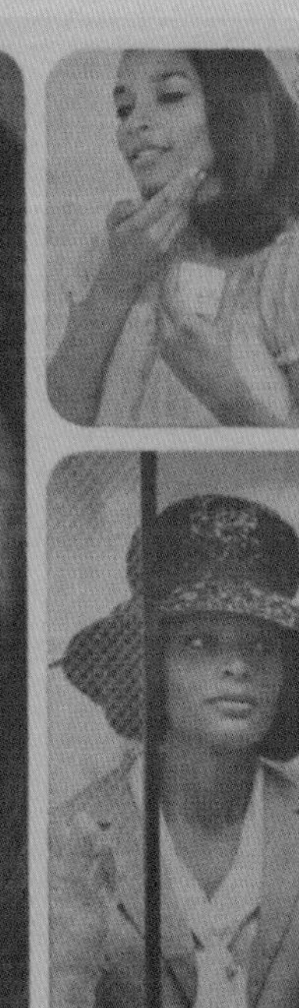

For happy days sake—use Nadinola Bleaching Cream

Nadinola starts its beautiful work the moment it touches your skin. And, in just a few weeks of use, a new radiance becomes you. Your skin looks brighter and lighter, feels softer and smoother, too. Nadinola with special ingredient A-M is mildly medicated and contains creamy conditioners so pleasant to use. It actually combats blackheads, blotches and other such surface blemishes to give you more even-toned new beauty. Whichever you choose—Nadinola DeLuxe or Regular—your money back if you're not completely satisfied with the beautiful way Nadinola improves your complexion.

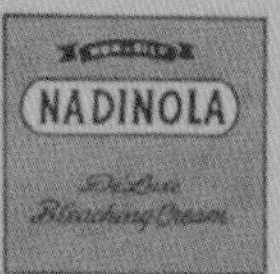

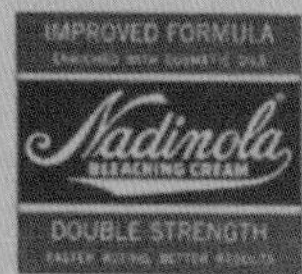

Nadinola DeLuxe—for oily skin, 75¢ to $2.00 • Nadinola Regular—for dry skin, 49¢ to $1.25

Brighten your skin
Brighten your life with NADINOLA

NADINOLA BLEACHING CREAM, CHATTANOOGA, TENNESSEE 37409

American advertisement for Nadinola Bleaching Cream. Photograph, 1966. © Alamy

A New Beauty Model

Fashion models were also flag bearers of beauty, and in the 1940s and '50s the industry was tolerant of Black women; models such as Ophelia DeVore and Dorothea Townsend were popular as they were on the right side of Black – fair-skinned with Eurocentric facial features including straight hair or a willingness to wear their Afro hair straight. The modelling industry was – and still is – only barely tolerant of Afro hair. However, midway through the twentieth century it was clear that whilst racism was still rampant, the white grip on who and what society considered beautiful was loosening. A shining star was the darker-skin-toned model Helen Williams, who led mainstream and editorial ads for the likes of Budweiser and Sears.

Black people had been physically granted freedom from slavery, but they were still very much slavishly bound to the white aesthetic. White beauty standards were the impossible benchmark that Black women were held up to, so much so that mainstream brands didn't think of creating any separate beauty and cosmetic products for them. Considering the thoughts, feelings and opinions of Black women wasn't the done thing, and brands didn't have to do it. Nor was there any impetus for change; Black women were too busy trying to look white to survive. Outside the US, people of the British colonies romanticised England as the Mother Country and that held them in mental bondage, feeding misplaced beauty ideals and unattainable European aesthetics.

White beauty standards were the impossible benchmark that Black women were held up to.

part two

managing black skin

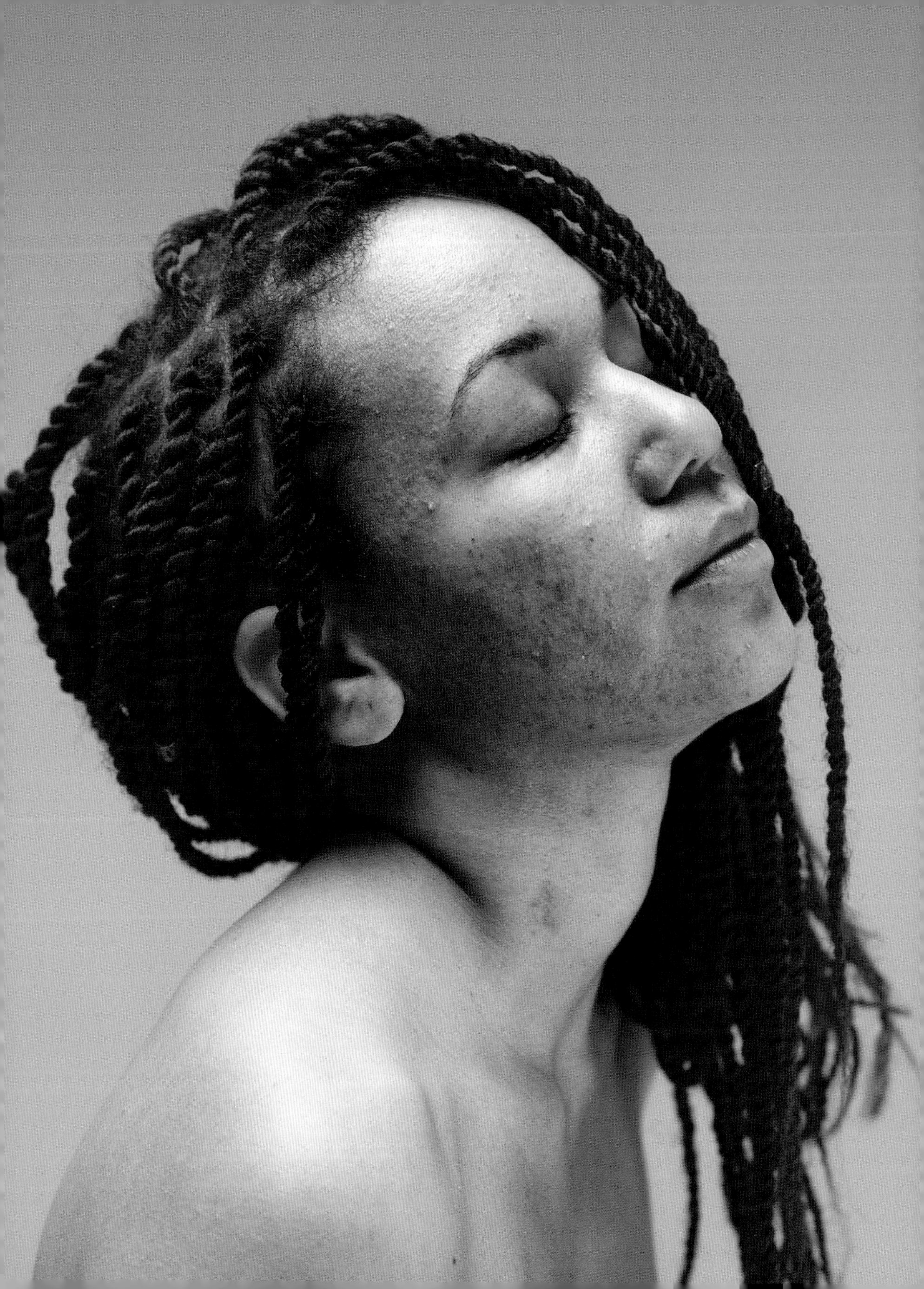

06.

common skin conditions

common skin conditions

IN life and in skincare, I believe you should control the controllables, and what I've learned over the many years of doing skin health consultations is that the condition of your skin is largely controllable. When the condition of your skin suddenly changes, it can throw you into confusion and dent your confidence, so it gives me immense pride to help you find your footing again.

The key to taking charge and looking after your skin lies in what you know, though. You need to know the basics about common skin conditions, how you can treat them and when to seek help. With correct advice and management, most skin conditions should, hopefully, be a passing situation caused by lifestyle factors. Careful tweaking and monitoring should return your skin to a more balanced state.

Sometimes, skin conditions can stem from a longer-term issue such as illness or disease or hormonal changes; in these cases your skin can be managed and supported to be in the best condition possible. For most people, once things settle down again, with a bit of a tidy up their skin will bounce back. That said, let's look at some of the common skin conditions we're all prone to and, importantly, how they show up in Black skin.

The key to taking charge and looking after your skin lies in what you know.

acne *vulgaris*

Simply acne to you and I, this is a very common inflammatory skin condition that can strike at any period in your life. In the past, it was largely seen as a rite of passage for teenagers in the throes of puberty, but now adult acne is a very real thing.

According to the NHS, 95 per cent of people aged 11–30 will experience acne at some point in their life, and 3 per cent of adults over 35 will experience adult acne. The *Journal of the American Medical Association* reported that in men and women over the age of 25, up to 54 per cent have some degree of acne; 12 per cent of women have acne persisting into middle age, while for men it's 3 per cent.[14]

I think it's likely that these figures are much higher; official statistics only record people who have visited their doctor or hospital dermatologist. There are so many people, especially Black women, who attend private clinics like West Room Aesthetics and these consultations are definitely not reflected in statistics.

Acne develops when the tiny hair follicles we have all over our skin become clogged and blocked with oil, old skin cells and the *Cutibacterium acnes (C. acnes)* bacteria which already live on the skin. The blockage causes congestion and inflammation, which if left untreated can proceed to blackheads, whiteheads, pimples and nodules underneath the skin. The main locations for acne are the face, chest, back and shoulders – areas where there are plenty of hair follicles and sebaceous glands that produce oil.

Lifestyle and environmental factors, such as your stress levels, the quality of your diet and sleep, exposure to pollution and the sun, and your skincare products and routines you follow (or don't!) also influence acne. They may not cause acne directly but they certainly have an impact, and these tend to be the factors that you can control.

Acne can also have hormonal roots. As well as during puberty, it's very common to get acne during your menstrual cycle, when using (or stopping) birth-control pills, as well as during pregnancy and the menopausal years.

It is also possible to develop acne as a result of an allergy, an untoward reaction to something, or even to food. I have clients who only have to look at dairy or gluten for acne to flare-up. I know that the research on the relationship between food and acne is inconclusive, but by my reckoning if you repeatedly eat certain types of food and you repeatedly suffer an acne breakout, I would say you need to watch what you eat, research evidence or not! Listen to your body.

Psst... Fungal acne – it's not a thing!

This is a phenomenon that started on social media to describe a condition that looks like acne but is definitely not acne. In fact, it is an uncommon yeast condition called *Malassezia folliculitis* that is treated with topical or oral anti-fungal medication. You'll find typical acne treatments don't work on this condition, so instead of frustrating yourself, seek a proper diagnosis from a skincare practitioner.

Acne has many descriptions – comedones is a standard one and it simply means a clogged pore or a spot. Blackheads and whiteheads are types of non-inflammatory spots, a blackhead being one that is open and blackened because it is exposed to air on the surface of the skin. Whiteheads, on the other hand, are closed spots that are still within the skin.

Papules are small bumps on the skin that can feel fleshy and hard. If they become filled with pus after a few days they graduate to pustules, which can then progress to becoming nudules – large, swollen and painfully deep within the skin. They take longer to heal, and the risk of scarring is quite high. Nudular acne needs a dermatologist!

Cystic acne is also a serious form of acne that can be tender, painful and pus-filled, originating deep within the skin. The risk of scarring is also quite high and proper dermatological management is required, especially if large areas of the face and upper body are affected. It is possible for acne to progress to rare forms, such as acne *conglobata* and acne *fulminans*, if due care and attention aren't taken.

Amongst my Black clients, I also tend to see acne that's a result of cultural influences. Using shea butter and cocoa butter (or butters in general) to moisturise the skin is generally fine, but on the face, these heavier fat-based textures can further clog your pores. Whilst we are here, you should also stop moisturising your face with coconut oil. There's always going to be one person who gets on fine slathering on these heritage skincare products, but if that person isn't you, accept it and find what works for *your* skin.

Certain hair products like pomades and gels that contain petroleum, mineral oil and heavy waxes can cause something called 'pomade acne' along the hair line. If you like 'laying down your edges' on your forehead and temples, you have to be mindful to give your skin a good wash every evening as leaving hair gel on the skin for long periods is setting up a breakout breeding ground.

There's such a thing called 'steroid acne', and this is common in people who bleach their skin for a lighter skin colour. Some of these products have high levels of corticosteroids in them, which make the sebaceous glands more prone to inflammation and infection.

Black skin also tends to suffer more pronounced effects of hyper-pigmentation, so there is a tendency to use heavy make-up and concealers to mask dark marks and scarring. Make-up is largely made of fats and waxes, so if you don't have a good skincare routine that properly removes these products from your skin, congestion and clogged pores are the next destination.

Acne is *very* individual and that also makes managing it a very individual process. There is no magic cure, so the best thing you can do is consult with a skin health professional who will help you put measures in place that control your acne. If your acne is mild, then seeing an aesthetician is a sensible first step, and it may save you time waiting for an NHS referral to a dermatologist or the costs of private treatment.

For severe acne, I do advise going to a dermatologist. They have the powers to prescribe acne medication such as Isotretinoin and Spironolactone, as well as to commission blood, allergy and hormonal tests that will all help in treating and controlling your acne. Doctors don't provide acne management or medication.

A typical treatment plan for managing acne may involve using an oral or topical retinoid, antibiotics, good-quality skincare products, lifestyle modifications, taking supplements, and professional skin treatments such as chemical peels and micro-needling. The treatment possibilities are endless, and I am pleased that as professionals we have so many tools at our disposal. Sadly, for some people acne can be a life-long skin condition that flares up from time to time, but with careful management it can be controlled. In Black skin, although it's secondary to the acne itself, the risk of developing hyperpigmentation always has to be considered and treatments must take this into account.

Black skin also tends to suffer more pronounced effects of hyperpigmentation.

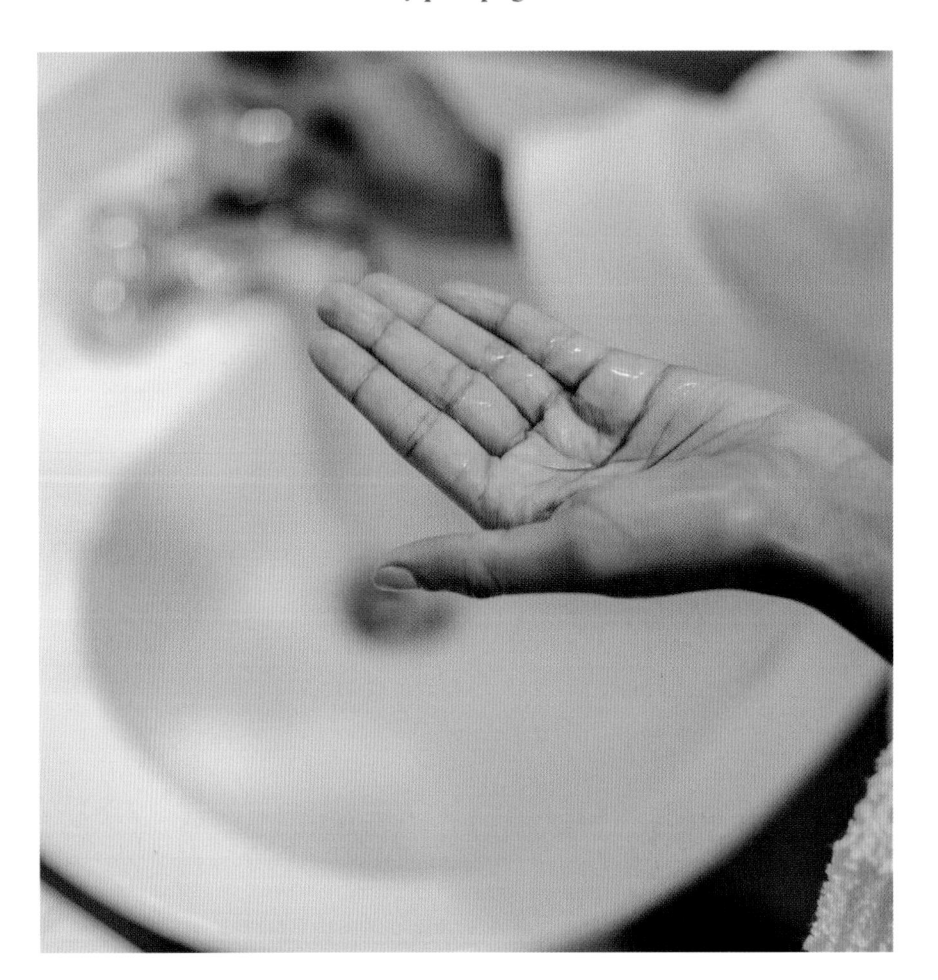

The golden rules for managing acne

- Only cleanse your skin twice a day using products suited to your skin type. Don't be tempted to wash your face more than this; acne is not there because your skin is dirty.
- Avoid using harsh skincare products like black soap that strip your skin of oil and much-needed moisture. Despite what your village people say, black soap does not solve *all* skin complaints, and your skin will clap back by producing more oil.
- Don't skip moisturiser; a lightweight oil-free serum or lotion with ceramides, cholesterol and peptides is enough to replenish the moisture level in the skin.
- Focus on gentle exfoliation to encourage optimal shedding of old skin cells.
- Don't pick at your skin as this spreads inflammation and causes scarring.
- Manage your lifestyle and diet, especially your gut health. Eat a colourful plate, get enough rest, stress less, drink water and mind your business.
- Use sunscreen to prevent hyperpigmentation from worsening.
- Toothpaste and Sudocrem are *not* appropriate spot treatments. It worked once for Folake in 2015 and it was a fluke.

dehydration

Black skin, regardless of whether you are an oily or dry skin type, is prone to dehydration because naturally it has a weaker ability to hold water. Your skin will be dry and itchy, lined and wrinkled, and looking particularly dull and ashy with no 'zhuzh.' If you have dehydrated skin, your hyperpigmentation will also look worse. Your skin will act like a sponge, drinking up anything you apply – serums, moisturisers, foundations. The latter will always end up looking a patchy hot mess.

> **FACT** Dehydrated skin and dry skin often get mixed up, but remember: dehydrated skin is a condition where your skin lacks water; dry skin is a skin type where your skin lacks oil.

Dehydrated skin is annoying but easy to treat: you need to help your skin keep in as much hydration as possible. Consider including a hyaluronic acid serum in your skincare routine to provide moisture to the upper layers of your skin, and also use a good moisturiser with fatty acids, glycerine and ceramides that will seal moisture into your skin.

Also make sure you're keeping your body adequately hydrated by drinking enough water and eating a diet that includes lots of water-rich foods.

Black skin, regardless of whether you are an oily or dry skin type, is prone to dehydration because naturally it has a weaker ability to hold water.

psoriasis

This is a long-term autoimmune condition where the skin is dry, discoloured, itchy and scaly because the cell turnover is super fast. Instead of the typical 21–28-day cycle in normal skin, the cell turnover with psoriasis is 3–7 days and natural exfoliation can't keep up. Skin cells start stacking on top of each other, causing roughness and discolouration ranging from a grey/silver appearance to dark brown and purple.

Psoriasis is very common on the scalp, but also occurs on knees, elbows and backs. For safe and effective management you will need to see a medical professional.

eczema

Whilst I have never personally suffered from eczema, I bear the scars of a mum up all night consoling a scratching baby who had extensive eczema where his skin was super itchy, cracked and inflamed. It can be painful to touch, and the skin can feel rough and crusty. Eczema flare-ups can be triggered by any and everything – in our case food allergies, but also hayfever, dust, pollen, asthma, washing powder, hard water, changes in seasonal weather and even skincare products.

Keeping the skin sufficiently moisturised using a mixture of lotions, creams and ointments is crucial. I cannot emphasise that enough. Even if it means setting an alarm to remind yourself every few hours. I've always had good experiences with the Aveeno skincare range for kids and grown-ups. The Dermexa range uses oats and ceramide complexes, which are well known to be deeply moisturising. Prescribed steroids in short bursts are also helpful. For some people they can cause very mild temporary skin lightening, but your skin colour does come back. In my personal experience, and from speaking to dermatologists who see a large number of Black patients, steroid ointments are better than creams for Black skin. Ointments are greasier and have more staying power on the skin, and therefore provide more long-term relief. If your doctor is reluctant to provide anything other than steroid cream, push for a referral to a dermatologist as they can provide more options, including ointments.

rosacea

Yes, Black people get rosacea too! There's always a look of surprise when I suggest the possibility of rosacea to a client because it is so associated with white people.

There is a persistent facial redness or deeper flushing, and inflammation around the forehead, nose, cheeks and chin, with or without spots filled with pus. You may also experience telangiectasia, where delicate blood vessels can also be visible on the surface of the skin. Annoyingly, rosacea isn't caused by any one particular thing; there can be so many triggers – sunlight, extreme heat or cold, strenuous exercise, spicy food, alcohol, even stress.

On Black skin, rosacea is easily missed and classified as acne. So, if you've been on acne treatment for a significant period and are getting nowhere, it's worth asking whether it could be rosacea. Especially if you are constantly flushed a deeper colour or red across the centre of your face, with breakouts on your cheeks that aren't budging.

There are four main subtypes of rosacea, and you can easily have one or a combination. I realise they are all a bit of a mouthful but I'm a firm believer that if you're ever going advocate for your health properly, it's important to be aware of the proper names of conditions. So here goes!

Erythematotelangiectatic: flushing and constant redness across the middle of your face, with or without telangiectasia.

Papulopustular: the above but with spots and breakouts.

Phymatous: the skin becomes thickened and misshapened and there is irregular texture on the nose, chin, forehead, cheeks or ears.

Ocular: feeling like there is something in your eye; you may also experience burning, stinging, sensitivity, dryness, itching, blurry vision, swelling and visible blood vessels.

Unfortunately, there is currently no cure for rosacea. It's all about control and managing the condition, starting by looking at lifestyle factors that can easily be changed to avoid triggering a flare-up. Your doctor can prescribe medications such as retinoids, azelaic acid and antibiotics if necessary.

From a skincare point of view, your watch words are *gentle*, *support* and *restore*. Key ingredients to have in your skincare arsenal include ceramides, cholesterol, gluconolactone, lactobionic acid and maltobionic acid. My go-to brand for rosacea clients is NeoStrata Restore – it's never let me down. Sunscreen is non-negotiable and you may find mineral sunscreens more tolerable. It is possible to also use in-clinic services like laser and LED therapies to treat and strengthen the skin, but you want to make sure you see not only an experienced practitioner but one that is a dab hand at using a laser on Black skin.

When it's all said and done, rosacea is a poorly understood condition on Black skin and, sadly, you may find yourself having to push against a practitioner, or even a medical professional, who doesn't recognise the condition on Black skin. You have all my support, and my advice is to remain steadfast, consistent and persistent in your requests for medical attention and further referral. Another crucial point to note is the importance of seeing an ophthalmologist for any eye-related concerns, as rosacea of the eye can affect your sight.

On Black skin, rosacea is easily missed and classified as acne.

keratosis pilaris (KP)

Keratosis pilaris is very common. It's a harmless, though sometimes unsightly, skin condition that develops on the top of arms and the back of thighs; I've also seen it on the cheeks. According to the British Skin Foundation, up to 70 per cent of adolescents and approximately 40 per cent of adults have keratosis pilaris. We've nicknamed it the 'chicken skin' condition because it looks and feels rough and goosebumpy, like chicken skin. It is caused when old skin cells block the opening of hair follicles, causing brownish/blackish bumps that can sometimes be raised and irritated. The size and amount of the bumps can change, increasing and decreasing with hormonal changes, such as with pregnancy. KP is another condition that hasn't got a total cure, but you can make it look better: dry body brushing is useful, as are sugar scrubs and exfoliating body washes, and hydrating/moisturising lotions that prevent dry skin from developing in the first place.

If you shave, be vigilant as your blade may nick areas of KP, especially on the thighs. This hurts like crazy and it leaves hyperpigmentation in its wake.

vitiligo

This isn't necessarily more common in Black skin, but its appearance is more stark and it can cause a lot of psychological distress, including depression and suicidal thoughts. Vitiligo is a genetic condition in which the body either doesn't produce melanin or destroys the melanin you already have, leaving you with no skin colour.

In some societies, diseases like vitiligo that affect pigmentation can mark sufferers as 'other' and leads them to be ostracised by their communities. Treatment varies, in type and in success, but can include topical steroids, skin grafts, melanocyte transfer, cosmetic camouflage, and even the medical removal of the remaining melanin if vitiligo is already widespread. It is rumoured that this is what Michael Jackson had.

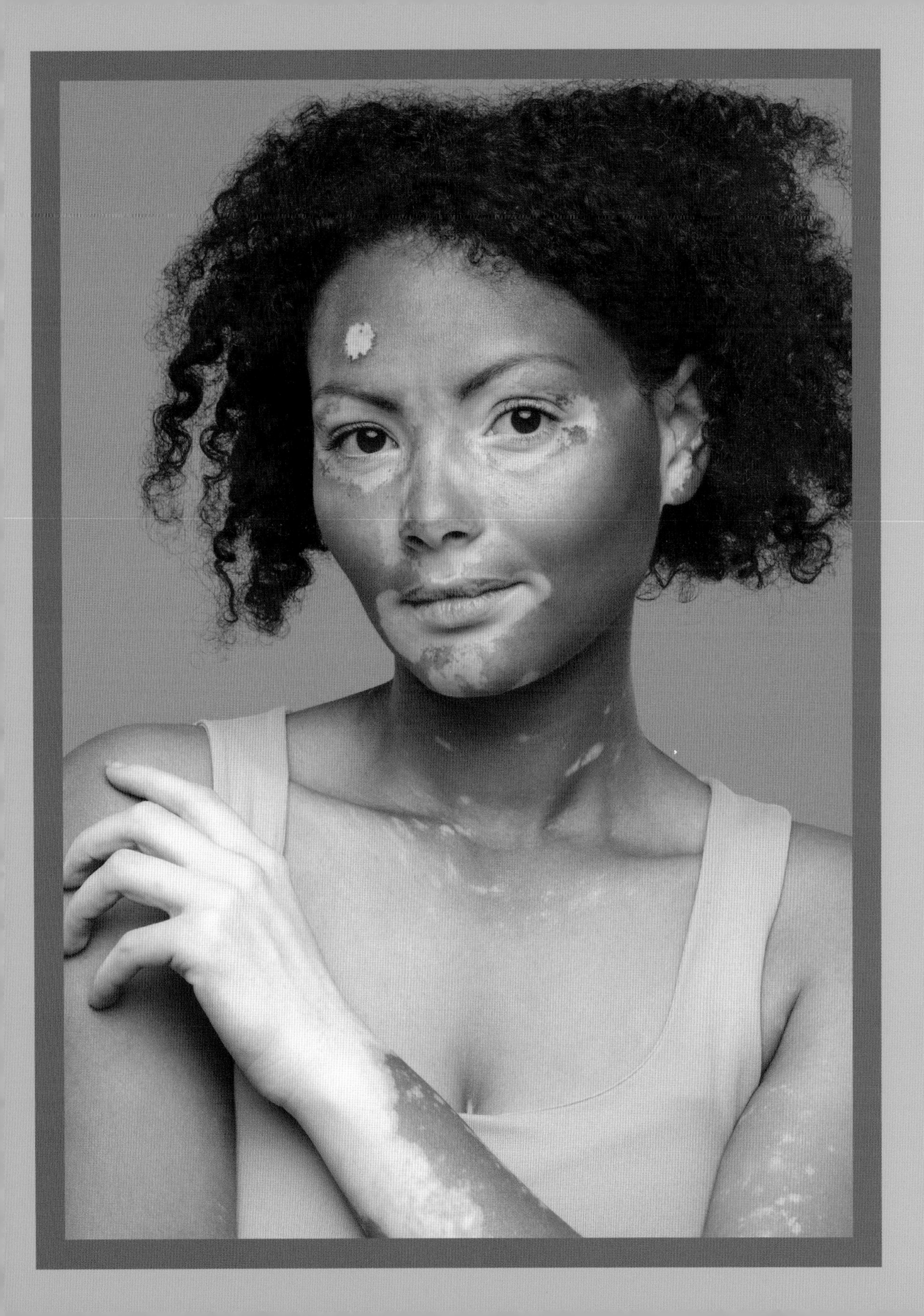

pseudofolliculitis barbae (PFB)

Also known as razor bumps or ingrowing hair, pseudofolliculitis barbae can be very problematic for Black skin, especially if you have thick curly or coily Afro hair. When Afro hair is cut the ends are sharp and blunt and the curly growth pattern means they can grow back into the skin, causing painful inflammation and infection, swelling of the hair follicle and hyperpigmentation.

It's predominantly Black men who experience this condition, as they shave and cut their hair more frequently than women. The usual areas affected are the nape and lower face/neck. Women can also experience PFB on the chin, jawline and cheek area if they suffer from male pattern hair growth and are also shaving. Ingrowing hair is also common on legs and the bikini area after hair removal where the hair is aggressively pulled from the skin, so waxing and sugaring as well as shaving are culprits.

Truth be told, it isn't always possible to avoid getting razor bumps, but you can certainly reduce the occurrence. Exfoliate regularly to keep skin smooth and free from dry skin build-up, as this can also contribute to the problem. Also, a single-blade razor like Bevel is best for Afro hair, as this is gentler on the hair.

If inflammation or infection has set in, then antibiotics are your next stop.

dermatosis papulosa nigra (DPN)

Forever mistaken for something else...I've heard them referred to as blackheads, warts, skin tags and moles, but dermatosis papulosa nigra is really just a fleshy bump that can develop on Black skin. Actor Morgan Freeman has the perfect display of DPN on the face, though it's more common in women than men. It starts off as a dot the size of a pinprick but will undoubtedly grow over the years, reaching anything from 1mm to 8mm, and protruding up to 3mm away from the skin. DPN is usually found on the face and neck, but it is not unusual to also find it on other parts of the body. You may have one or you could have a hundred (or a thousand).

The bumps are harmless, but I get that they can be cosmetically undesirable and many women will look for ways to get them removed. Safe treatment options include using laser, electrotherapy or cryotherapy to freeze them off, though take heed that all treatments can result in some form of skin discolouration. I have two on my left cheek which I think are quite cute. I may change my tune if I get more.

Most skin conditions come with an uninvited 'plus one': hyperpigmentation and it's a concern that crops up repeatedly on Black skin, so much so I've dedicated the next chapter to this very common complaint.

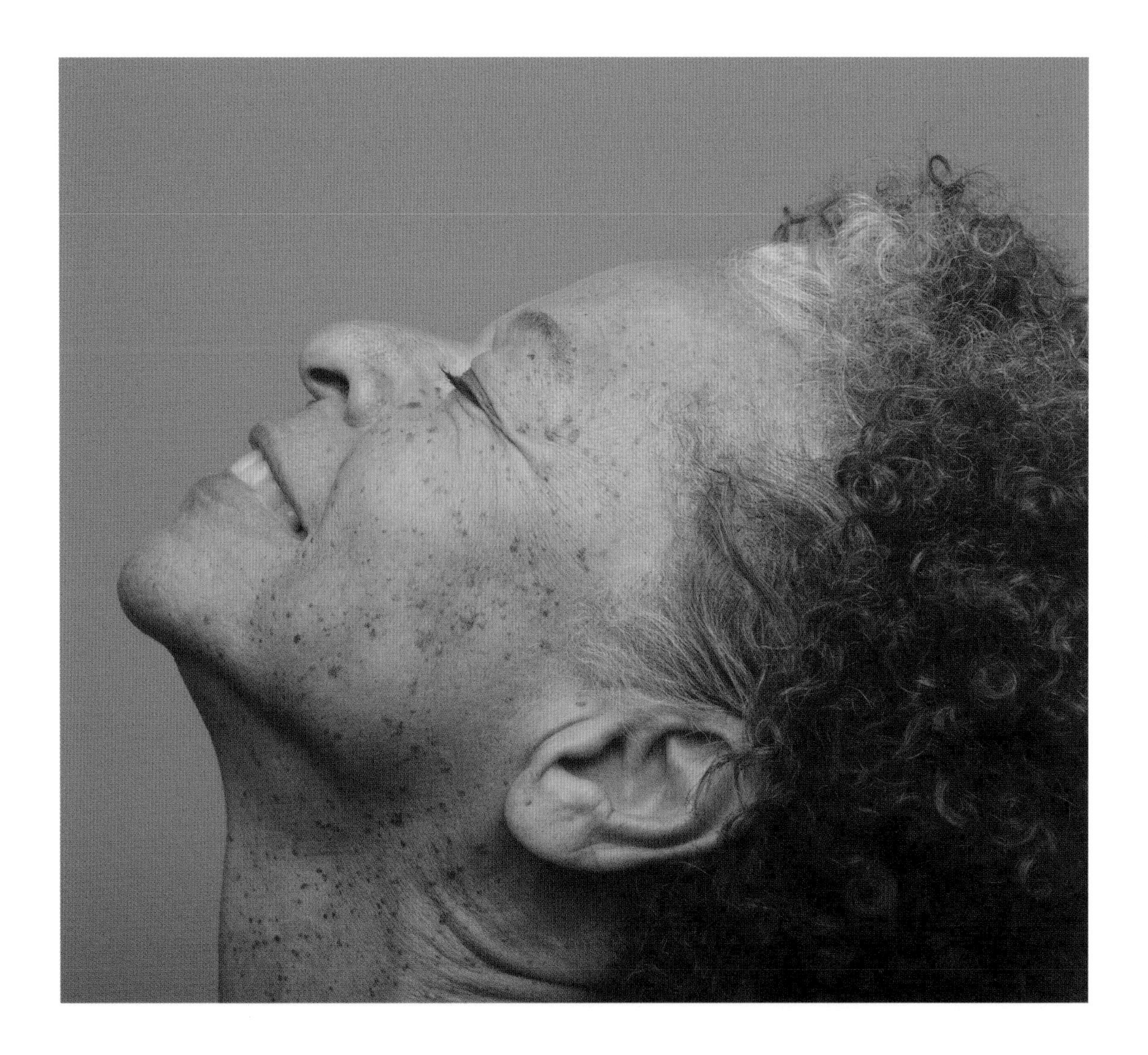

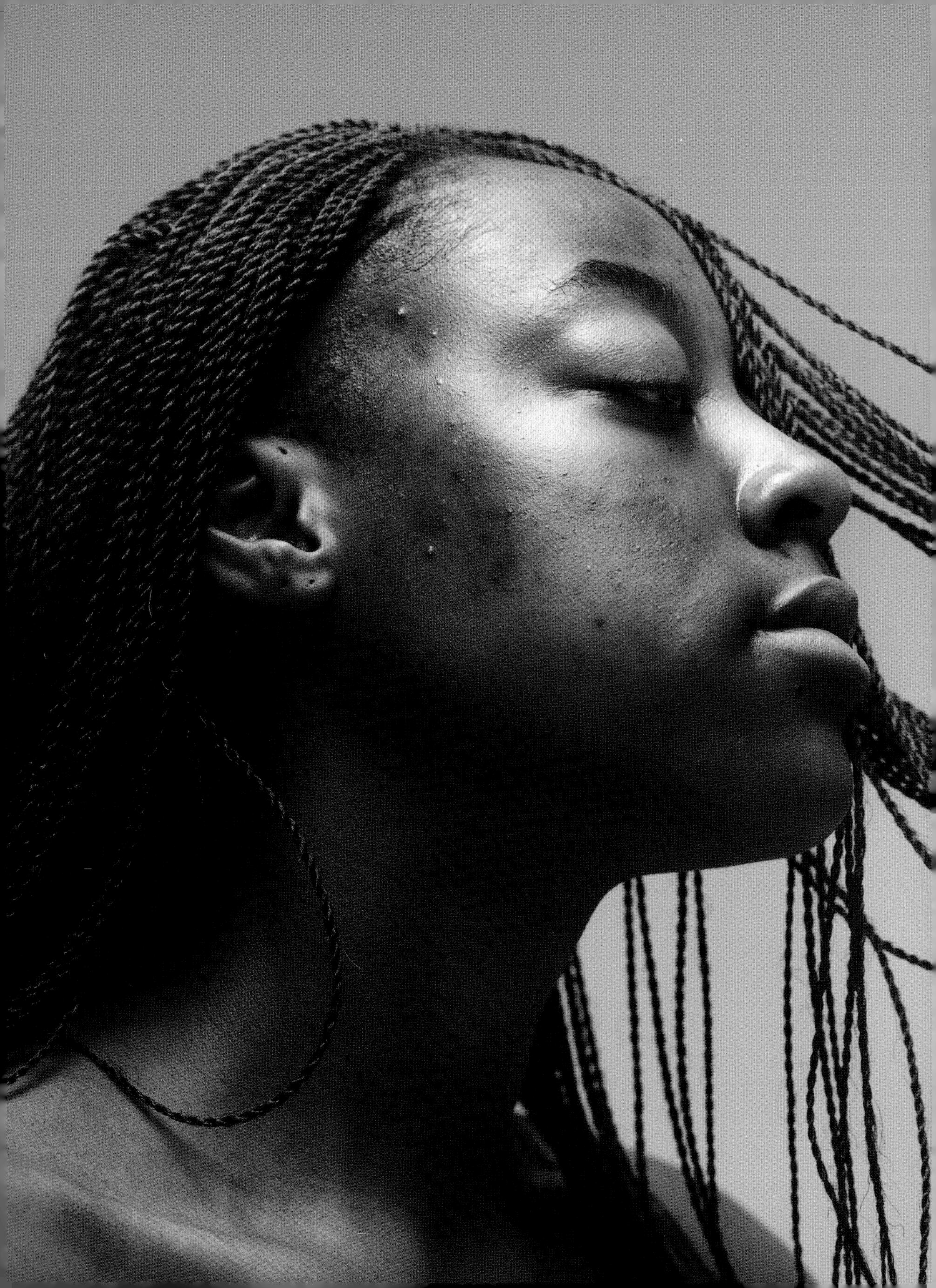

07.

hyperpigmentation

hyperpigmentation

THERE is no way I could write this book and not dedicate an entire chapter to hyperpigmentation. I mean, come on...skin discolouration is the top complaint I deal with in clinic and get asked about on a daily basis, even on social media. Google search data and clinical research also puts it up there in the top 5 issues that affect Black skin, and don't I know it?! Like a lot of Black women, I have my own personal struggles with hyperpigmentation, too.

First things first, let's settle the matter of what really is hyperpigmentation. Generally, it is an undesirable dark patchiness of the skin, where there are areas of increased melanin creating an uneven skin tone. I use the word hyperpigmentation interchangeably with discolouration and it can be anywhere on the face or body, though most of the complaints I deal with are on the face.

> **Hyperpigmentation itself is not a skin condition. It is the outward symptom of a skin condition.**

It may surprise you to know that hyperpigmentation itself is not a skin condition. It is the outward symptom of a skin condition, e.g., acne or an injury. Skin discolouration is always triggered by something else. It doesn't just turn up on its own. And it can cause so much distress. So much! Sometimes more than the condition that caused it. Even though it's back-to-front thinking, I have seen women with acne more concerned about how to get clear skin than how to treat their breakouts.

causes of hyperpigmentation

When the skin is injured or inflamed in any way, extra melanin is produced. This is what causes the increase of colour. Skin conditions such as breakouts, acne and eczema are all inflammations of the skin that trigger the melanin cells to over-produce melanin. Physical injury to the skin also results in hyperpigmentation, so cuts, wounds and grazes are also triggers. Likewise, melanin cells can be stimulated to produce more melanin as a protective mechanism to shield the skin from damage, as in the case of sun exposure. Extra melanin is produced to guard the skin cells from damage created by UVB rays. This is why sunscreen is so important and why a tan isn't something to be celebrated.

Illness and medication can also stimulate increased melanin in the skin. Lupus is a disease that affects predominantly Black women, and one of the symptoms is that the skin becomes darker. Medicines such as anti-malarial tablets are also melanin stimulating.

Hormones play a big role in stimulating melanin production. Pregnancy and birth-control pills are big culprits. In the last trimester of pregnancy, it is very common to see Black women go temporarily much darker in the face, a phenomenon called 'the mask of pregnancy.'

How we treat our skin on a daily basis can also trigger discolouration. Using incorrect skincare products that scratch and scrape your skin or which aren't suited to your skin type, or subjecting your skin to harsh and aggressive treatments, can cause inflammation. As can the overuse of certain ingredients like hydroquinone and steroids; they eventually lead to discolouration that is almost impossible to resolve.

How we treat our skin on a daily basis can also trigger discolouration.

types of hyperpigmentation

Post-inflammatory hyperpigmentation (PIH) is extremely common. This is what we see left over on the skin after spot breakouts, injury or inflammation and it tends to be superficial, hanging around on the upper layers of the skin. This also means that it tends to fade on its own or, with concerted efforts, we can help it along quickly.

Sun damage, aka photo-ageing, solar damage, photo damage – many words all meaning the same thing: skin that has been overexposed to the sun and is now unevenly mottled and patchy, with or without individual age spots or clusters. I see this in much older and fairer-skinned clients, who more than likely grew up in Africa or the Caribbean and have never taken heed of the sunscreen message.

Dark eye circles are a common complaint amongst Black women and there is always a genetic, age and lifestyle link. The skin around the eye is much thinner and more delicate than any other area of the body, which makes it particularly vulnerable to increased pigmentation. Lifestyle is a big contributor: late nights, screen time, stress, smoking, bad sleep and poor diets – especially those high in salt – can eventually leave our skin looking worse for wear, with the eye area being the most revealing.

Hay fever sufferers tend to suffer with irritable eyes that cause them to rub and scratch, ramping up the melanin production and discolouration around the eyes. Some people hold a lot of fluid around the eyes, which causes puffiness and discolouration too. It is worse if you add dry skin into the mix, too, as that makes the eyes look even more tired and lacklustre.

There is also such a thing called tear trough depression, and you'd know if you have this because the under-eye area will be sunken and it causes a dark shadow, making you look permanently tired as well. It also pays to take a look around your family and if you can see relatives with dark circles too; genes are the culprit and (sadly) there may be little you can do if it is a family trait.

Melasma is a very common type of patchy discolouration that mainly women experience, though men can get it too. I see it a lot in mature women approaching the menopause, but every so often I see it in younger age groups too. It's more common on dark skin because we naturally have more active melanin-producing cells that can become hyperactive and produce more melanin in certain areas: the forehead, cheeks, chin, upper lip and nose. It always tends to occur in a symmetrical pattern, mirroring both sides of the face.

The main triggers are hormones and sun exposure, and they go hand in hand. Fluctuating hormones play a big role, hence why pregnancy, birth control and hormone replacement medication are common triggers. The sun tends to exacerbate these triggers. Not only do UV rays worsen melasma, but heat and visible light also play a role in either firing it up or worsening it. Melasma is a challenge to treat and sadly has no cure, but it can be managed so that its appearance on the skin is improved.

Chloasma is the proper name for what we refer to as 'the mask of pregnancy', caused by the hormonal changes when you are with child. It typically shows up late to the party, anytime from seven months on in the pregnancy. It's very similar to melasma, but for most people it fades after birth.

A large proportion of the complaints I deal with about hyperpigmentation on the body are to do with darker joints – knuckles, elbows and knees, discoloured armpits and differing shades between the neck and chest. I've even had to counsel about discolouration in the intimate areas! These are all areas that experience a lot of use and friction, e.g. from shaving and waxing, plus the way melanin deposits in different areas of the body vary, so it's highly unlikely for anyone to have the same skin tone all over.

Hyperpigmentation can be anywhere on the face or body.

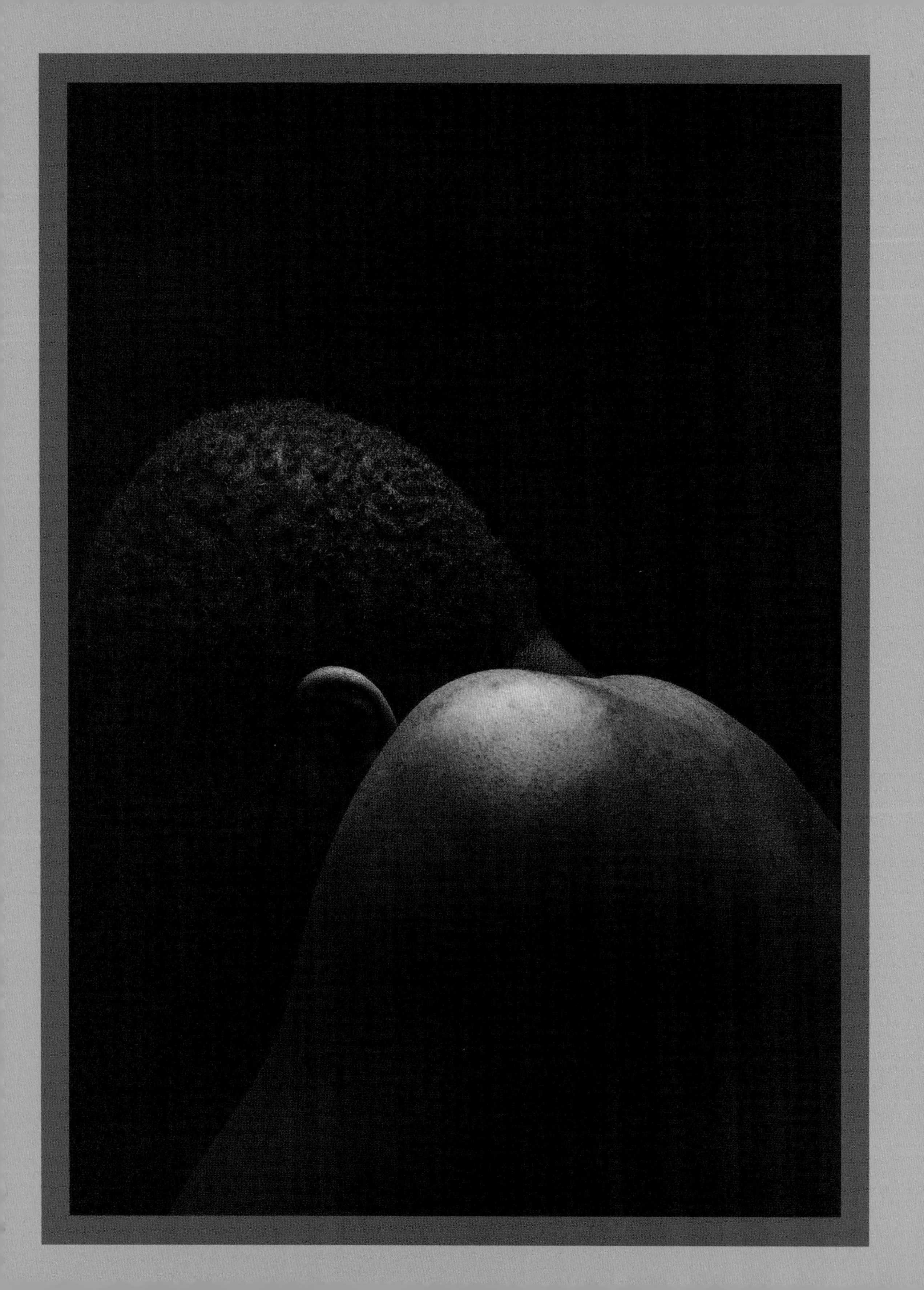

treating hyperpigmentation

The easiest, cheapest and best thing you can do for your hyperpigmentation is to invest in a good broad-spectrum UVA/UVB sunscreen that is a minimum SPF30. This will prevent future discolouration and prevent current hyperpigmentation from getting worse.

Secondly, your daily skincare should include a pigmentation evening serum. This is a must because if you want an even complexion, discolouration is something that must be tackled every day. The way Black skin is set up, hyperpigmentation can occur at any time, so it's best to stay on the defensive with a robust skincare plan that protects, inhibits and clears hyperpigmentation before and after it rears its bothersome self. Flip forward to the section on tyrosinase inhibitors in Chapter 9 for the full low down, and Chapter 13 for my favourite hardworking pigmentation serums.

Thirdly, include professional treatments in your skincare repertoire. Chemical peels, micro-needling and lasers are all suitable treatments to combat hyperpigmentation and deliver clearer skin. I know a lot of people tend to associate laser treatment with hair removal – which, yes, it is great for – but laser therapy is also fantastic for skin rejuvenation, so don't overlook it. All these professional treatments boost exfoliation so that patches of pigmentation fade quicker, and they improve your skin's healing processes so that discolouration doesn't become a thing.

Psst!... Talking about hyperpigmentation

It's also worth noting that hyperpigmentation will always come and go; I hate to be the bearer of bad news but the chances of never ever being affected by it are very slim, so with all the love in my heart I'm telling you now that you need to have a certain amount of realism and stay on top of your skincare routine to keep discolouration under control. Also invest in a good concealer – it is a handy tool of disguise. I'm partial to Urban Decay Stay Naked Quickie Concealer for fast, everyday make-up. If I want to go to town then I call upon Nars Radiant Creamy Concealer, which corrects, brightens and blurs pesky dark marks. It's a ten across the board!

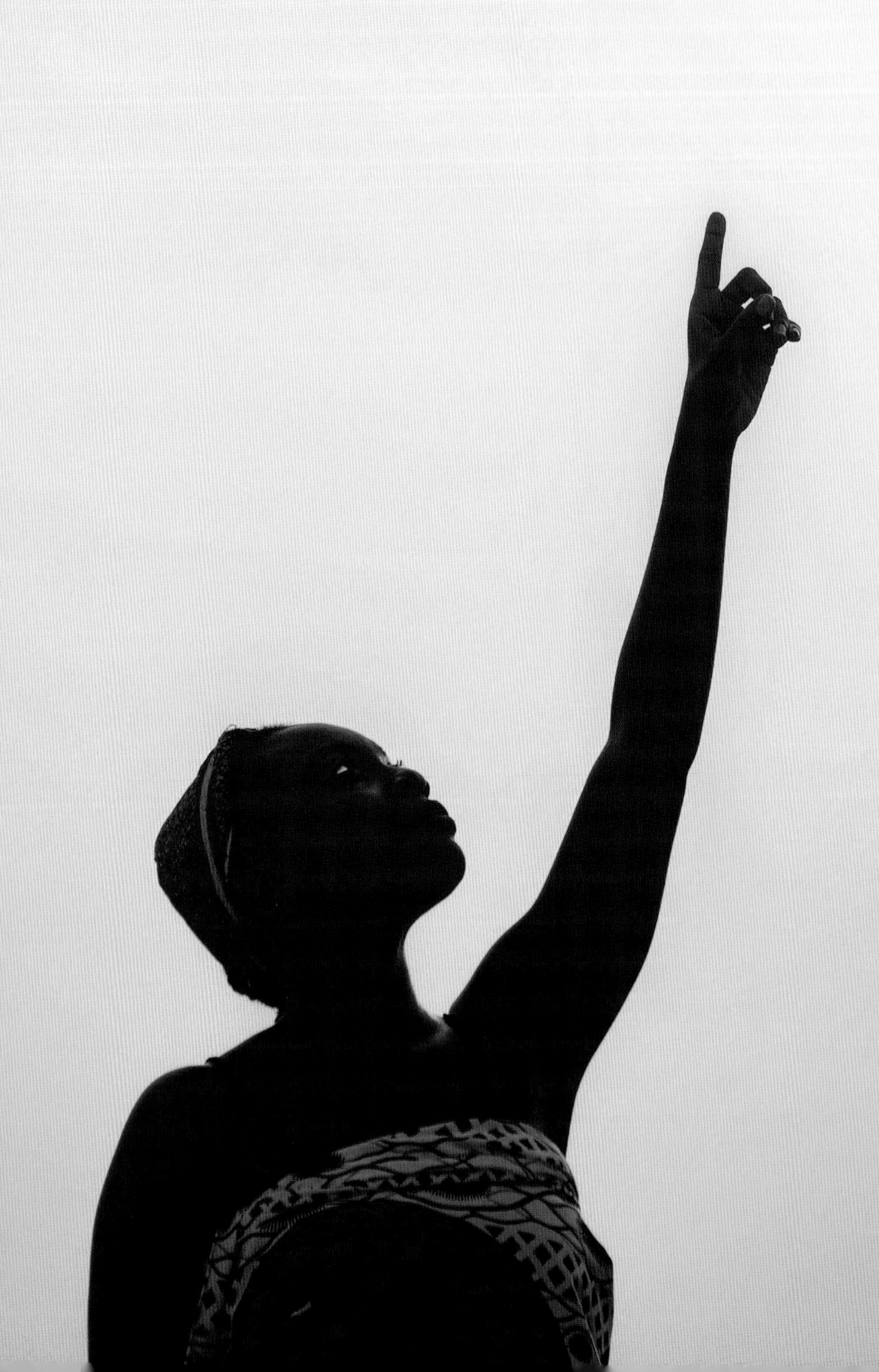

08.

the sun and black skin

the sun and black skin

THERE is plenty of misinformation about the effects of the sun on Black skin. Over the years, the health messaging, the lack of advertising, lack of suitable products, and poor formulas have meant that the Black community has largely been left out of this conversation. To be frank, up until the last decade, sun protection was very much seen as something for white people. To top it off, there are many within the Black community who openly disregard and/or do not believe in the need for sun protection. The first thing to get out of the way is that, yes, melanin does protect Black skin from the sun. On average melanin provides a natural SPF of approximately 13, but that is not enough to offer universal protection against all the damage that the sun can do to our skin.

The main damage from the sun comes from UVA and UVB rays, and even though we can't see them with the naked eye, they wreak havoc on our skin if left unchecked. UVA rays are the longest, accounting for some 95 per cent of the UV radiation that reaches the Earth. They are responsible for ageing your skin because they penetrate deep into the dermis to break down collagen and elastin, and they darken the skin, so worsening any dark patches you have already. These rays are pretty much the same strength throughout the year, regardless of season, and they can penetrate through cloud and glass, which is why it's important to protect your skin even when indoors.

FACT Sunburn can happen even on a cloudy day. According to Cancer Research UK, 90 per cent of the sun's rays can get through light clouds. You're also likely to be less sun aware on cloudy days and take fewer preventative measures, so the likelihood of you getting sunburn is higher.

Conversely, chronic exposure to UVA rays can also cause what I call 'reverse freckles' on Black skin, where you get a scattering of lighter patches slightly larger than pin pricks. I see these more on mature skin and a lot of people worry that they are the beginning of vitiligo. For the vast majority of people this discolouration is simply a result of too much sun and underscores why sun protection is so important for us all. Melanin will protect collagen and elastin to a certain extent, but it offers no protection for hyperpigmentation and hypopigmentation or other melanin-driven conditions such as melasma, dermatosis papulosa nigra, or even age spots. These will just get worse with unprotected sun exposure. Research also shows that the closer you get to the Earth's poles, the higher the concentration of UVA rays, which means Black people living in Northern European countries like Britain really do need to be mindful in protecting themselves against these powerful rays, more so than people living in sub-Saharan Africa, for example, who conversely have a higher requirement for UVB protection.

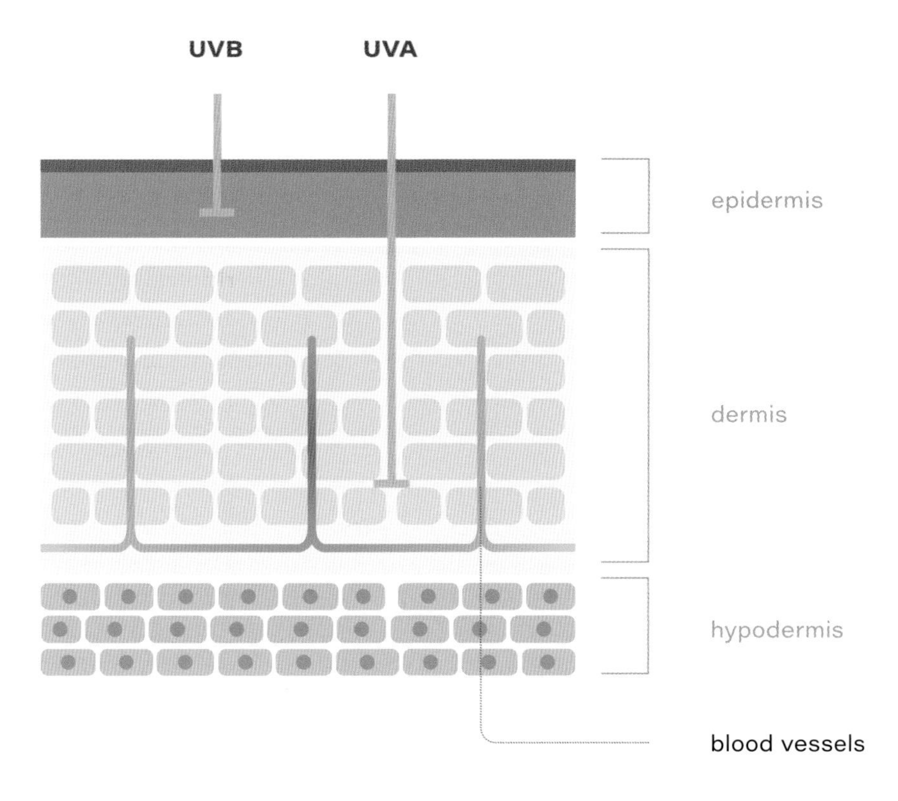

> To be frank, up until the last decade, sun protection was very much seen as something for white people.

UVB rays only reach the bottom of the epidermis and they are mainly responsible for burning the skin, which can lead to the development of skin cancers like melanoma. Granted, Black people are much less likely than white folk to get this sort of sun-induced melanoma, but 'less likely' doesn't mean 'not at all', so it's still important to protect your skin. There are many reports of Black people developing sun-induced cancer.

Burns can also be very uncomfortable. The skin will be flushed, even taking on a reddish, inflamed colour, blistering and peeling – all leading to hyperpigmentation.

FACT There's a lot of talk about blue light reflected from mobile phones, computer screens and televisions affecting Black skin. One (sensationalised) study showed that it increased hyperpigmentation in Black skin by the amount equivalent to receiving up to 2½ hours of direct sunlight. To get the same exposure in blue light you would need 2,000 hours and have the light up close. Long story short, you don't need to worry about blue light, especially if you have a robust skincare regime with antioxidants and sunscreens.

UVB rays are able to damage the skin all year round, but their intensity varies with time of day, geographical location and the season. UVB rays are more damaging at high altitudes, and in snowy/icy conditions – think skiing – where the rays can bounce back from the snowy surface and penetrate the skin twice, intensifying the damage they do. They can also bounce off water and sand at the beach.

Psst… We all love a golden tan, but…

There's nothing I love seeing more than rich, golden Black skin, but truth be told I prefer the version that comes from a bottle. To be specific, a Tan-Luxe bottle. The tan you get from lying out in the sun for too long is actually DNA damage that forces the skin to produce more melanin so it can protect itself. That's the type of tan that can lead to skin cancer.

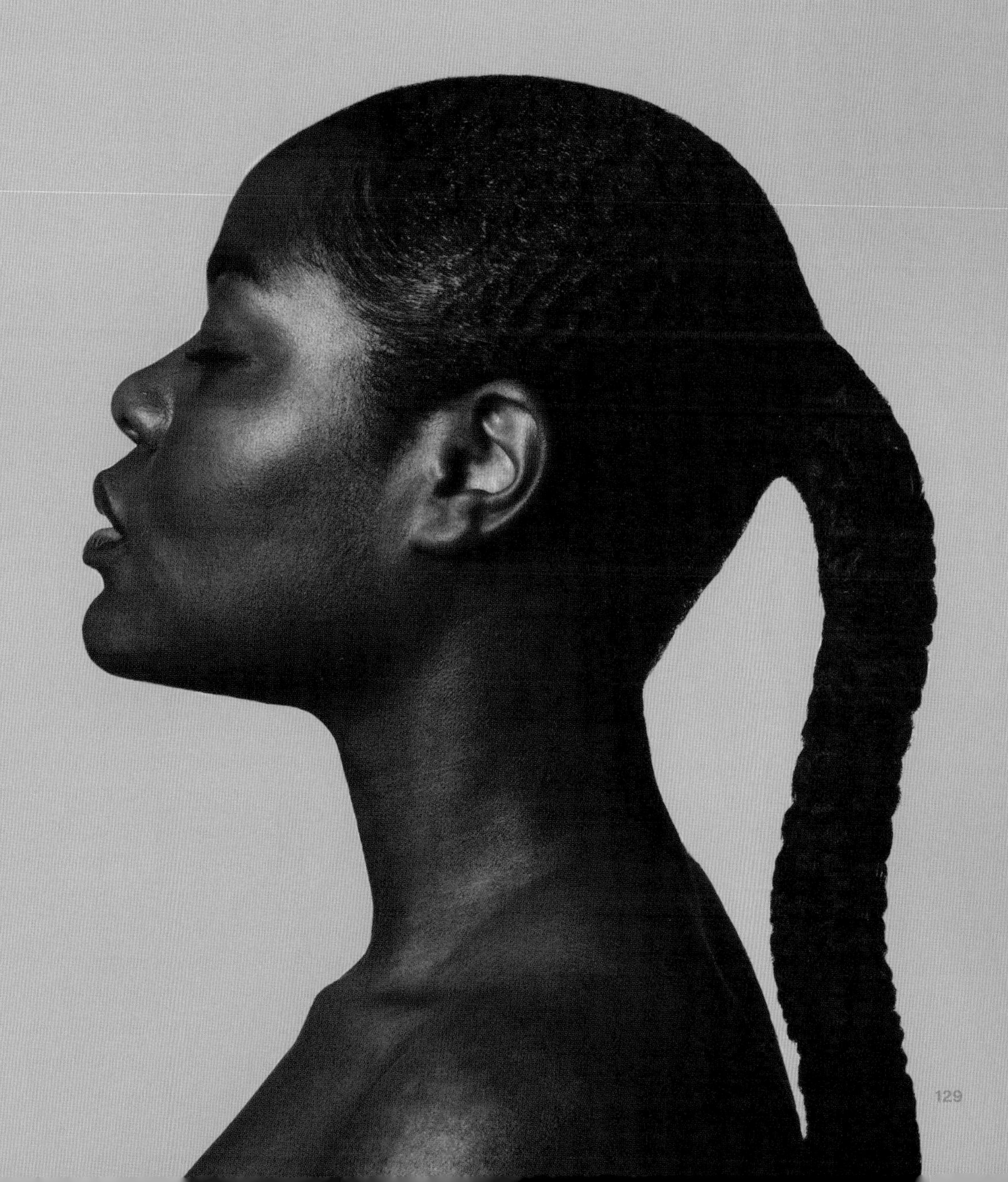

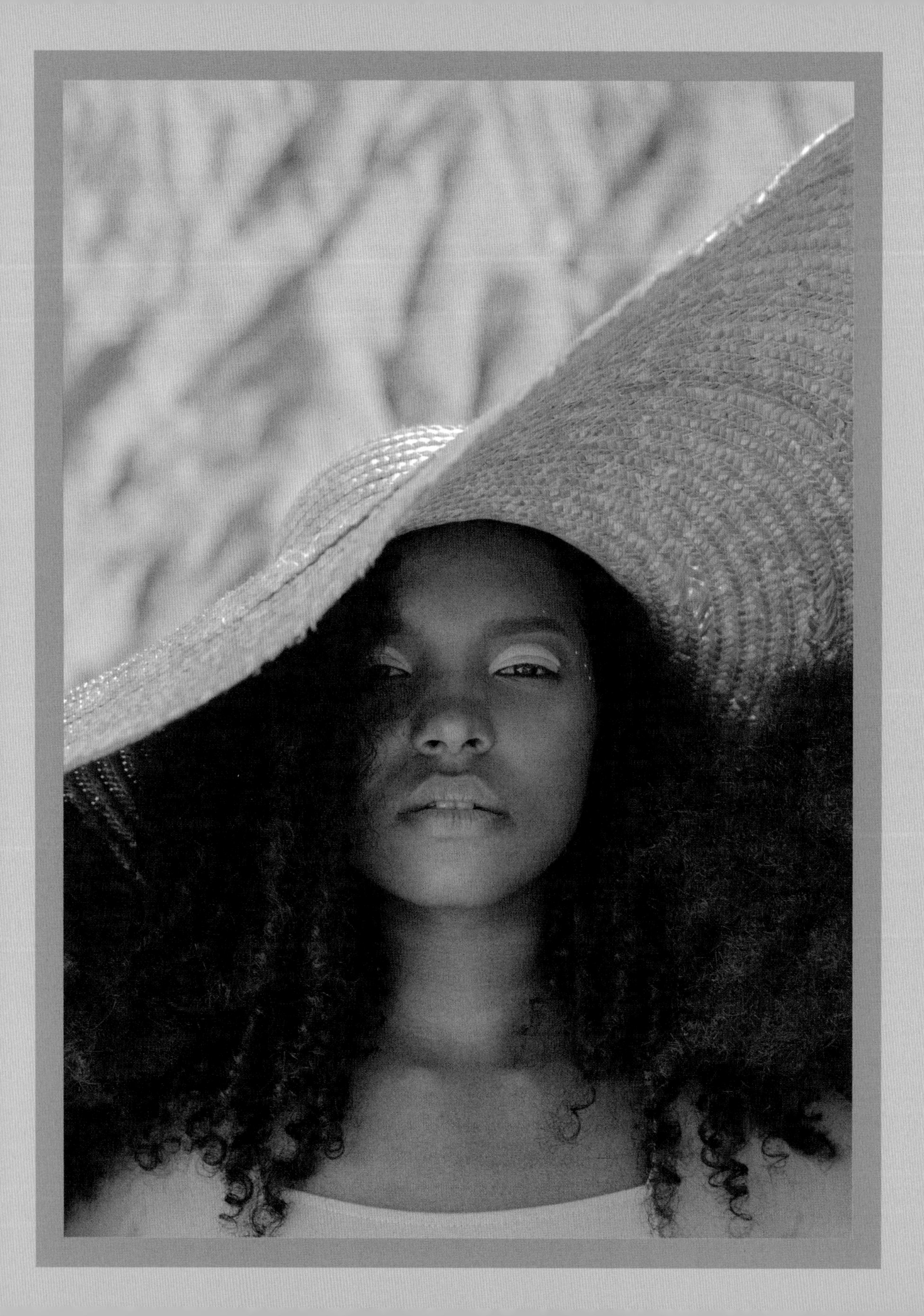

When it comes to treating sun damage, prevention is always best, so using a minimum SPF30 broad-spectrum UVA/UVB sunscreen is key, alongside frequent re-application. You could also step up your protection by wearing wide-brimmed hats (the larger and floppier the better) and lightweight clothing that covers the arms and shoulders that tend to get the brunt of sun damage. On really hot days, it may be bougie to spring open an umbrella to block the rays but it will never be a bad idea. Extend your fashion statement with over-sized sunnies because these will guard the already very delicate eye area.

The sad news is that sun damage cannot be reversed, but your skincare routine will play a massive prevention role (see Chapter 12), and treatments (Chapter 15) will help to improve the appearance of sun damage. The best thing to do is avoid sun damage in the first place.

FACT SPF is short hand for Sun Protection Factor and the number tells you how long it would take for your skin to burn when you have sunscreen on versus when you don't have any on at all. For example, if you apply an SPF30 sunscreen, it would take approximately 30 times longer for you to experience a burn, than if you didn't apply any sunscreen at all. Look for an SPF30 or above to give you the best protection.

When it comes to choosing sunscreen, my mantra has always been, 'The best sunscreen is the one that you are happy to use every day.' It really is as simple as that. Sunscreen is also very personal, and you may have to try a few before you settle on one you really like.

Also, it's best to have a few different sunscreens to suit different activities and occasions: Are you wearing make-up? Indoors all day? Exercising? Going bare faced whilst running errands? Just had a facial treatment? Knowing what you need the sunscreen for makes it easier for you to pick the right one and will help you build an appropriate sunscreen wardrobe.

There are two main types of sunscreen – physical and chemical. Physical sunscreens, also known as inorganic or mineral sunscreens, have active micronised mineral ingredients, mainly zinc oxide and/or titanium dioxide, that sit on top of the skin to partially deflect and scatter harmful UV rays away from your skin. They also absorb the rays and turn them to heat. Physical sunscreens have long had a complicated relationship with Black skin, because they have an undesirable white cast that makes Black skin look grey and corpse-like once make-up goes on top. Not to mention they can be quite thick and gloopy, making them time consuming to use. The whiteness is from the zinc oxide, the same thing cricketers mark up with – so if it looks bright white on white skin, it's not going to look any better on Black skin. However, in the last decade physical sunscreens have come on in leaps and bounds to suit darker skin tones, so they shouldn't be totally discounted, especially if you have a fairer skin tone.

Chemical sunscreens have organic filters that protect the skin from UV rays by converting the rays into heat before releasing them from the skin. Common filters are oxybenzone, avobenzone, octinoxate, mexoryl SX, octisalate, octocrylene, homosalate, tinosorb S, tinosorb M and mexoryl XL. Their consistency is much finer, and they have an added advantage of being perfectly colourless on Black skin.

Psst… Remember your rays

When thinking of UV rays, remember UVA is for ageing and UVB is for burning.

I often come up against the argument from Black people who don't see the point of sunscreen, that Black people in Africa don't apply sunscreen and they seem to get on fine. Likewise, even clinicians argue over the need for sunscreen for Black people. Whilst there may be disagreements, there are a few things I know for certain: I have seen Black people with sun-induced melanomas; there are very few skin cancer registries in Africa and, sadly, their data isn't robust enough to either prove or disprove this argument; and also wearing sunscreen isn't a death sentence. It's more like an insurance policy that protects you from being that one in a million Black person with a melanoma. The jury is still out, but the majority of skin industry folk worldwide believe that some degree of sun protection is needed for everyone, so the best thing you can do is to apply it.

Another often poorly cited argument is that sunscreen stops Black skin from being able to produce vitamin D after exposure to the sun. Vitamin D helps the body to absorb calcium and so helps prevent bone disease. With melanin already being a natural barrier in the absorption of vitamin D for Black people, especially in the Northern Hemisphere, some people think that applying sunscreen adds another hurdle that can lead to a vitamin D deficiency.

The solution lies in eating a vitamin D-rich diet, with food such as mackerel and salmon, fish oil, eggs (especially the yolks), liver and butter. Some foods like cereal and bread are also fortified with vitamin D. Medical professionals also advise a daily supplement of 10mg (micrograms) of vitamin D.

If you want to have healthy, robust skin, it is important to protect it from the sun. Take good care of your skin and it will look after you too.

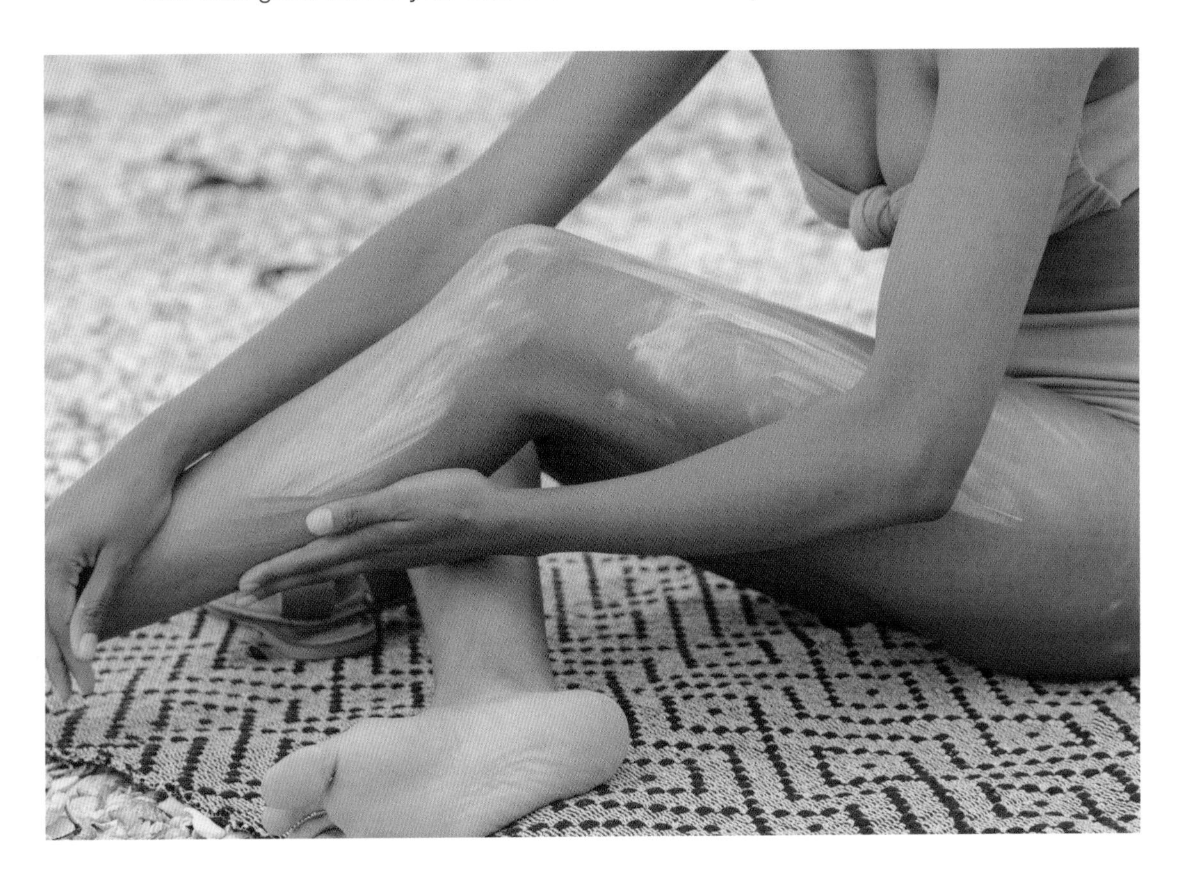

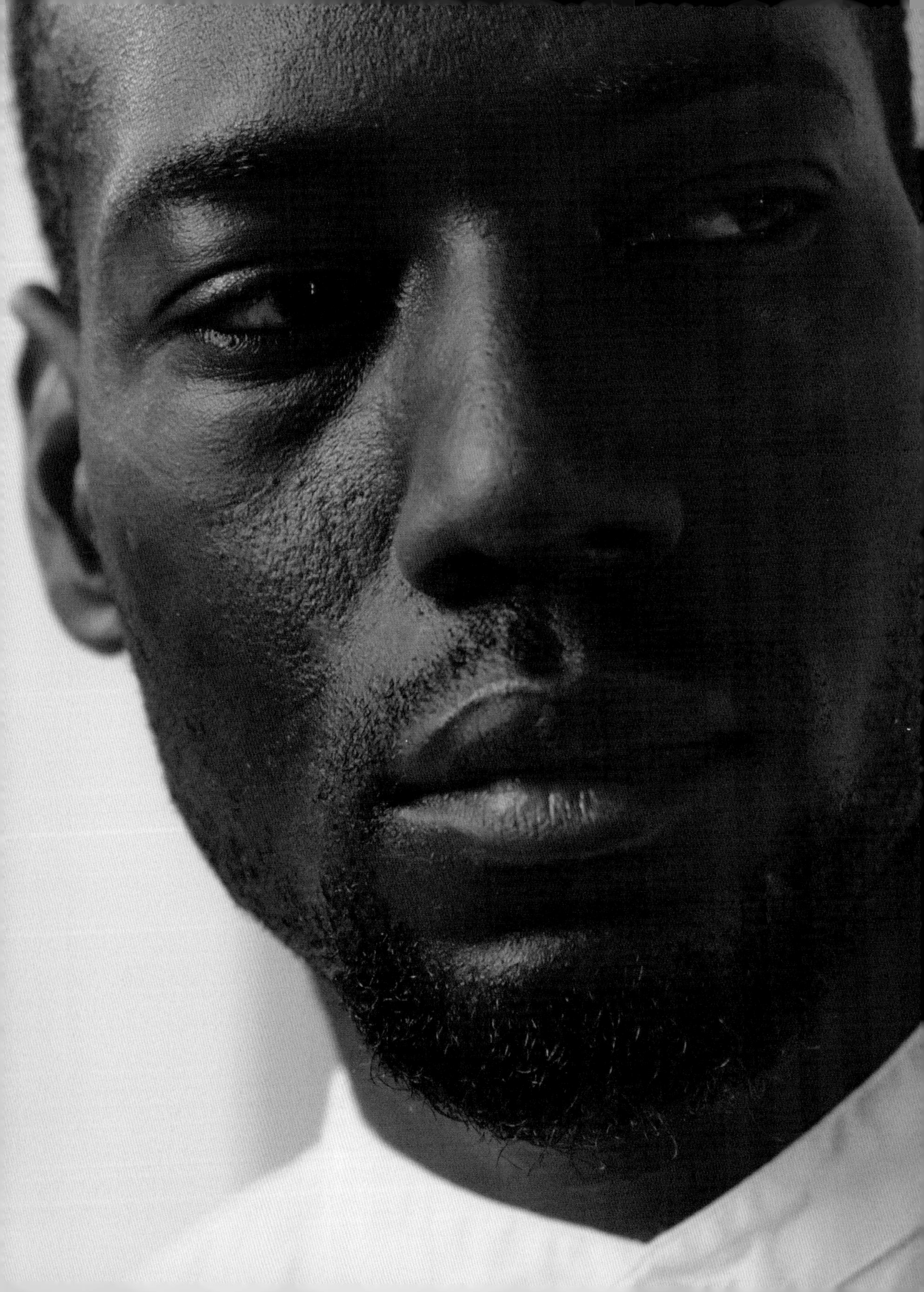

09.

men, teens and children

men, teens and children

WHILE this is very much a book for Black women, because I wholeheartedly believe that we have been left out of the beauty, skincare and grooming conversation for too long, I also believe that Black men have been left out in the cold for far longer. Society has feminised the beauty narrative so much that men are ostracised from it and viewed suspiciously should they dare go down these halls where we discuss moisturisers and sunscreens. Men don't have the carte blanche that we women have to care for ourselves and our well-being, and Black men certainly aren't afforded that privilege.

Some of the best aestheticians I know are male – Andy Millward (in the UK), Sean Garrette (US), Psalmuel Joseph (Nigeria) and Jordan Samuel (US) – and they do a great job putting male skincare on the map. Likewise, we have content creators like Gary Thompson and Ola Awosika, who are very much into grooming and will happily share pictures of themselves having a facial and applying make-up. Whilst I may not be the biggest fan of Fenty beauty (too much fragrance for me personally), I loved that when Rihanna burst onto the skincare scene she included Black men in the narrative from the get-go, featuring A$AP Rocky and Lil Nas X in the adverts. This definitely helps to make skincare and grooming more accessible, especially to Black men who currently feel very left out of the narrative. I am here for this type of barrier breaking.

Judging by the way I mentioned to my husband about a spot the other day and he said, 'Just dab some of my vitamin A on it, babe.' (I'll be honest, it took me a while to separate my jaw from the floor because, look who's giving me skincare advice!) And the way my brother never goes without his antioxidant (he's an outdoor runner) and sunscreen because he doesn't want the sun to 'fry his beauty,' I know the tables are turning and men want to be more clued up on how to have their best skin.

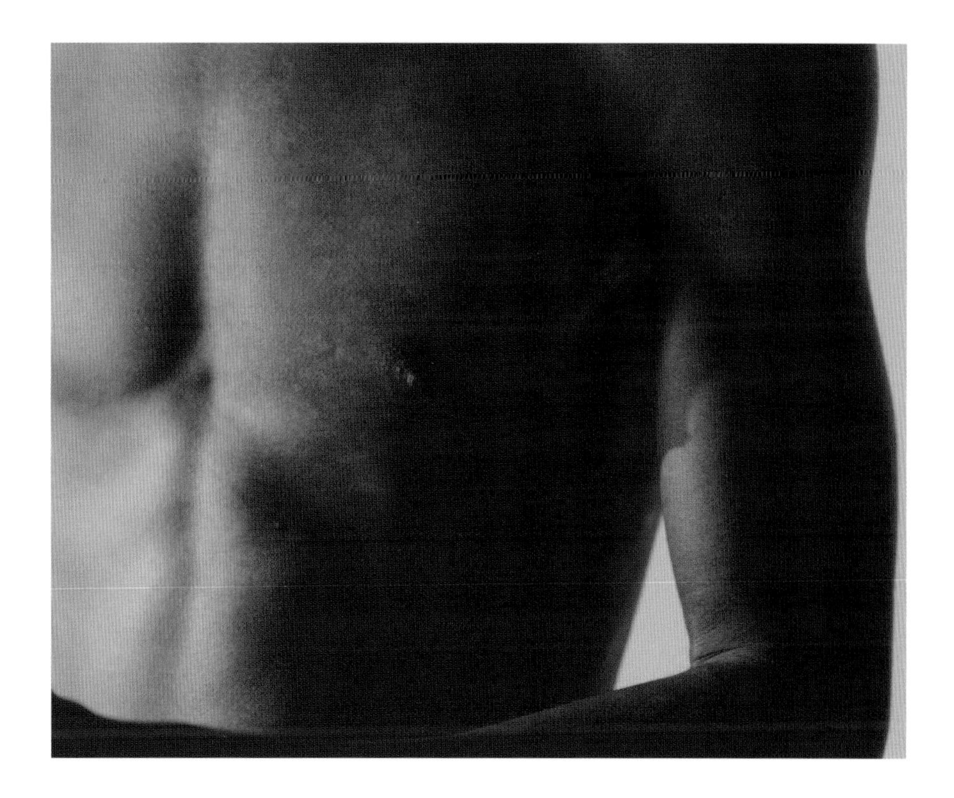

male skin

Black men are interested in grooming and skincare, but they don't always have access to the tools and resources to help them on this journey. This is why this chapter is dedicated to the men in your life, and I truly hope that you will include them in your skincare conversations – and that they will also realise there is no need to front; lotions don't use themselves up, we know they are helping themselves to our stash!

Whilst the physical structure of the skin of men and women is the same, higher levels of testosterone in men mean that their skin is 25 per cent thicker than female skin.[15] You can see evidence of this in the upper layers of the epidermis, where their skin has a visibly rougher texture, larger pores and more oil.[16] Men are also blessed with more collagen, which they lose at a slower rate than women, but this doesn't give them an advantage in the ageing process because men (especially Black men) are much more likely not to protect their skin from sun exposure, which massively speeds up premature ageing and worsens hyperpigmentation and skin discolouration.

Men are also blessed with more collagen, which they lose at a slower rate than women.

When men brave the threshold to come into the clinic, either of their own accord or having been dragged in by their partners or friends, the main concerns are:

Acne can be quite bothersome especially when it starts to interfere with shaving and causes discolouration of the face.

Pseudofolliculitis Barbae (PFB), also known as razor bumps, is very common in Black men, with up to 85 per cent of them being affected. It is caused when freshly cut Afro hair curls back and penetrates the skin.[17] This creates an inflammatory reaction that causes sore and painful bumps on the skin – hence the term razor bumps. Shaving is a major cause of this condition as it leaves the tips of the hair sharp and easily able to stab and pierce back into the skin.

Acne Keloidalis is common in men who have low fade haircuts and it typically affects the nape of the neck where the scalp has been irritated by clippers and razors for the much-loved 'shape up.' Some men are really prone to irritation in this area, which can lead to dryness, itching, PFB, patchy hair loss, scarring and, subsequently, keloids. I know how devastating this can be having watched my husband experience it. Thankfully, it's under control now, but it needed aggressive steroids, antibiotics and retinoids.

Skin discolouration and hyperpigmentation in its many guises, is also a concern, whether it be from sun damage or dark marks left from spots and breakouts.

General lack of routine I've lost count of the amount of black soap and shea butter men that come through the doors. They want better skin but don't know where to start to make the relevant changes in order to improve their skincare.

When it comes to caring for the skin, the first thing to do is to establish a basic but effective skincare routine – what I call the 'Ease in gently, no-fuss routine' that includes a skin-type-appropriate face wash that will cleanse, condition, exfoliate and decongest the skin; an antioxidant to protect and defend the skin from the environment; and a lightweight moisturiser and sunscreen. Because of the increased oiliness of male skin, I like to include a deep pore cleansing ingredient such as salicylic acid in the routine from the off. Over time it will reduce the amount of oil on the skin, and also minimise the size of the pores.

Unless discolouration is a concern, there is no need for a separate pigmentation serum (see Chapter 11). A good antioxidant like SkinBetter Science Alto Defence Serum will also brighten and even the skin tone. If dark marks are a concern, though, pigmentation serums that even the complexion are a must-have.

In the evening, an exfoliating night moisturiser, such as Paula's Choice Daily Smoothing Treatment 5% AHA with glycolic acid, or a retinoid treatment after cleansing, is a good option to keep the routine short and to improve all-round quality, texture and oil control. This also reduces the build-up of old skin cells, which influence the development of PFB.

If you are prone to Acne Keloidalis and PFB, then do extend your skincare routine to include the back of your neck and also your throat.

Whether or not you have professional treatments is up to you and the condition of your skin. However, there are very few men that aren't suitable for treatments such as facials to rejuvenate the skin, chemical peels to exfoliate, and microneedling to plump up collagen. If you want to take your skincare to the next level, then regular in-clinic treatments are most definitely the next step. This is a way to keep on top of your skin health, especially if you're acne- or ingrowing hair-prone. If extractions are included, that's a bonus, because you can sit back and let the pro squeeze out all that congestion and tweeze out trapped hair without damaging your skin.

Treatments are skin-type and skin-concern specific, and there is no difference between the treatments men can have or women can have – though if you have a beard, we have to modify the treatment slightly, such as using gauze instead of cotton pads. A fluffy white beard is not a good look!

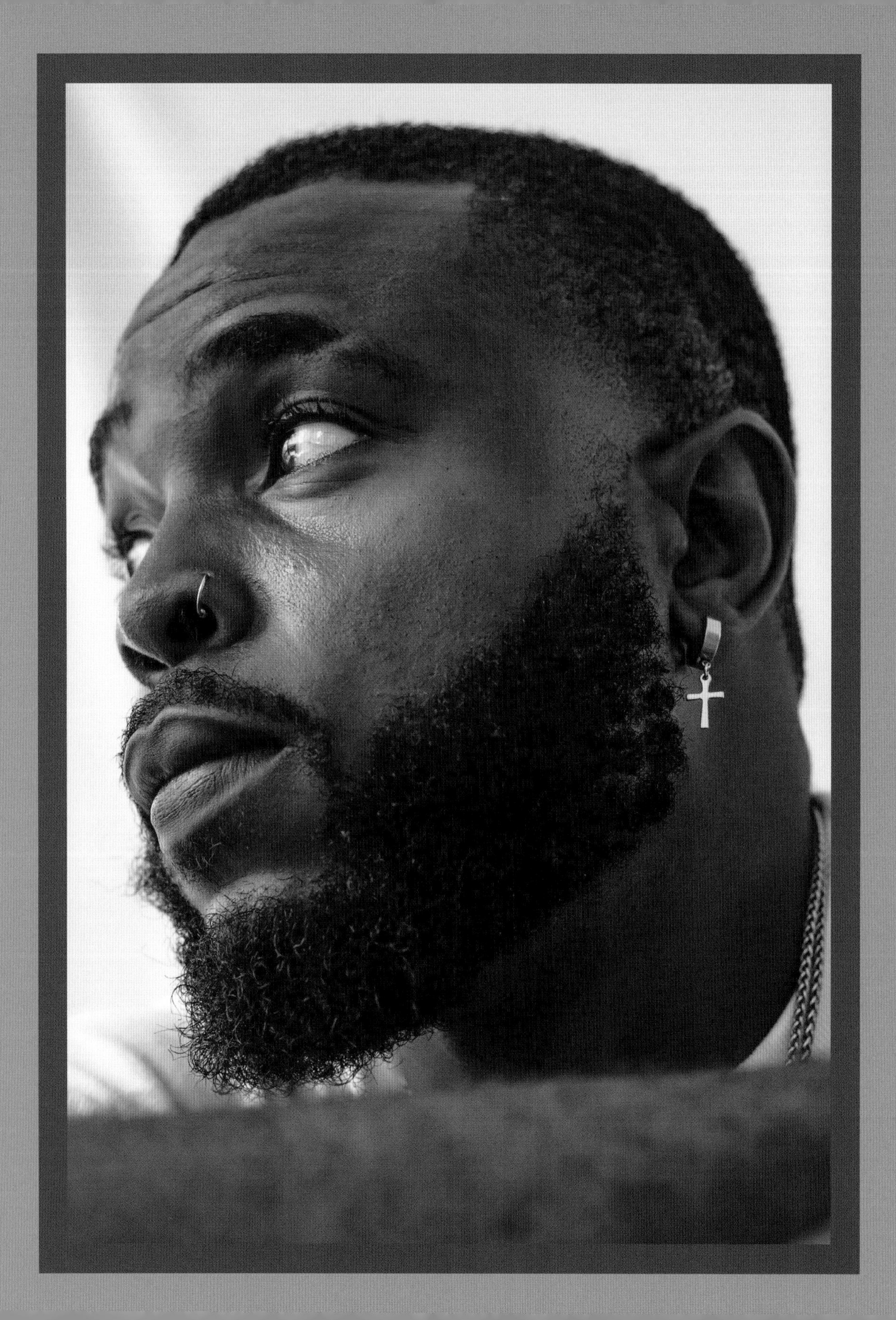

My Top Shaving Tips

- To avoid ingrowing hair and razor bumps, prepare the skin before shaving: a steam will soften your skin, open pores and loosen skin cells. If you cannot do a hot shower, then putting a hot flannel over your face will do a similar job.

- Wash the face with Dermalogica Skin Resurfacing Cleanser or apply an exfoliating mask such as Cosmedix Pure Enzymes Cranberry Exfoliating Mask to remove old skin. Wash off after 5 or 10 minutes; the longer you leave it on the better. You'd be amazed that some men think nothing of shaving a dirty face! Not you though.

- Use a single-blade razor like Bevel to shave in the direction of the hair growth.

- Make sure your blade is sharp so you can do a good job first time round, as you don't want to be repeatedly shaving the same area over and over again. That creates friction, which leads to irritation and then hyperpigmentation. Not a good look.

- After shaving, apply an antioxidant and a gentle moisturiser to condition the skin and encourage healing. Don't forget your sunscreen.

Psst... Beard Gang Crew

Yes, a full and lush beard is something to be admired but stop coating your beard in oil every day to keep it shiny and glossy. You sometimes forget you have skin underneath that tends to be oilier, thicker and rougher. Oils can block your pores, leading to breakouts, which leads to hyperpigmentation.

If you are using oils, thoroughly wash your face in the evening to avoid stacking up future problems, and apply a proper moisturiser to your skin before a few drops of oil to keep your beard glossy and tame the stray hairs.

teen skin

Clearasil. If I could sum up my teenage skincare experience, this would be the word, or rather the product. This is what I used and it's what all my friends used. We knew of nothing else. Whilst I don't remember whether or not it worked for me, I do remember the tightness of my skin, but in those days that was taken as a sign that the product was working. There was no one to tell me that if a product makes your skin feel stripped then it's too much for you.

Also, there wasn't much skincare talk in my house, bar the usual 'Have you had a bath?' But no one took any interest in my skin or the state of it, not the way I fuss over my daughter's and niece's skin. A large part of it is that, mostly, my teenage skin life was uneventful, but I do recall some really big juicy spots from time to time that I had no idea what to do with. Do I try to burst them? Leave them alone? Apply something? If so, what? What about this Black stain the spot left in its wake?

As a teenager I also didn't see any representation of myself in the media and magazines either. I read *Sugar* and *Bliss* and, whilst I enjoyed them, there was nothing in there I could relate to from a cultural or heritage point of view because the default was white. Boys didn't even have a magazine to start with, let alone a magazine that was intended for Black boys. There was nothing available for Black teens really, nothing, nada, niente!

This was 20-odd years ago, so when my 13-year-old niece asks me the same question in 2021, I am a little taken aback because I honestly thought times had changed, especially given that information is literally at our fingertips and, with the touch of a button, anything we've ever wanted to know about teenage skin will appear on a screen in front of us. And herein lies some of the confusion for teenagers, because there is such a thing as too much information, and for a lot of the teen skin complaints I see, most of the clients have been victims of skincare information overload.

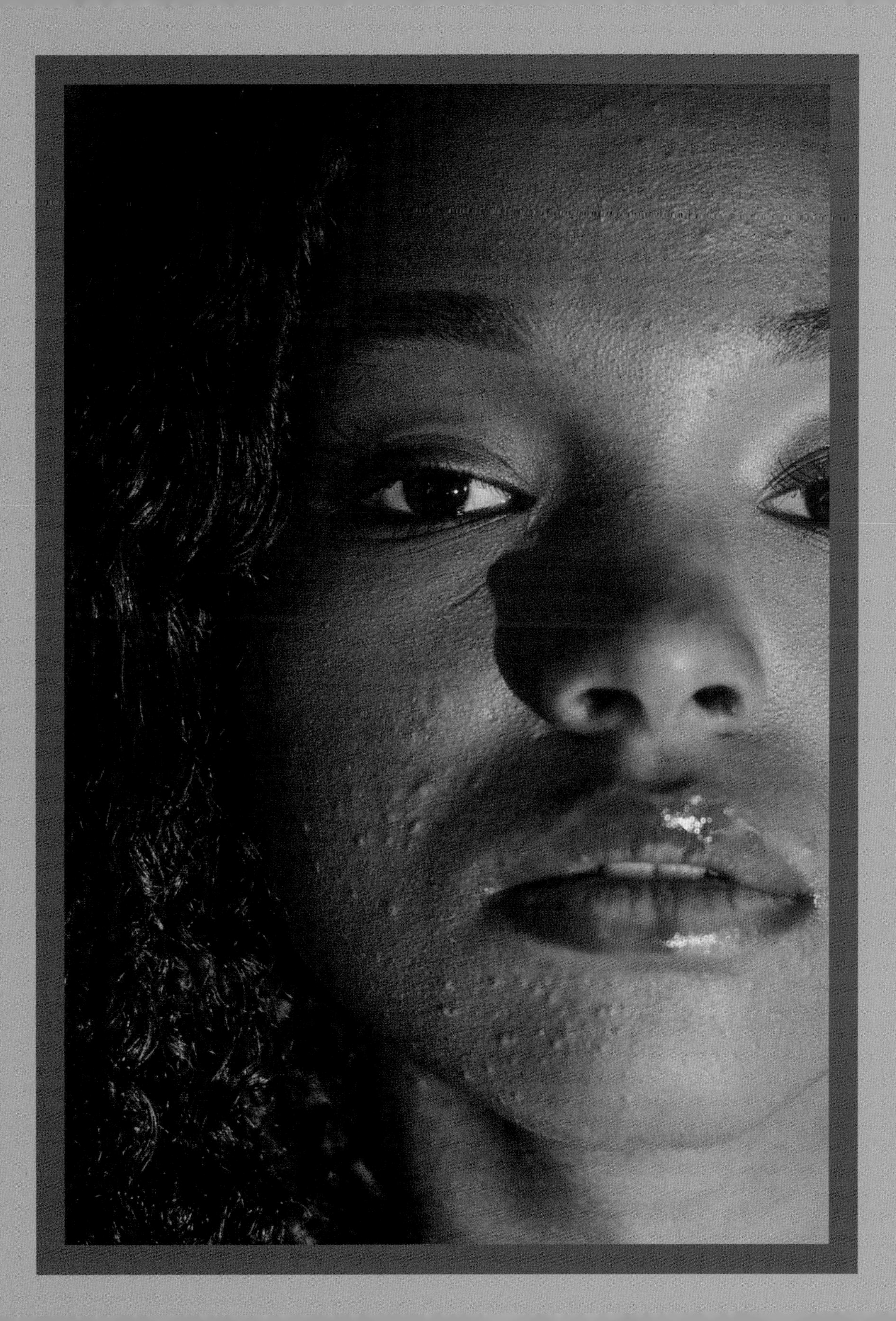

Let this section be your fount of skincare knowledge. I sit at the intersection of knowing how much information Black teens lacked about their skin in the Nineties when I was a teenager, to seeing the abundance of information that is now readily available on the interweb, from brands to influencers and even skincare specialists like myself! I can see why your questions still have question marks and your head is spinning from the lack of answers, even if it appears there is a lot of noise. Fear not, I have filtered and condensed all the available information into everything you need to know for your healthiest and best skin.

How your periods affect your skin

Days 1–6

All hormones low

Your skin may be dry and dull so the focus should be hydrating; those products containing hyaluronic acid are great.

Days 7–14

Oestrogen hormones are high

Your skin is settled and radiant. Maintaining this calm with gentle exfoliation and moisturising is key.

Days 15–28

Progesterone & testosterone take over

Your skin responds by being oilier, greasy and spot prone. The key thing here is to control and treat using ingredients like salicylic acid.

Teenage skin is that period when your skin is not quite a child's delicate skin but it's not yet mature, grown-up skin. By age 12 your skin is structurally the same as an adult's; however, you're also experiencing puberty, when the body goes through significant changes with the rush of oestrogen, progesterone and testosterone hormones.

Testosterone has a massive effect on your skin because it stimulates the oil glands to produce more oil and the skin can become sweatier; throw old skin cells and *C. acnes* bacteria into the mix and this is the setting for congestion and breakouts. Some teenagers are more prone to breakouts and acne than others and your family history will have something to do with it.

For girls, when you start menstruating you may also notice another pattern in your skin: that you start experiencing more breakouts around the time of your period and how hormones affect your skin throughout the month. See the diagram on the opposite page.

Something else that can fuel oiliness and spots is stress. Not only do you go through bodily changes in the teenage years, but there are also psychological changes that can impact your skin. Mental health, exams, boy/girl worries can all increase the amount of stress you're under and this can become a double-edge sword. The body reacts to stress by producing more oil, not only making you feel and look greasier but also increasing the likelihood of spots and acne.

When I was a teenager, the day was not complete without an after-school trip to the Patel News corner shop for the holy trinity of snacks: a Snickers chocolate bar, Walkers Cheese & Onion crisps, and a can of Coke. Many teens are still the same and your diets are high in sugar and carbohydrates. Whilst I won't outright say stop, because a small part of me thinks it's a rite of passage, I will say that if you are concerned about your skin, then think about cutting back and making high-sugar snacks a treat rather than the norm.

Through various pathways in the body, excess sugar stimulates the production of more testosterone, which – as you already know – plays a key role in oil production, acne and breakouts. Not to mention that this food category is also highly inflammatory and weakens the skin, which makes any conditions you have, like acne or even eczema, so much worse.

There are four main concerns that usually come up with teenage skin:

Acne is a major one – an inflammatory condition that cause pimples, spots, papules and pustules due to the overproduction of oil combined with clogged pores, old skin cells and the *C. acnes* bacteria. These spots and pimples can be individual, in clusters, on the surface or below the skin. Depending on location and depth, they can also be painful and can sometimes be filled with pus.

Whiteheads and **blackheads**, which are also basically spots. At the surface of the skin, exposure to air oxidises the spot and causes it to turn a dark brown/black colour. You can usually find blackheads in the areas of your skin that are most oily – the nose and chin. Whiteheads, on the other hand, are closed spots still within and under the skin but with a creamy white head.

Dark marks are also an issue, and these tend to happen after you've had a spot or some other inflammation of the skin. The general term is hyperpigmentation. Black skin is melanin rich, and during the skin-healing process melanin will flood the area, and the extra deposit of pigment is what we see on the surface of the skin causing the dark mark, which does eventually fade (though sometimes it can be quite stubborn).

Dry skin, although this is very rarely a major concern as many people feel they can handle this successfully by themselves.

A quick 10 minutes on social media will have you thinking you need a cabinet full of products (and expensive products, too) to keep your skin in tip-top condition. You don't. You can keep things simple and within your pocket money/Saturday job range.

By simply keeping on top of your skincare you will make the experience of breakouts a lot less painful and tiresome.

Teen Skin Kit

Eye make-up remover (If you wear lots of eyeshadow, liner and lashes – if not, leave this out.)

Cleanser This is a super-important step because it sets the tone for everything else you do for your skin.

Liquid exfoliant (Only if you experience spots and breakouts regularly. A lactic acid–salicylic acid combo would be great to help get rid of the old skin cells and decongest oil from your pores.) No matter what TikTok says, you do not need glycolic acid just yet...

Moisturiser Oil-free and lightweight for oilier skin types, or choose something more nourishing for dry skin. You can use the same one morning and night.

Sunscreen Use a minimum SPF30 to keep your skin protected. Sunscreen is the key to preventing hyperpigmentation and dark marks from getting worse. Getting into the habit of using sunscreen now will preserve your skin well into the future.

Lip balm Self-explanatory really, but lips don't produce any oils to keep them lubricated, so if you want to avoid dry, chapped or sore lips then lip balm is a necessity.

Suggested Routine

MORNING	EVENING
Face wash	Eye make-up remover + make-up remover
Liquid exfoliant (every other day)	Face wash
Moisturiser	Moisturiser
Sunscreen	

I'm often asked by teenage clients, *'How do I get good skin?'* First off, there is no such thing as good skin. When I hear this, my brain translates this to mean how do I have clear skin? How do I not get spots? Even with the best skincare routine, you may still experience the occasional pimple or breakout. There's not much you can do about it, but I can tell you that by simply keeping on top of your skincare you will make the experience of breakouts a lot less painful and tiresome.

You can prevent breakouts by doing the following:

- Follow a decent routine of cleansing twice a day, morning and evening. This is the art of doing the least to gain the most.
- Be gentle with your skin. It's not a fight, and you're not at war.
- Change your pillowcase as least once a week. Not only do they harbour bacteria but also oils and dirt from our hair.
- Stick to lightweight oil-free products. Your heavier body products, such as pure shea butter moisturisers, are not for your face.
- Have a spot treatment with salicylic acid or benzoyl peroxide to hand for those breakout days.
- Seek professional advice when in doubt about your skin, especially if it's starting to affect your mental health, whether it be from your doctor or by popping into a local beauty salon. Just promise me you'll avoid Dr Google, Dr TikTok and Nurse YouTube. Even if you see something on there you think is right for you, check with a professional first.
- Avoid comparing your skin to your BFF or fave social media influencer. There is so much that determines the quality of your skin – genetics, lifestyle, diet. Outside these influences, there's also technological factors such as filters and ring lights that can dramatically change the way in which skin is presented. Be mindful that what you see on your screen may not be the real truth.

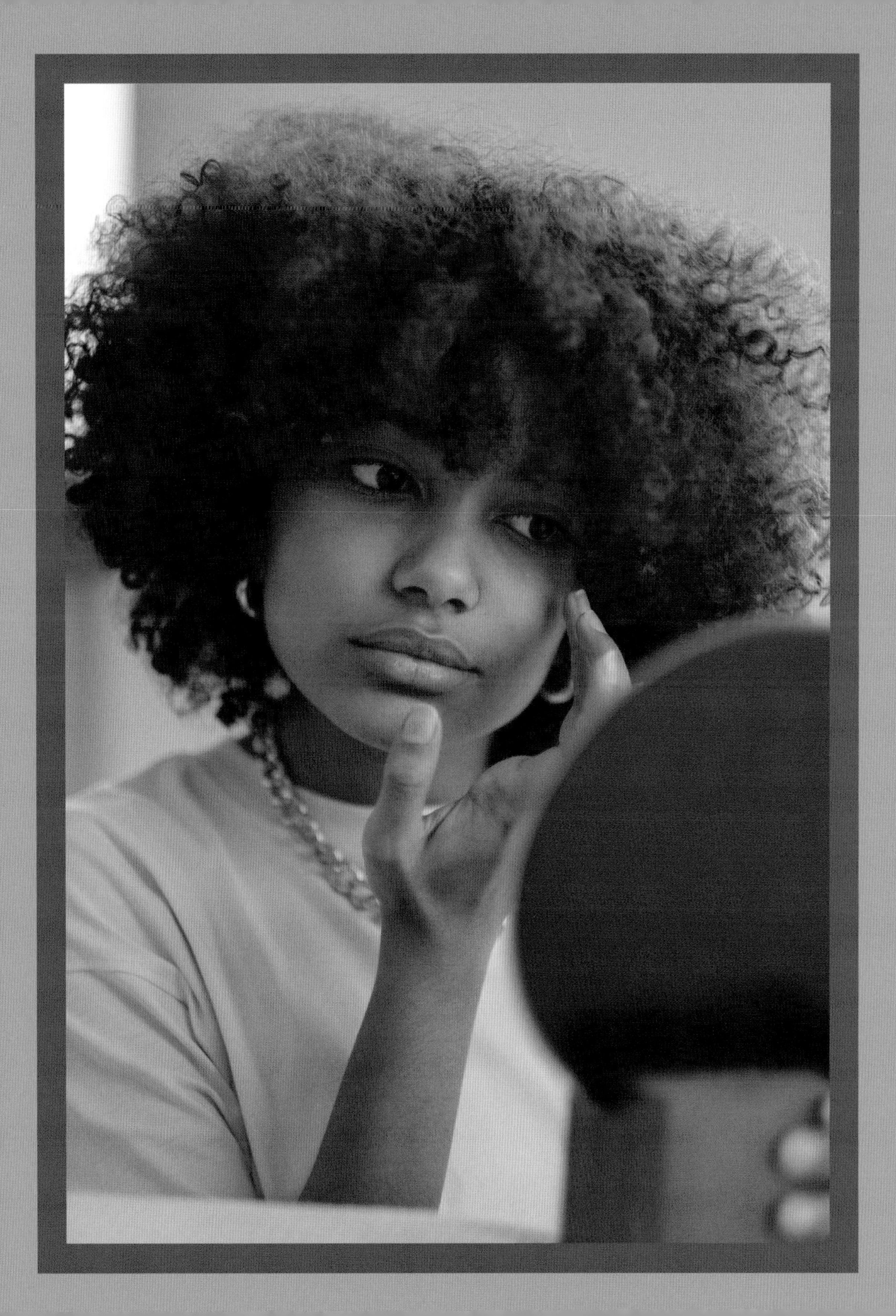

On Black skin, one of the key problems for most people is dealing with dark marks and hyperpigmentation. They are irritating. Period. Your skin can be smooth and soft like a newborn's, but dark spots will end up making it look patchy. The good news is that as a teenager, your skin-cell turnover is very efficient, and you will have a new layer of cells coming to the surface roughly every 21–28 days. This means that dark marks fade super fast from the skin, so I'm always a little reluctant to suggest pigmentation serums for your age group. But I also know that you're trying not to hear that; so if you're finding that some of the dark marks are really stubborn, my top picks to help keep your skin clear are pigmentation serums from La Roche-Posay, The Ordinary and Naturium. Apply immediately after cleansing and before your moisturiser for the best results.

It's also important you know a little bit about how dark marks are formed, as that will help you avoid them in the first place. Check out Chapter 7.

On Black skin, one of the key problems for most people is dealing with dark marks and hyperpigmentation.

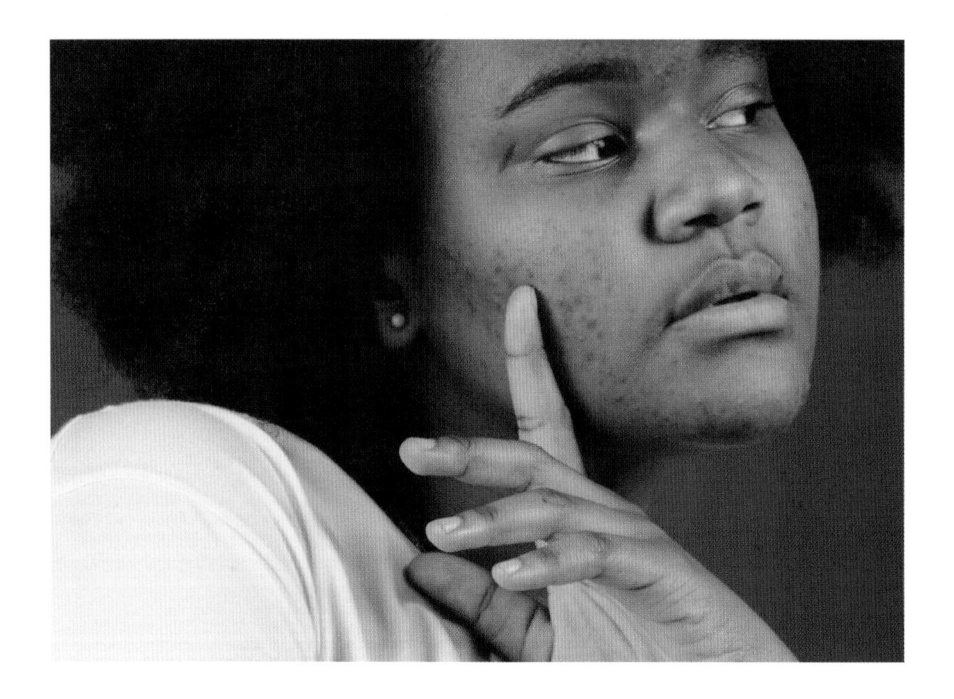

Favourite Teen Skin Brands

- CeraVe
- La Roche-Posay
- Vichy
- Sam Farmer
- REN
- Dermalogica
- Avène
- Zitsticka
- The Ordinary
- Dermalogica Clear Start
- Eucerin
- The INKEY List
- Glossier
- Starface
- e.l.f. Skincare

If you're going to try these brands, it's also important you have some idea of your skin type, so refer to Chapter 3.

For most teens, temperamental skin is a hallmark of puberty and you will get through without many knocks and bumps and your skin confidence will remain intact. More so if you follow the advice in this chapter, and in this book in general. As a Black woman, I'm well aware of the scrutiny and harsh gaze that is sometimes cast on you as young Black girls. The need to have 'dewy, juicy, flawless skin on fleek' can put quite a bit of pressure on, so I want you to extend grace to yourself and stop seeking perfection, because you're good enough as you are. Even if you have a breakout from time to time.

Remember that spots are common and will come and go, and that not all skincare advice applies to you, so be selective who you listen to. Sometimes it's worth asking yourself, 'What's this person's qualification?' The answer will tell you whether they are worth taking solid skincare advice from. Don't be led, you are not a sheep. It's important that you develop a healthy attitude towards your skin, and this involves looking at the people you follow on social media as well. Not everyone is a good influence, so take back your control by unfollowing anyone that makes you feel bad or less than.

Also, take time to understand your skin. It's not going to happen in one day, so be patient. Observe your skin over the course of 2 or 3 months, because when you know your skin, you will be able to treat it better and more kindly with a skincare routine that works and gives you the results you are after. Knowing your skin also helps you find out your breakout triggers – is it stress? Too many late nights? Are you inconsistent with your skincare routine? Sugary food? Once you can spot these patterns you will be able to look after your skin better.

Use your voice and know when to ask for help. It's usually when you can't think about anything else other than your skin. If you're waking up an hour early every day to do your make-up before school, you need to ask for help.

Finally, remember that you will have your skin for life, so how you regard and treat it now will determine how it looks in the future. Be kind to it (and yourself).

**Take time to understand your skin.
It's not going to happen in one day, so be patient.**

If you're a parent or other responsible adult reading this, please understand that for us as grown-ups we know that there is more to living than skin and our appearance, so it's easy for us to dismiss teenagers' concerns and preoccupation with looks. But I urge you to cast your mind back to your teenage years and remember that it was a period filled with much confusion and anxiety, and we didn't even have an online world pushing false images of perfection to contend with too.

As much as life is easier for our teenagers now, life is also more challenging in certain respects. So when your teenager starts expressing concerns about their skin, please take them seriously – book an appointment with the doctor, find a reputable skin therapist, or consult a dermatologist. Left unchecked, teen skin concerns can unnecessarily spiral into a big deal. The earlier skin complaints are addressed, the better both the mental and physical outcomes.

children's skin

When it comes to children's skincare, if you are in doubt about anything at all, your first stop should be your doctor. That said, being a mum of two I know just how handy it is to have something to refer to that can put your mind at ease.

We fret over their skin. A lot. I guess how they turn out is a reflection of us and our parenting skills. I grew up in the era where if your face didn't gleam like a new coin, you were surely trying to embarrass your mum. Smooth, shiny and glossed skin was a marker of you being clean and healthy, and that you came from a caring home with responsible adults.

I get asked a variety of questions about children's skin on a daily basis, from what to use for dry skin to whether steroids really are safe for eczema and what to use for an 8-year-old who's started getting spots that leave dark marks.

Children's skin is very different to an adult's. For starters, it's immature skin; the very top layer of the epidermis is thinner and they have fewer of the components (fatty acids, cholesterol, ceramides) that create a waterproof barrier on the surface of the skin. This means that their skin finds it more challenging to balance moisture and hydration, leaving it open to sensitivity, irritation and dryness.

General dry skin issues are amongst the top three concerns I come across. I have experienced extremely dry skin on both my children, and with Black skin being naturally prone to moisture loss, this can be a double whammy. In these situations, the skin will peel, flake and chaff, leaving the babas feeling raw, sore and downright miserable.

A layered approach to moisturising the skin is the solution. I've never been let down by Aveeno and I add a sachet of the Soothing Oatmeal Bath Treatment For Itchy, Dry Skin to the bath water to soften it. This is the same as adding a sock of Quaker oats to the bath, just a lot less messy! Oats have anti-inflammatory properties that soothe and reinforce moisture in the skin. La Roche-Posay Baby Lipikar Syndet AP+ Cream Wash is also very good, as is Salcura Bioskin Junior Face & Body Wash, which is suitable for bodies prone to eczema, psoriasis and the usual dry skin conditions.

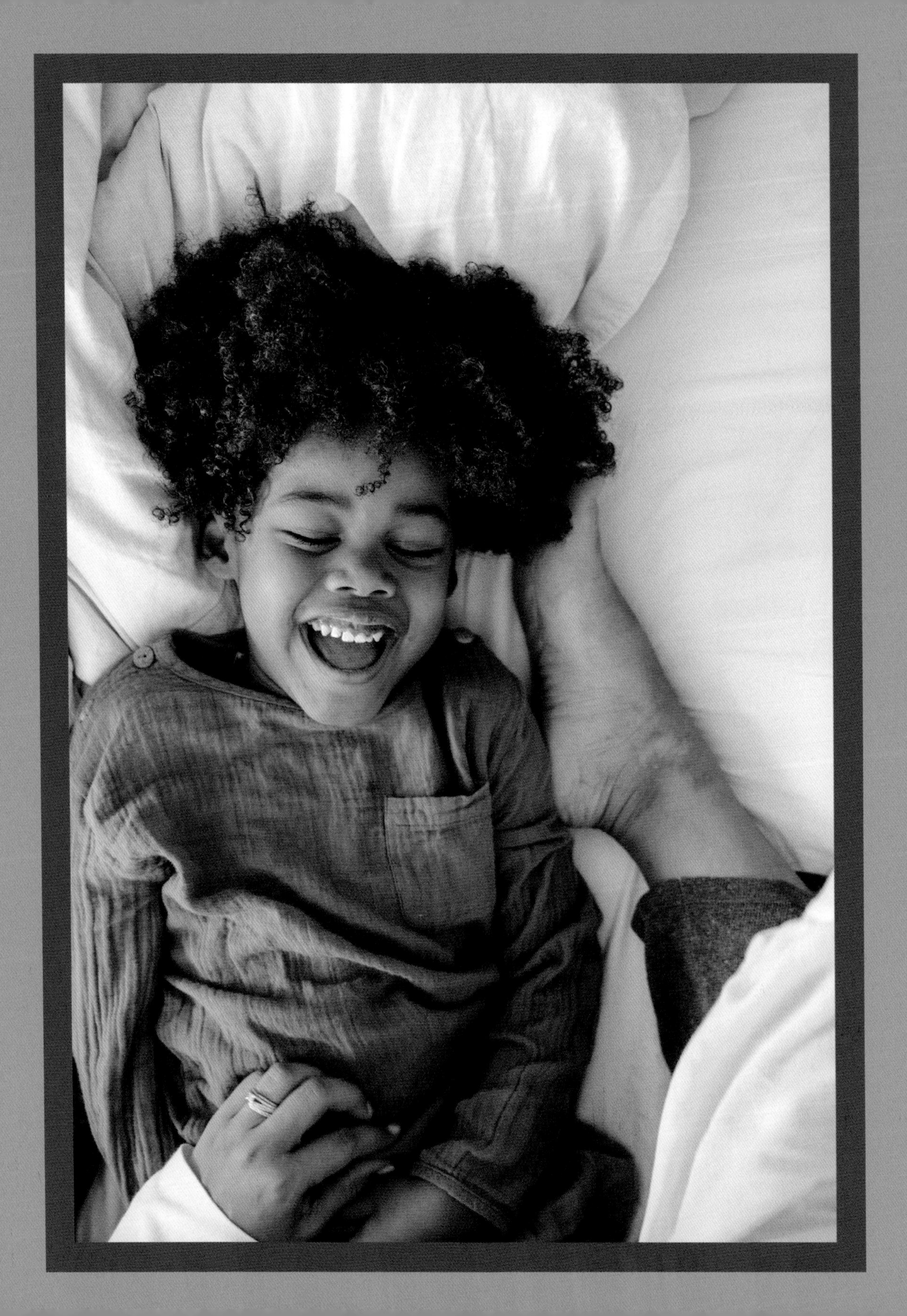

After bath time, and whilst skin is still damp, I go straight in with a lightweight hydrating moisturiser such as Aveeno Dermexa Daily Emollient Cream, or La Roche-Posay Baby Cicaplast Baume B5 Repairing Balm. The most important aspect of this routine is the third step: to seal all this moisture in. For that I swear by the 50:50 ointment. Sometimes I even apply a hyaluronic acid before the moisturiser to give the skin more hydration. I discovered this was a very effective solution for dry-skin flare-ups when my son got a bout of terrible dry skin on holiday in France. Unfortunately, the baby bag had been stolen earlier in our trip and we'd lost our usual skin soothers, so I went to a pharmacy to see if I could find some replacements and in my 'Frenglish' explained my predicament to the old lady behind the counter. She jumped up, went over to one of the sections and shoved La Roche-Posay Hyalu B5 Hyaluronic Acid Serum into my hands. She was the no-nonsense type and reminded me of my grandmother, so of course I did as I was told and it worked a treat. Since then I've also tried Medik8 Hydrate B5 Serum, and both have been lifesavers!

I've seen lots of mums pull back on products when their child has dry skin and opt for a moisturiser like pure shea butter. Shea butter is great, but again it is a sealant, not a moisturiser, so still apply a water-based hydration layer on the skin first.

Atopic eczema is also something that pops up quite a lot and I am very familiar with it; my son developed eczema from just a few weeks old, when I noticed his face and torso were flushed, sometimes reddened, with a raised sore-looking rash. At the time, we couldn't figure out the cause – his skin was just angry at the world. We rewashed his clothes, changed his toiletries over to my tried and tested Aveeno – my oldest started off with dry skin so I've been on this rodeo before, and Aveeno saved the day – but for him none of these changes made a difference.

FACT 'Atopic' means sensitivity to allergens. The exact cause of atopic eczema is unknown, but it's clear it is not down to one single thing alone. It tends to develop before the first birthday and most children grow out of it before their fifth birthday.

Whenever my son had formula milk, his discomfort would be worse, so we stopped formula and upped the breast milk. His eczema reduced but not completely. So I decided to investigate what would happen if I stopped dairy and – kaboom! Over a number of days his skin was smooth like butter. Win for him, but sadly for me it ended my life-long love affair with cheese. (I would subsequently go on to discover that my son's eczema was also triggered by gluten and eggs. With his sister having a severe allergy to nuts, I didn't even go down that road with him.)

A small child with eczema is tough on everyone, but there are quick fixes, and sometimes medication is the only thing that brings relief.

FACT Steroids are anti-inflammatory medicines in cream, gel or ointments that are used to calm inflammation like eczema and reduce irritation. Sometimes steroids are even concentrated into bandages that you can strap to the skin.

We followed a dry-skin routine for my son, but a product I found really helpful was the Aveeno Baby Dermexa Good Night Emollient Balm, which we used round the clock layered over lightweight moisturiser. With eczema, the skin barrier is really compromised so the aim is to support and build it back up, so that it's able to retain moisture. The balm has similar properties to the fats and waxes that make up the skin's natural barrier and is fortified with avenanthramides made from oats, and is really soothing for dry skin. We use this so much, I always joke that Aveeno needs to give me some shares in their company.

The other range that eased eczema flare-ups was Cetraben – the bath additive was a game-changer for us to keep his skin cocooned and moisturised whilst he got clean. In 2018, research published in the *British Medical Journal* said that bath additives were of no real clinical benefit to children with eczema, though there was some small evidence that showed they were beneficial to children who bathed 5 or more times a week. My son has a bath every day, so it makes sense that it works for him.

In the winter, when skin is naturally drier, using the heavier Cetraben Ointment as a final layer to lock in moisture is a good shout.

One particular area that I find Black mums reluctant to explore is the use of topical steroid. I appreciate the fears around thinning the skin and potential de-pigmentation; however, steroid use is very transient and, in my opinion, they are a worthwhile component to your arsenal if offered by your doctor.

Psst… A word about fragrance

This is really down to preference. For children I prefer to avoid using it, especially if the skin is already showing signs of sensitivity. But, in the grand scheme of things, fragrance shouldn't be a deal breaker.

We follow the 'short-term contact use' for steroids, meaning that we only use them when needed, i.e. when a flare-up is so bad that we can't sleep through the night. Our average length of use is 3–4 days, applying a thin layer (a finger-tip unit) on affected areas, twice a day. Once the area is calm, we go back to following the dry-skin routine. Because Black skin is drier, we've always preferred steroids in an ointment rather than a cream, as it has more staying power.

Your doctor or dermatologist will guide you, but so long as you aren't using steroids more than twice a day, and using only a thin layer for a few days at a time, Black skin will remain intact and with colour. I want to encourage you that at a time where you're at your wits' end with very little sleep and an unhappy child, please do consider using a steroid to bring relief to all of your household.

On top of this, it seems like children are starting to experience spots and breakouts a lot earlier nowadays, and not a week goes by when a mum doesn't ask me about their under 10's skin.

My first question is what is your child putting on their skin? My daughter went through a period of a spotty forehead and it took me a minute before I realised that she was moisturising her body with shea butter before applying her face moisturiser, and this action was congesting her skin, breaking her out in small pimples and rashes. Once she learned to moisturise her face first, with no oil residue on her hands, it was spots no more. It was as simple as tweaking the routine.

If you love styling those baby hairs into curls and swirls on the forehead, bear in mind that, because the face is warm, oils in hair gel can seep further down the face, leading to congestion and spots. Lay those edges for sure, but make sure the gel is washed off properly every evening so your child isn't going to bed with hair gel on their face.

My friends are always surprised that my 8-year-old has a skincare routine. It's really simple, with a face wash, moisturiser and sunscreen. Same thing in the evening but without the SPF. You can never start grooming too early in my book, and I really rate the CeraVe range as a good starting point. Equally, Sam Farmer and Avène are great options. See pages 142–152 for more guidance on managing teens' and tweens' skincare.

When it comes to looking after children's skin, the goal is to always keep it simple, concentrating on cleansing and moisturising and, when necessary, short-term intervention with more concentrated and potent products.

Looking after children's skin, the goal is to always keep it simple, concentrating on cleaning and moisturising.

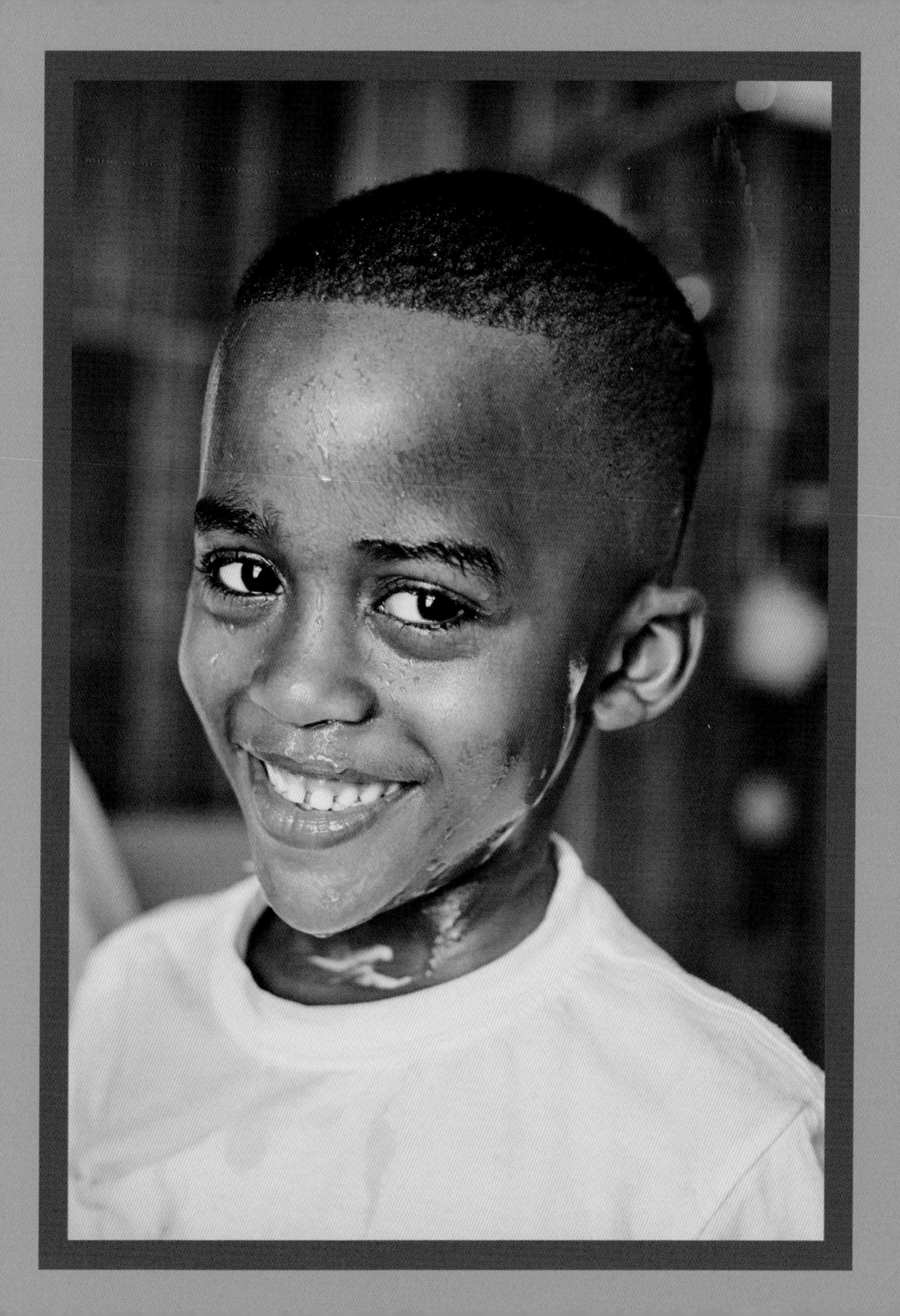

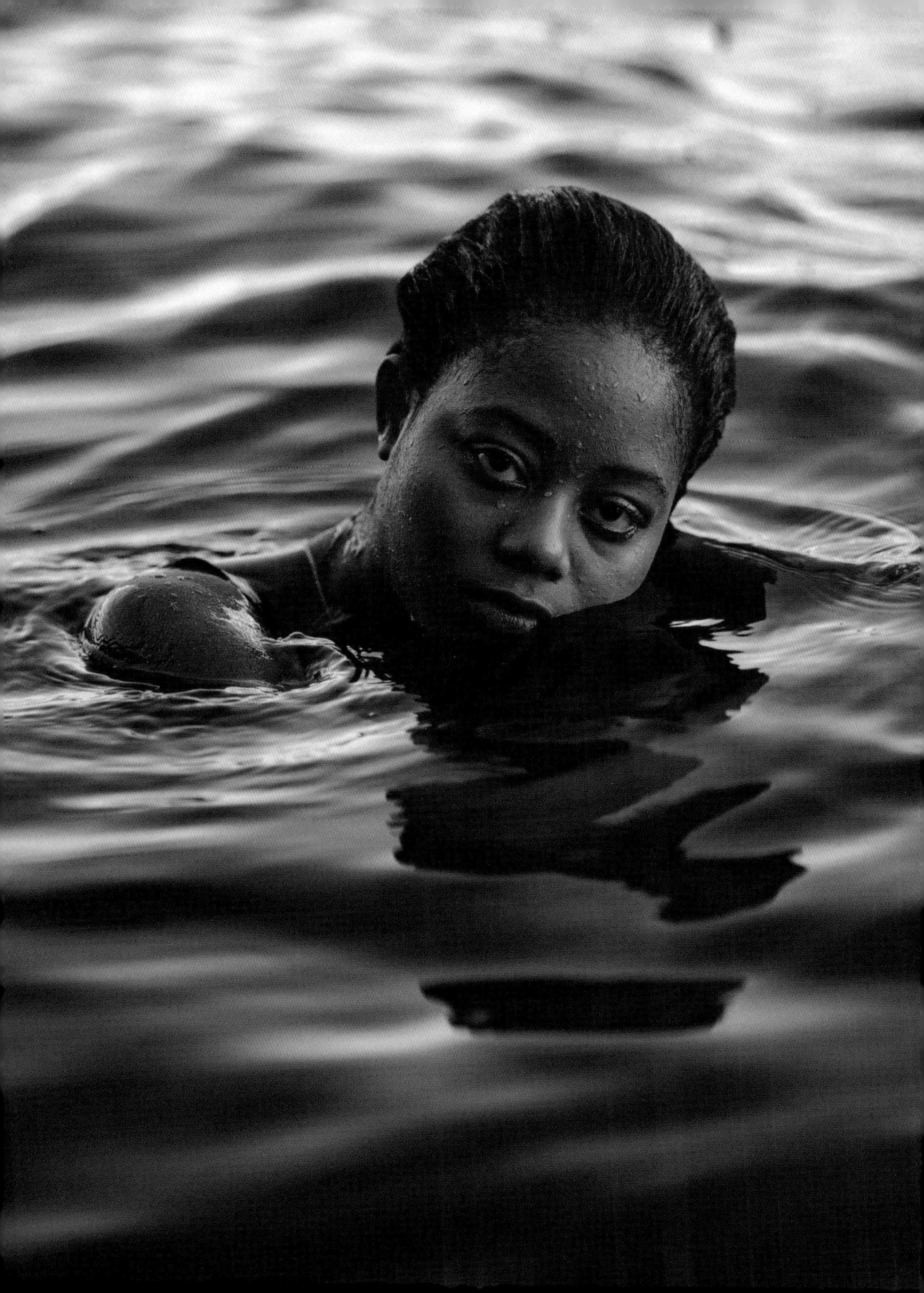

10.

unpacking black skin myths

unpacking black skin myths

ONE thing that stops Black women from accessing the best information, treatments and products to care for their skin is the number of myths and misconceptions about Black skin that litter the beauty and skincare world. These create unnecessary fear and confusion, so it's time to settle the matter once and for all.

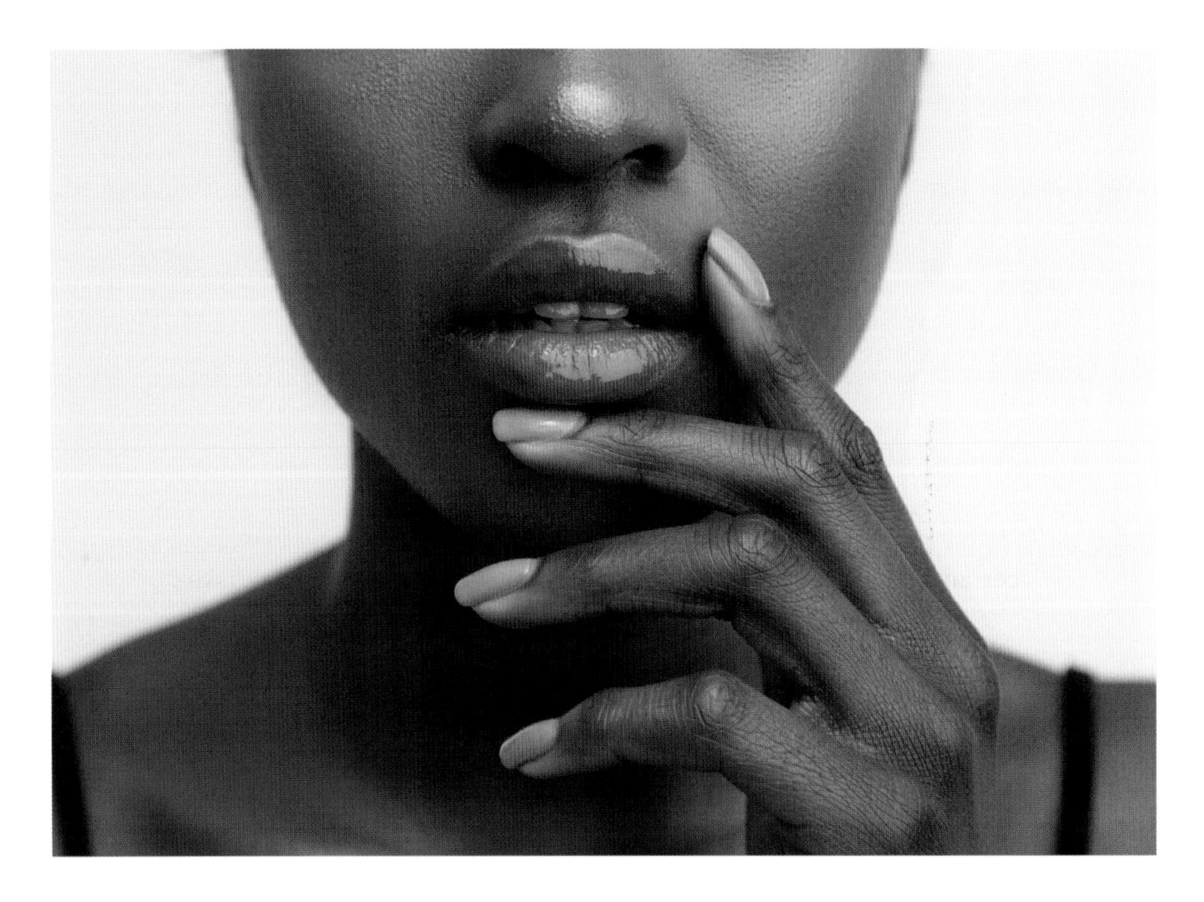

'Black skin doesn't need sunscreen'

Yes, it does! The sun speeds up premature ageing and will make hyperpigmentation worse, so don't be a stranger to your broad spectrum SPF30 UVA/UVB sunscreen.

'Black people can't get skin cancer'

Black people can get skin cancer, including the type caused by the sun. Albeit at a lower rate than white people, but that is not a hall pass to be less vigilant about sun protection. Experts say that Black people are more likely to die from skin cancer because we spot the signs a lot later than white people, because we are not used to monitoring our skin for changes.

'The sun charges melanin to keep Black skin black'

False. Melanin isn't produced by the sun and neither does it need charging. Over-exposure to direct sunlight without sun protection can lead to burns and hyperpigmentation.

'Hydroquinone is bad for Black skin because it bleaches and lightens the skin'

Hydroquinone is only bad for the skin when used incorrectly and without medical supervision. It's actually a great ingredient for solving hyperpigmentation concerns, but it's unfairly got a bad rep because certain groups use it carelessly for bleaching and lightening their skin.

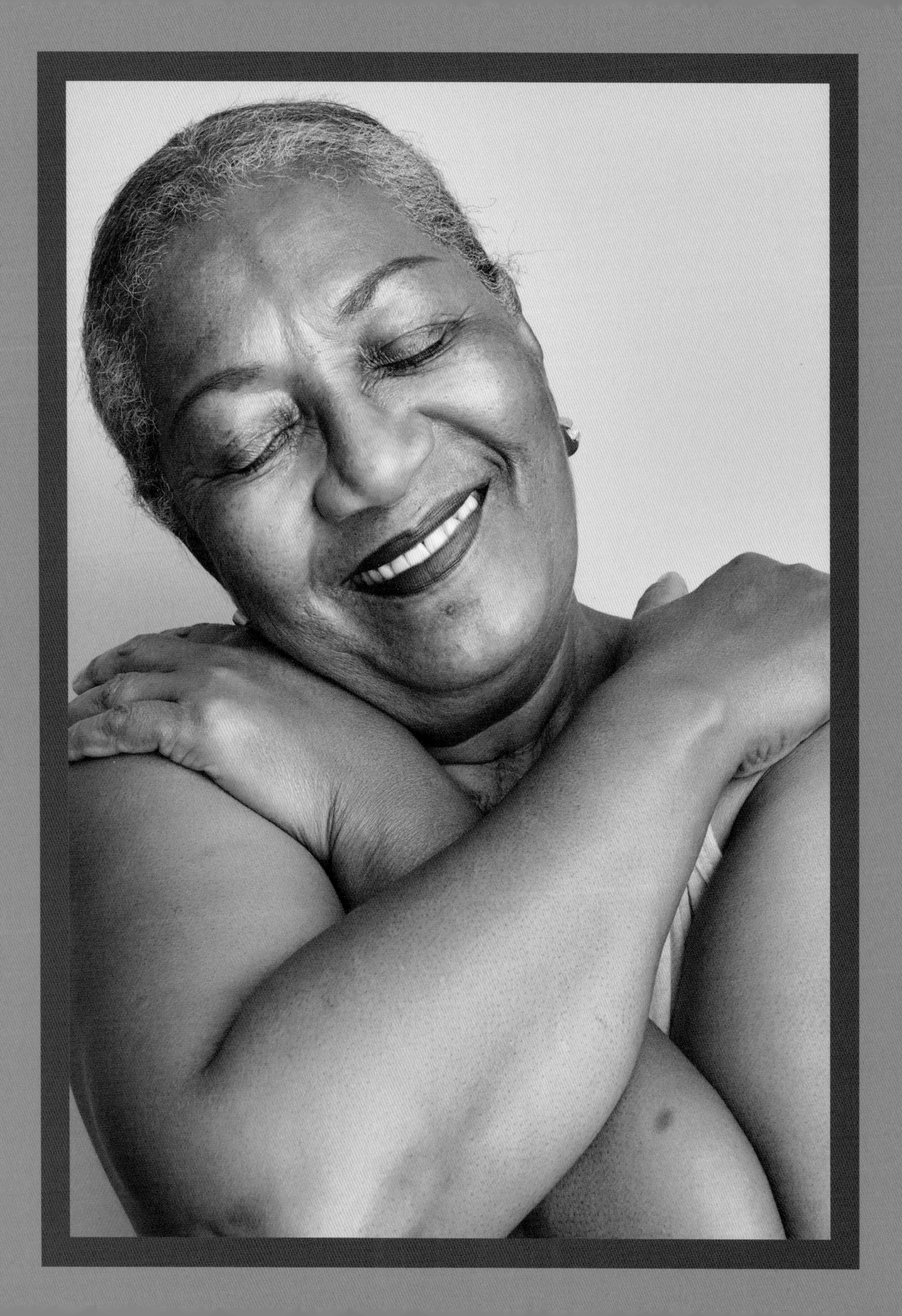

'Black skin can't have advanced treatments such as chemical peels, micro-needling or laser treatment'

This is incorrect. Black skin can successfully have all these treatments. Just ensure your practitioner is qualified and experienced. Treatments are always improving, and some can be easily modified to suit Black skin, so don't be put off.

'Black don't crack'

We love to say this, but Black will crack if you slack. Black skin is not immune from 'cracking', i.e. fine lines and wrinkles; it just happens at a slower rate than white skin. Black skin having more melanin is not an excuse not to look after it or protect it from the sun and other types of environmental damage like pollution. Apart from lines and wrinkles, discolouration is also a sign of ageing.

'Black skin needs specialist skincare'

False, Black skin can use readily available skincare. You just have to be conscious that there are some ingredients, such as tyrosinase inhibitors (see Chapter 11) that work better for darker skin because of their interaction with melanin. On the whole, it's skincare according to skin type just as much as skin colour.

'Shea butter is the best moisturiser for Black skin'

False. Shea butter, and any butters or oils in their pure form, can clog your pores and will form a seal over skin, stopping it from getting rid of natural waste, sweat and toxins. In addition, they stop the skin from being able to attract and absorb moisture from the environment.

'Glycolic acid is unsafe and unsuitable for Black skin because it causes hyperpigmentation'

Totally incorrect Glycolic acid is both efficient and effective in exfoliating the skin and fading dark marks. It is a complete misconception that it is unsafe and unsuitable for Black skin. You just have to select the right one, at the right strength, and use it appropriately for your skin type. Sadly, most problems that arise with glycolic acid are down to user error.

'Mandelic acid is better than glycolic acid for Black skin'

False. Both are equally suitable for Black skin. Glycolic acid is excellent for exfoliation and mandelic acid is great for oil control.

'Black skin should avoid chemical sunscreens because they cause hyperpigmentation'

No truth in this. Sometimes, like any product, some ingredients in chemical sunscreens may not agree with you and can result in a rash-like reaction that may cause temporary hyperpigmentation. It's simply a case of trying another sunscreen.

'Black soap dries up acne and oily skin'

Not at all, black soap actually dehydrates the skin and strips it of oil, especially on the face. This forces the oil glands to produce more oil to compensate, and in the long run this creates more acne.

black skin

a history

'I'm Black and I'm proud!' The Identity Fightback

The thirty years between 1960 and 1990 were tumultuous, with world-wide social, political and economic changes. The Black experience was characterised by the identity clawback and an attempt to embrace African roots. The air was thick with protest, revolution and change.

The American Civil Rights Movement was in full swing and having a considerable impact on the perception of Blackness. The Sixties were passionate and centuries of pent-up Black frustration and rage flowed, galvanised by leaders such as Martin Luther King, Malcolm X, the Black Panthers and Angela Davis. Black music was in its heyday, led by the Motown record label and The Supremes, Marvin Gaye and Jimi Hendrix. Black sports stars such as Muhammad Ali, Wilma Rudolph and Arthur Ashe were winning despite the odds. Significant strides were being made in the modelling and fashion world too: Naomi Sims became the first Black supermodel after many years of being turned down by agencies saying she was too dark, and Donyale Luna was the first Black woman to be on the cover of *Vogue* magazine, 74 years after its launch in 1892. Diahann Carroll had her own television sitcom. In the UK, celebrities such as Shirley Bassey and the publisher Margaret Busby were influential for their brains and their beauty. Black people, Blackness and, by extension, Black beauty was arriving in a big way.

In 1965 Flori Roberts launched the first range of cosmetics and make-up specifically for Black women, and it was the first brand that was sold in major department stores for women of colour. This was a major turning point that said to Black women: 'You matter and deserve the same treatment that white women have been afforded for five hundred years on the basis of their skin colour.'

Tennis - Wimbledon Championships - Men's Singles - Semi Final - Rod Laver v Arthur Ash © Alamy

SUPREMES Promotional photo of American pop trio about 1965. From left: Diana Ross, Mary Wilson, Florence Ballard © Alamy

Angela Davis speaking at a rally against the death penalty outside the state capitol building in Raleigh, North Carolina, 4 July 1974. © Alamy

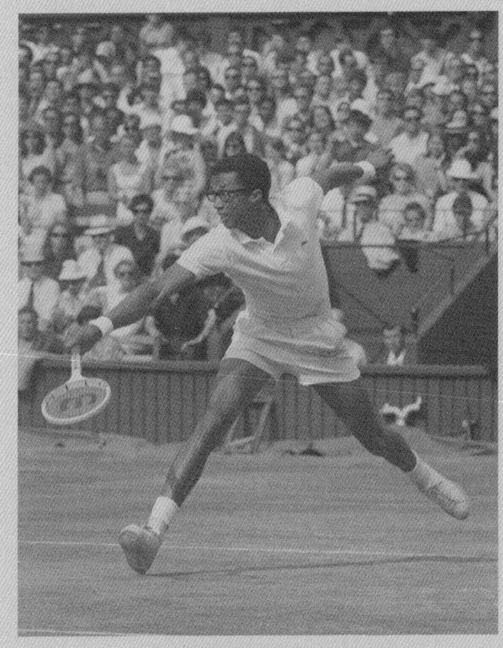

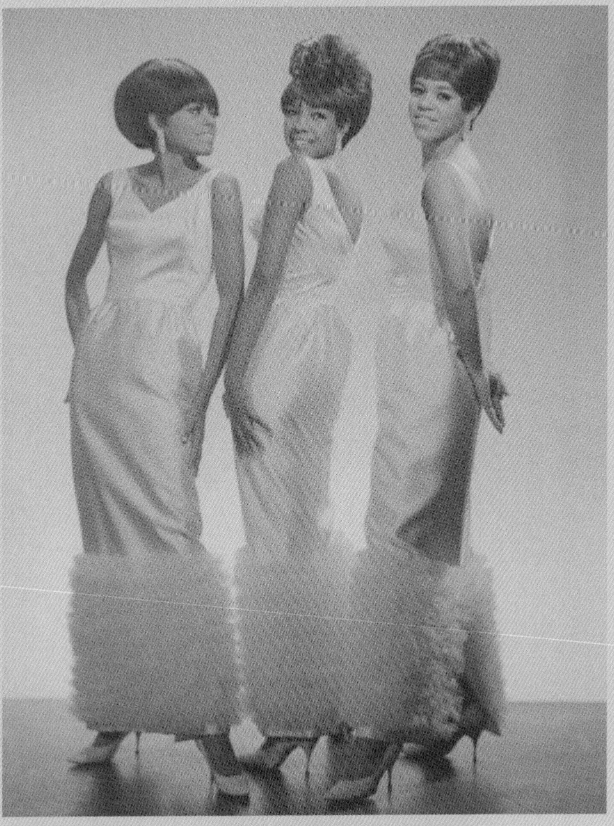

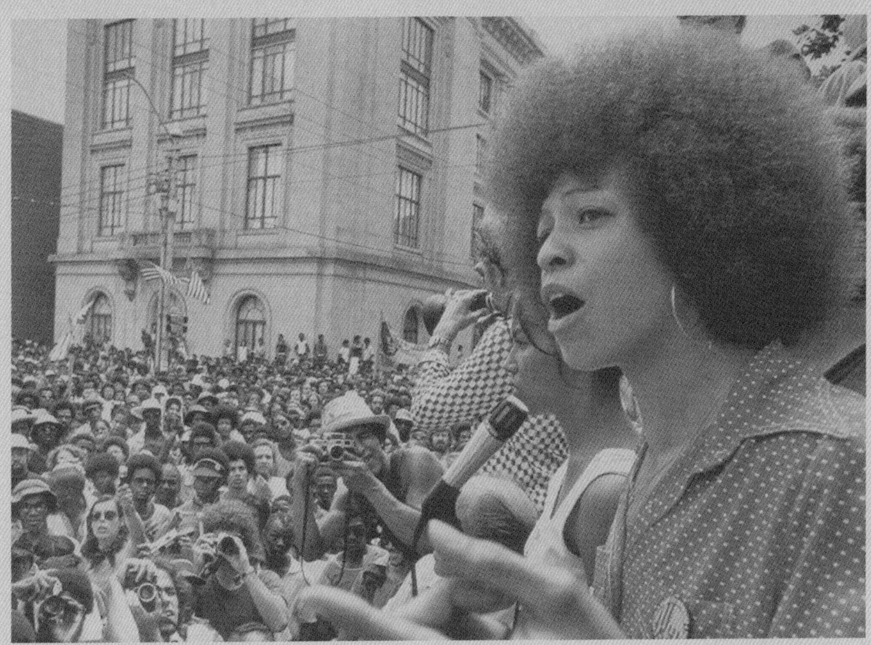

Radical Black Beauty

> 'Our noses are broad, our lips are thick, our hair is nappy – we are black and beautiful!'
>
> Stokely Carmichael, Civil Rights activist

The Civil Rights movement sparked and inspired Black people to make physical changes to their appearance and embrace their Blackness. Malcolm X and Stokely Carmichael were the most outspoken about Black beauty. Malcolm X, though quite forceful in his views, wanted Black people to row back from the self-hate and loathing that had been instilled during slavery, and he centred Black women in his speeches.

The Blank Panthers declared Black power and ownership of Black beauty meant radical self-love and respect; and even music and pop culture rallied Black people to love themselves. James Brown asked folk to say it loud, 'I'm Black and I'm proud!' Jazz singer Nancy Wilson crooned 'Black is Beautiful', and that phrase went on to become a national slogan that birthed an entire movement based around Black pride and celebrating Blackness. It was empowering and the beginning of the end of descriptions such as 'Negro' and 'coloured', which held so much shame and pain for Black people. In 1964, heavyweight boxer Muhammad Ali, who fought as hard in the ring as outside it for Black equality and for Black beauty, proudly declared: 'I'm so pretty; I can't hardly stand to look at myself!' In the early 70s, actress Pam Grier playing Foxy Brown (in the movie of the same name) hailed Black skin with the iconic phrase, 'The blacker the berry, the sweeter the juice.' These were pivotal rejections of the white standards of beauty.

During this same time, Africa was cutting ties with the colonial powers. Between 1960 and 1970, 34 African nations achieved independence, and there was an influx of African scholars to both America and the United Kingdom who were proudly African on arrival. The story goes that because the new arrivals didn't have the burden or shame of slavery in their psyche, they flaunted their Blackness and beauty in their dashikis and Afros without a second thought.

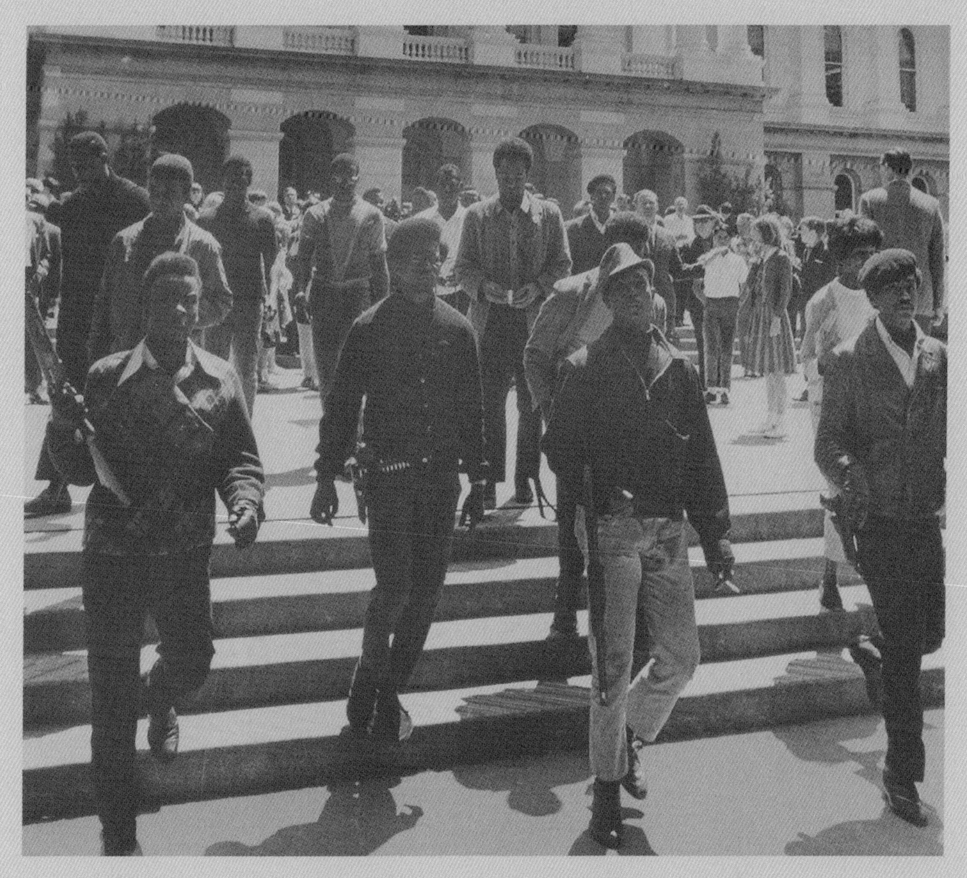

Black Panthers on the steps of the California state capitol, protesting a bill banning the carrying of loaded firearms, 2 May 1967. © Alamy

> 'Who taught you to hate the texture of your hair? Who taught you to hate the color of your skin? To such extent you bleach, to get like the white man. Who taught you to hate the shape of your nose and the shape of your lips? Who taught you to hate yourself from the top of your head to the soles of your feet?'
>
> Malcolm X 'Who Taught You to Hate Yourself' speech, 5 May 1962

My mother arrived on UK shores from Sierra Leone in 1965, and as a young woman in her early 20s living in Bristol, she found honouring and celebrating her beauty challenging. Beyond using Avon for make-up and Astral as a body moisturiser, her options were not only limited but involved going out of her way from Clifton to St. Pauls to buy beauty supplies from the Jamaican stores or asking relatives coming from back home for replenishments.

In 1966, when model Pat Evans shaved her head in protest at her agency demanding she straighten her hair she became even more in demand. Even *Ebony* magazine, which once championed a look that glorified proximity to whiteness, changed its editorial direction in 1968; there was a marked increase in showcasing very dark-skinned Black women, with natural Afro hair. This Black pride movement went on to birth *Essence* magazine in early 1970, to meet the beauty and lifestyle needs of the modern Black American woman. The first cover was a close-up of model Barbara Cheeseborough in a full-bodied Afro.

The 'Jim Crow' laws were finally dismantled in 1968, the same year that Beverly Johnson became a *Vogue* cover girl. This was the decade in which Black women (and men) really shook off the shackles and shame of slavery to freely proclaim the beauty and richness of natural Black skin, to make personal choices about how they cared for their skin (thanks to the provision of more cosmetics and make-up) and how they wore their hair. More importantly, there was a palpable rise in the ideological value that Black women attached to their beauty and how they demanded to be seen and treated by white people.

> Iconic phrases such as 'the blacker the berry, the sweeter the juice' were pivotal rejections of the white standards of beauty.

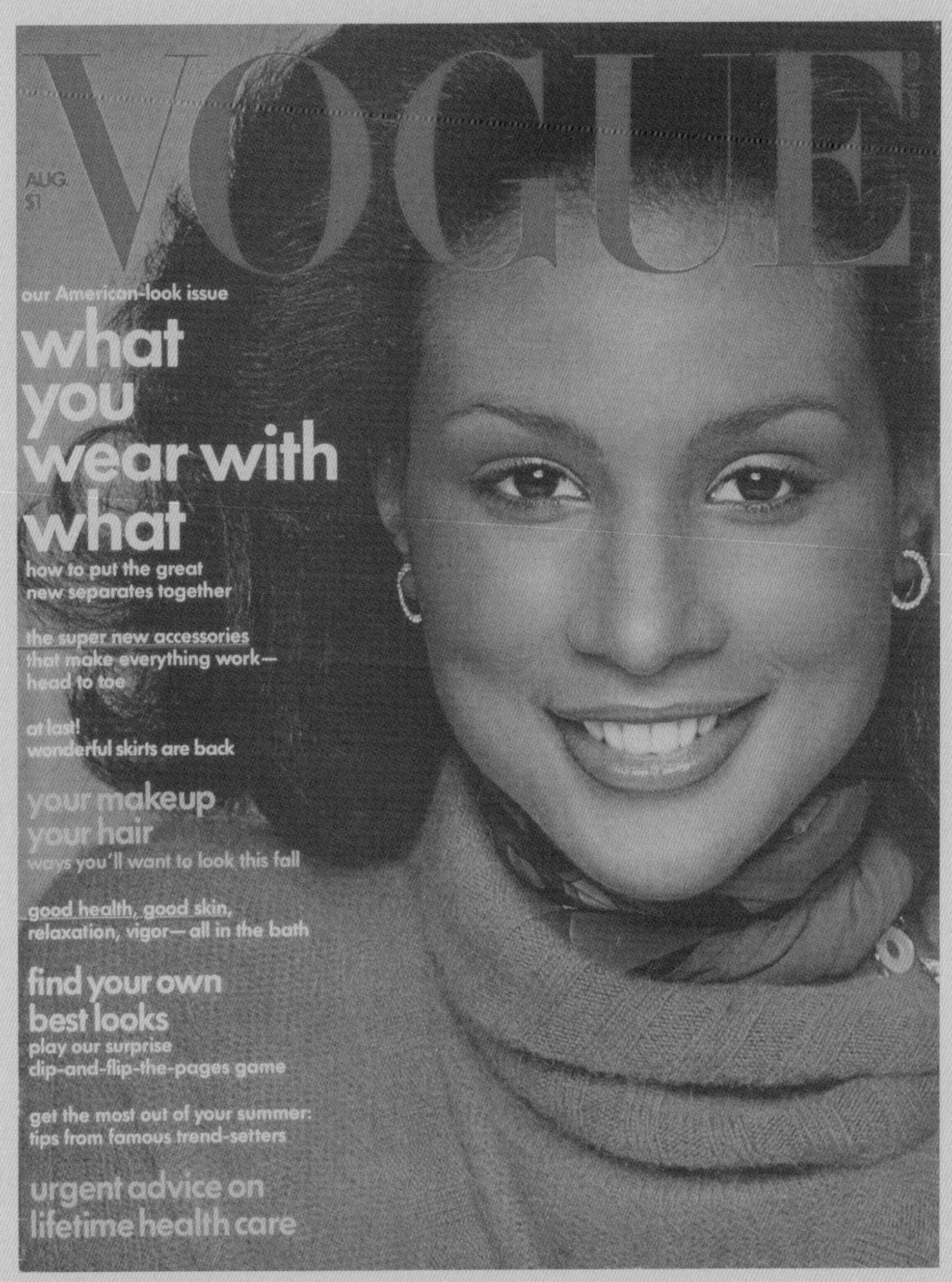

Photographed by Francesco Scavullo, *Vogue*, August 1974. Reprint from August 1974: The cover of American *Vogue* with model Beverly Johnson. ©Alamy

Just Not Beautiful Enough

In the years between 1970 and 2000 the 'Black is beautiful' message still existed, though it was less forceful and pervasive. Things would never go back to the way they were during the height of the Black power movement, but the undercurrent of white beauty standards was still present.

The beauty provision and options for Black women, though still basic in many respects, had improved. Make-up artists, however, still complained of having to mix foundations for Black women, something they didn't have to do for white models. Skin bleaching had morphed into 'skin lightening' and was now rampant in Africa in a way that was akin to the situation in America after the abolition of slavery.

In South Africa, for example, there was a marked increase in the use of skin-lightening products as citizens chased 'the American dream'. Skin-bleaching products were dangerous and still contained high levels of mercury, but Black Africans were very much sold on the idea that to gain the economic success promised by the American dream you had to be as close to white-skinned as possible.

In 1975, the *British Journal of Dermatology* described the problems associated with skin bleaching, which subsequently led to the control of component ingredients such as hydroquinone. In 2011, the World Health Organization (WHO) reported that Nigeria was the bleaching epicentre of Africa, with 77 per cent of women engaging in the practice. There are crude cottage industries where skin-bleaching products with names such as 'European Ultra Whitening' and 'Super Lightening' are mixed with high levels of hydroquinone, steroids, glutathione, mercury and acids.

Financial independence drove the acceptance of Black beauty; with Black women having more money to spend, consumer brands courted more Black models. Revlon was one of the first mainstream brands to start developing products for Black women. In another first, Somalian model Iman secured a $150,000 cosmetics licensing deal (still significantly less than that of white models); however, she was constantly asked to validate her ethnicity as people could not believe she was all Black or African. The idea being that for a Black woman to be that beautiful, she had to have some white ancestry in there. Black on its own just wasn't good enough.

Cinema also played its role. Bond girls were heralded as the epitome of beauty and brains, so Trina Parks playing the first Black Bond girl in *Diamonds Are Forever* in 1971 was another step towards beauty equality and the levelling up of skin colour. That said, in the entire franchise of 27 Bond movies, there have only ever been 4 Black Bond girls.

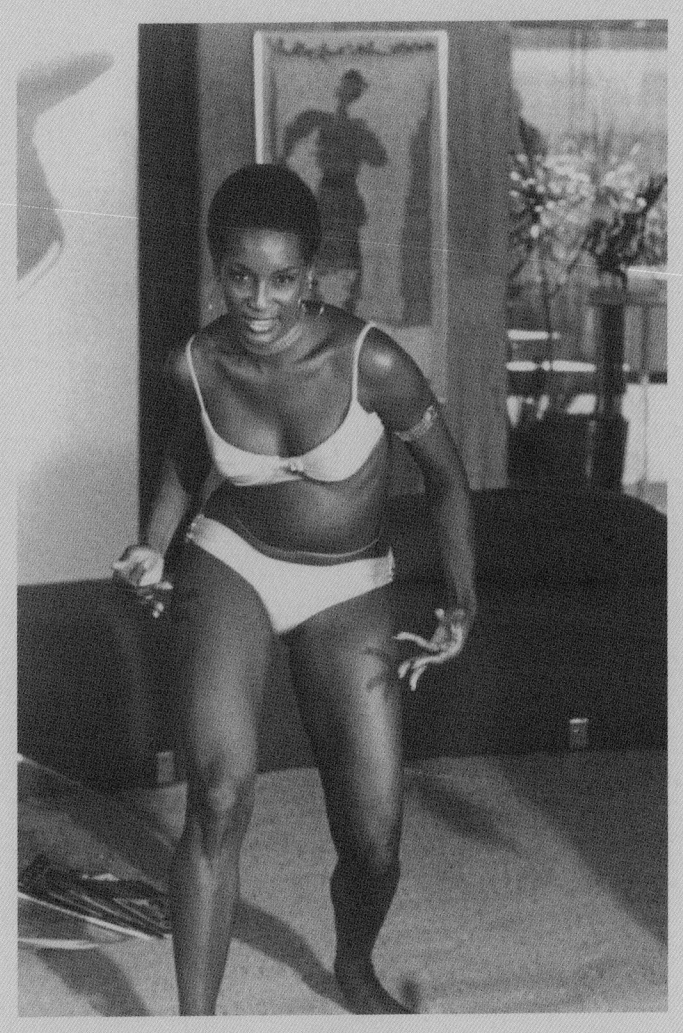

Diamonds Are Forever, Trina Parks, (as Thumper), 1971.
© Alamy

Another noteworthy year was 1984, when Vanessa Williams was crowned Miss America – the first Black contestant to win since the contest started in 1921. For the first 29 years of the pageant Black women were categorically barred from competing as all competitors had to be 'of the white race'. In 1985, Black supermodel Naomi Sims introduced her own skincare and cosmetics line for women of colour, providing more shades and make-up options for Black women. Overtly African features were still derided, though. There was such a thing as being too Black, or too African-looking, whilst white women with some hint of Blackness were celebrated: collagen lip fillers were taking on a new role to give white women fuller lips, whilst Black women were using the popular trick of using skin-colour lip liner to minimise the fullness of their lips.

Clearly, whilst doors were opening, there was a ceiling to the acceptability of Blackness, and it seems the Black aesthetic wasn't permitted to exist freely if white people could not capitalise on it. Being Black now took on a different financial value.

Revlon was one of the first mainstream brands to develop products for Black women.

The Commoditisation of Blackness

By the mid-1980s, society went from 'Black is beautiful' – a narrative owned by Black people – to 'Black is cool' – a narrative owned by conglomerates to sell products to the new Black Urban Professionals (Buppies) who had more money than Black people had ever had before.

Benetton launched the 'All Colours of the World' campaign using models from all ethnic backgrounds. Whilst it was impressive, the profits due to their capitalisation on Blackness were just as noteworthy. The coolest man in music, Michael Jackson, together with his brothers joined forces with Pepsi in a 10-year deal to bring the product to a whole new Black and ethnic audience and put rival Coca-Cola in the shade. And there was a marked increase in Black women signing endorsements, from RuPaul, Mary J. Blige, Lil' Kim, Veronica Webb, Tyra Banks, Brandy, Vanessa Williams and Halle Berry to Naomi Campbell and Alek Wek. This showed the marketability of Black beauty.

Beauty companies woke up to this Black financial power, and companies such as Estée Lauder that had previously left Black women out of the narrative, thanks to their impressions of what we could afford, started extending their ranges to include provisions for Black skin. Inclusivity was the *in* thing, and the early 1990s saw the market opening up for Black women. It is key to note that the new products were not separated but rather positioned within existing lines. Acceptance of global beauty standards meant the industry adopted a broader world view, to create multiracial products rather than products for completely separate market segments.

Beauty companies woke up to Black financial power.

The Fight for True Inclusion

Black people in the Western world have lived in a state of 'other' since slavery. Aptly described by sociologist W. E. B. Du Bois as 'double consciousness', where we look at ourselves through the lens of both African Blackness and a racist whiteness, we try to reconcile the two into one identity. For a long time, being Black was on par with being worthless, and Black people have had to fight (and die!) for equality. Black people have been defined not by who we are, our capabilities, dreams and aspirations, but by who we could never be.

Because of the strides society has made, double consciousness isn't front and centre of our daily experience today, but it is always lurking in the background and, in some instances, it is inescapable. And nowhere more so than in the beauty industry, which, by default, has to take skin colour into consideration if it is to meet the needs of the consumers.

As Black economic power has increased, society has sought to rebalance itself through diversity and inclusivity initiatives. A big part of my work is about ensuring the skincare and beauty industry meets the diverse needs of Black people. We have been talking and doing diversity in one form or the other since the 1960s but being *wholly* included has eluded us. It is my sincere desire that this book will add to the body of work pushing visibility for Black women, but that it will also arm white allies with the historical knowledge that strengthens our allyship. Initiatives such as Black Lives Matter (BLM) and Pull Up For Change are just as important now as the Civil Rights movement and anti-discrimination laws were important in the past. BLM provides a means by which anti-racism education can be delivered.

Brands have done well providing for diversity but true inclusion hasn't always happened. To be included means to be accepted as you are, made to feel welcome and unburdened. The beauty industry fails to be inclusive when clinical and consumer trials don't include Black people, when there are no senior Black team members, when provision for Black consumers is provided after the main product launch, when advertising and articles are a reflection of whiteness with no nuance for a non-white audience, when Black women are expected to be grateful for inclusion, and when companies employ the colour-blind theory, which ignores the way historic racism impacted and still continues to impact our experience, participation and enjoyment of the beauty industry.

Black people need their skin colour to be acknowledged as equal, not swept under the carpet like something that doesn't matter. To sweep it under the carpet is to deny us our identity and to say it is inconsequential. After centuries of being attacked and killed for being Black, to being told that Black skin is less than and not good enough, this lack of acknowledgement has real practical consequences.

It means the beauty industry then fails to consider and provide for the unique needs of Black skin. It means that education providers churn out therapists who don't know the fundamental differences between Black and white skin. It means therapists who are apprehensive of treating Black skin – thereby reinforcing 'otherness' and restricting access of service to Black people and restricting them from participating in the act of beautification. It means establishments that turn away Black women saying, 'We don't treat Black skin.' It means brands failing to take into account that their foundation shade ranges need extending to the deepest ebony, or that Black women may prefer products that tackle issues of hyperpigmentation.

In order to truly honour diversity and inclusivity, obvious differences need to be positively highlighted so that the needs of varied consumer groups are met.

Arise, Black entrepreneurs! Rihanna made history when she successfully launched Fenty Beauty in 2017 with 40 foundation shades – the highest number of shades ever – indicating to the industry that they had been sleeping on Black skin. With heritage brands stumbling to provide skincare and beauty options for Black women, Black entrepreneurs have always risen to the challenge. From Iman Cosmetics to Beverley Knight, Black Up, Emolyne, The Lip Bar, Uoma Beauty, Pat McGrath, MDMflow, Candour Beauty, 4.5.6 Skin, Melé Skincare and Rejuva Skin, this has been the drive of inclusivity and a way of showing heritage brands that Black women have money and are deserving of the same provision and luxury afforded to white women.

Reclaim Black Beauty

I am not surprised that so many myths and misconceptions exist about skincare, ingredients and products and how they interact with and affect Black skin. For the longest time the beauty industry didn't engage with Black women, and when they did, it came from a place that capitalised on selling inadequacy, marginalisation and misinformation that encouraged Black women to cling to ideals of beauty that aren't physiologically Black: the desire for a straight nose, lighter skin and straighter hair, or remain on the outside of what and who was considered beautiful.

Black people need their skin colour to be acknowledged as equal.

As we move forward with purpose, vigilance and a celebration of Blackness, I want every Black woman to feel seen and know that her worth and beauty is valued and will always be universally valid.

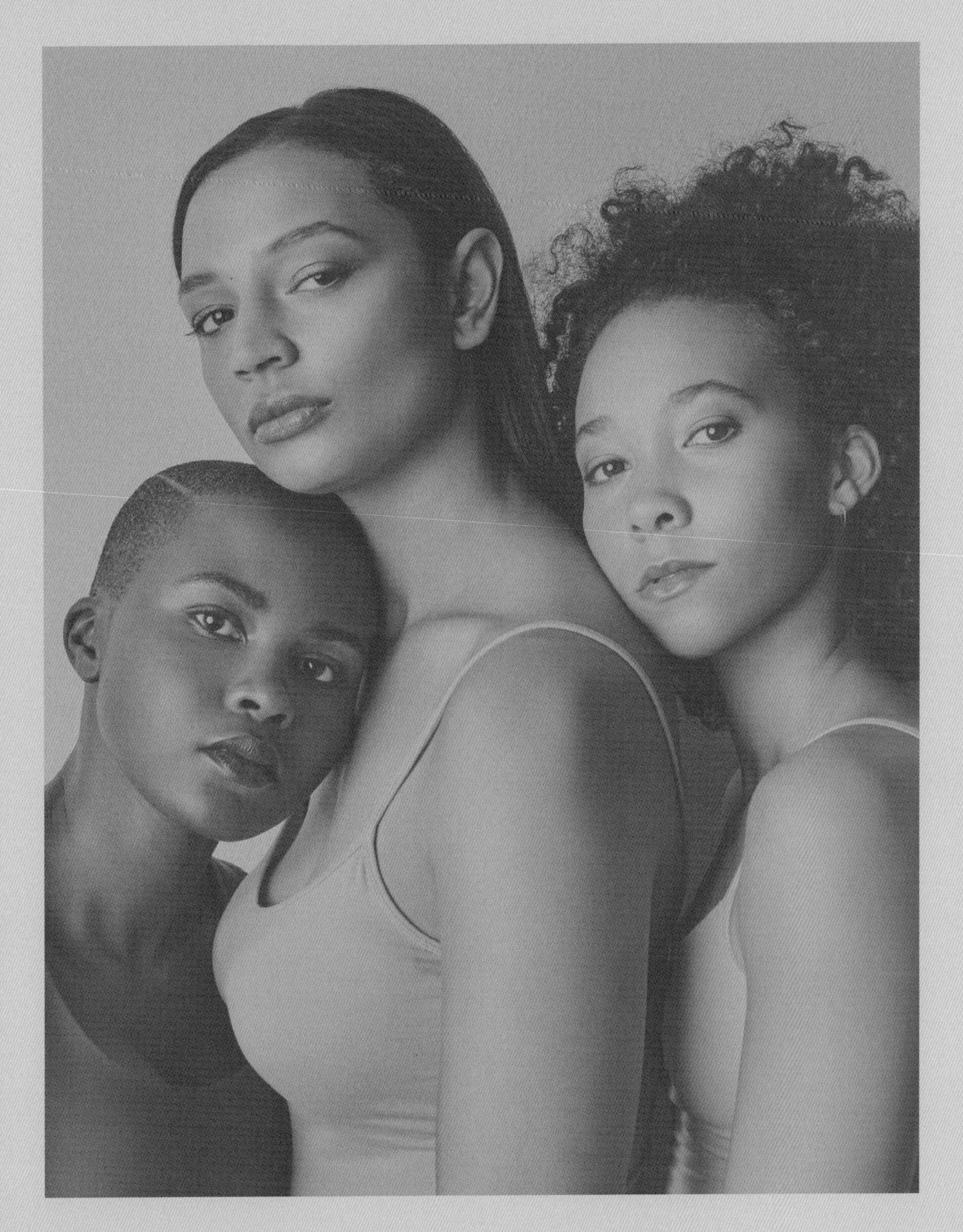

part three

finding your skin regimen

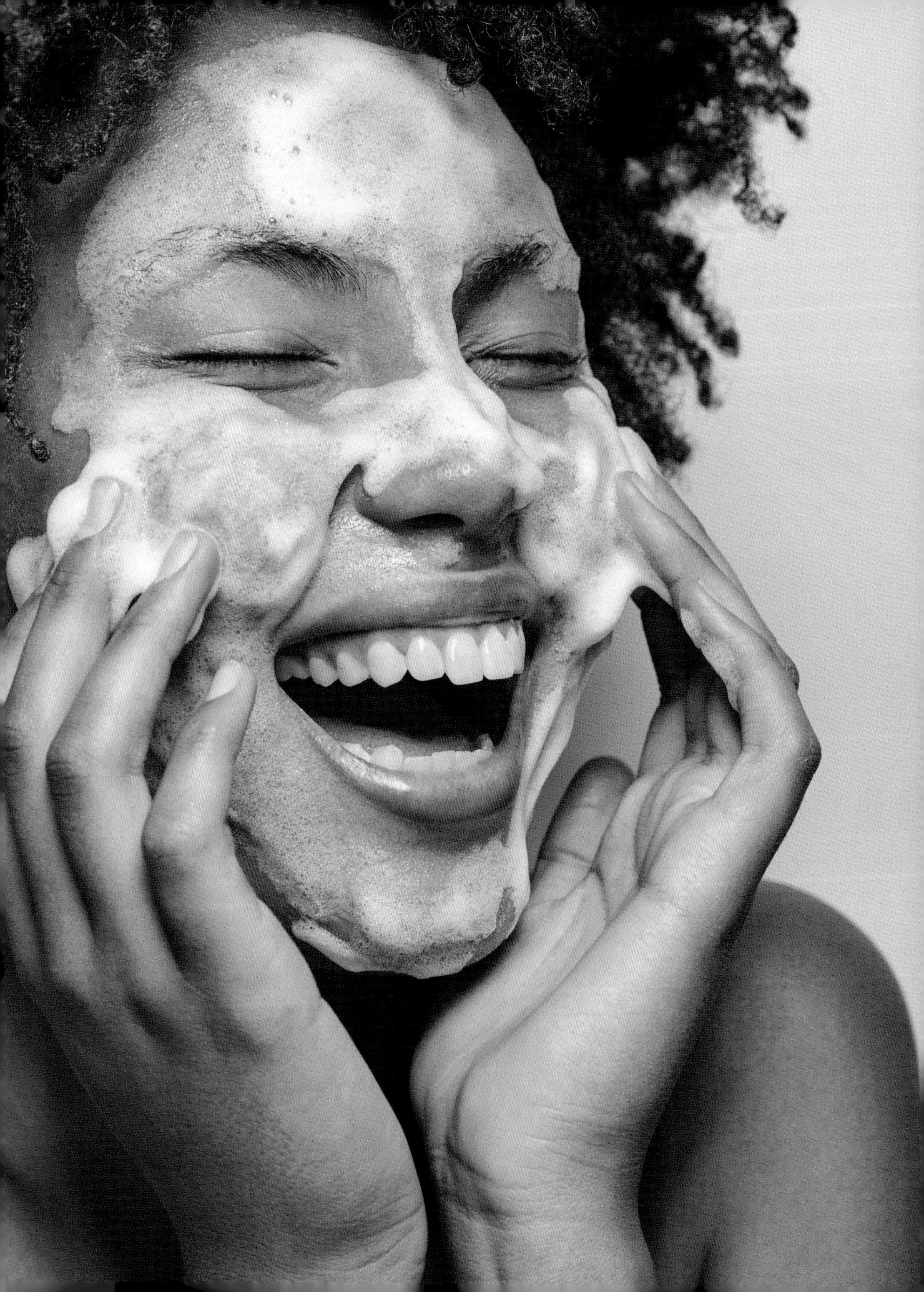

11.

key skincare ingredients

key skincare ingredients

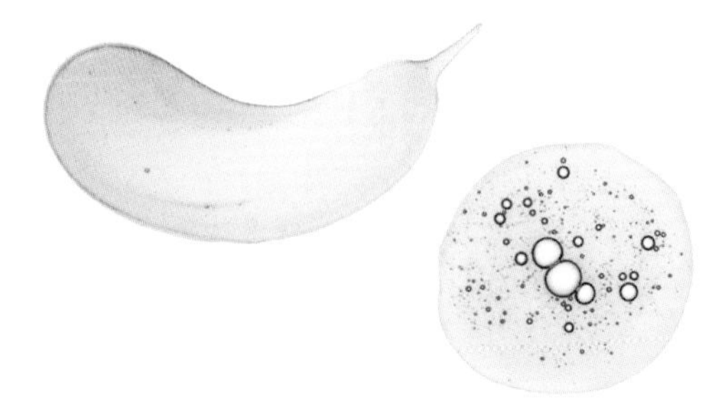

WE are blessed with so many amazing skincare ingredients and every year there are new ingredients being released. So much so, I could easily dedicate a tome to skincare ingredients alone, but that's for another lifetime. For now, I'm going to focus on classic ingredients and, even though some may be old school and not very sexy, I know they deliver great results. In any case they are the common ingredients you'll find in most products, so it makes sense to focus on them.

Pick up any product in your bathroom and look at the ingredients on the back; you're likely to be met with a list ranging from 4 or 5 items to 15 or even 20. It can be mind boggling: just how do you know what all these ingredients do and the role they play in the overall formula of your product? Given the number of ingredients that can go into any one product, I find we are increasingly more concerned and curious about what we are putting on our skin, and how we can use certain ingredients more effectively in our skincare routines.

With Black women, I find the questions to be more around whether an ingredient is safe for Black skin, or whether it has been tested on Black skin. These sorts of questions tell me that Black women are engaged and interested in discovering more about their products but there is a disconnect in the way ingredient information from brands is shared and advertised. There's a lot of apprehension and needless worry about some ingredients, driven by misinformation and scaremongering, so I hope this chapter helps to alleviate and solve some of these worries.

vitamin a, aka retinoids

The head honcho of all ingredients and one that seems to scare a lot of Black women, causing copious amounts of anxiety. The fear tends to come from various sources, from friends and family who've had poor experiences to Dr Google, always presenting worst-case scenarios. Of course, this is off-putting for anyone and the cautious thing to do is to avoid retinoids, but in reality it isn't necessary. They are not only safe but also beneficial for darker skin tones, delivering excellent results, especially for issues such as acne and hyperpigmentation.

Retinoids are a group of certified gold-standard ingredients that have been around since the 1970s. They are the workhorses of skincare and countless studies have proved their anti-ageing capabilities. They stimulate collagen so your skin is firmer and bouncier, minimise the appearance of fine lines and wrinkles, fade pigmentation for a more even skin tone, increase exfoliation for smoother skin, boost the skin's own natural moisture levels, and upgrade your natural glow. Retinoids are really *the* business.

FACT You might be familiar with the term retinol. Like Hoover became the accepted name for a vacuum cleaner despite being only one brand amongst many, retinol has become the accepted name for vitamin A despite it being only one type of vitamin A amongst many.

The confusion also tends to happen because there are so many different types of retinoids. I can give you a list as long as my arm, but it's easier if you just remember that, like human families, retinoids also have many different members that can perform different roles. Some retinoids are available only with a doctor's prescription and some can be purchased with just a few clicks of your mouse.

For retinoids to be useful, they've got to be in their most basic form: retinoic acid. This is the only way they can interact with your skin. Prescription retinoids like Tretinoin and Isotretinoin (sometimes referred to simply as Tret) are already retinoic acids and they come in various strengths, ranging from 0.025 per cent to 1 per cent, making them very powerful as soon as you apply them to your skin. The downside is that this immediate potency is more likely to irritate your skin, causing stinging, burning, flushing, redness, dryness, scaling and flaky skin. This is why they are prescription only, because they need medical supervision to be used effectively to manage conditions like severe acne.

FACT Retinaldehyde is also able to directly tackle bacteria, making it popular for breakout and acne-prone skin.

On the other hand, over-the-counter (OTC) retinoids, such as retinol and retinaldehyde, need to be converted by your skin cells into retinoic acid before they can be useful to your skin. Although their path to usefulness is slightly longer, the upside is that they are less likely to irritate your skin.

There's also retinyl esters, such as retinyl palmitate and retinyl acetate, which are not particularly effective on their own, so if you want real results for your skin don't waste your time or cash on any product that makes these their star ingredients. Instead make a beeline for retinol or retinaldehyde and you're sure to get more bang for your buck.

However, not all esters are made equally. These are a class of pseudo-retinoids that are worth knowing about:

Granactive retinoid The oil-based new kid on the block also known as hydroxypinacolone retinoate, which can get to work quickly without needing any conversion. The Ordinary, Skin Rocks, Garden of Wisdom and Sunday Riley use this version.

Ethyl lactyl retinoate An exciting combination of lactic acid and retinol for supercharged exfoliation. SkinBetter Science have an entire and very successful range based on this formula.

Retinyl retinoate The non-irritating offspring of an interesting marriage between the stronger retinoic acid and retinol. Medik8 have also successfully used it in their Retinoate range.

Whether your retinoid is prescription or OTC, I can't emphasise enough the need to start small and slowly build up your use over a number of weeks. Start by using twice a week, leaving a few days between applications. I normally opt for a Wednesday and Sunday. This is when you also need to appreciate what a pea-sized amount really means. You really only need a little bit, trust me.

Retinoids are best used at night and even though I prefer them to go straight on to clean skin after cleansing, you can apply a light moisturiser before and/or after your retinoid. This is known as buffering and can help to reduce irritation. Once your skin is comfortable, you want to cut out this step though. Your skin will be more sensitive to the sun, so this no time to be stingy with the sunscreen. Slather it on, and during the warmer months a front-facing cap or hat is always handy to shield your face from the sun.

Pay attention to your application technique as well; dotting your retinoid around your face can help even distribution, which is important to prevent hot spots. The skin around the eyes, lips, neck and décolleté is much thinner, so do them last.

FACT When your skin is acclimatising to your retinoid you may experience a little sensitivity, soreness and dryness, which is called retinisation. It soon passes, but you can avoid it by taking your time to build up your retinoid use.

Look for retinoids that are stored in opaque, airless packaging rather than in clear glass and/or with pipette droppers. They can be quite sensitive to light and air, which degrade their effectiveness.

It's not uncommon for me to get at least one message a week from a client cursing their retinoid and vowing to throw the whole thing in the bin because they've experienced retinisation. You have to remember, the journey to skin health is a marathon, not a sprint.

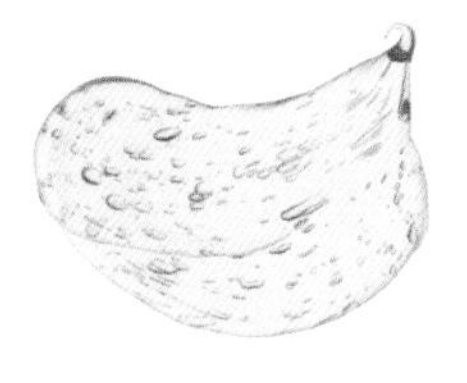

The ageing process starts setting in from your mid-20s, so that's a good time to start using a retinoid twice a week, ramping up your use over time once your skin settles. Funnily enough, the older you are the quicker you see results with vitamin A. Over 30s will start to see some results in 4–6 weeks. Don't try to speed things up by over-applying: you will undoubtedly cause yourself retinisation and that is no fun!

niacinamide

Niacinamide is part of the complex of B vitamins and is good for maintaining a healthy and strong skin barrier by helping the skin to retain water. For Black skin especially, niacinamide is also a brightening and skin-softening ingredient with powers to help curb hyperpigmentation. Definitely welcome it with open arms!

vitamin c, aka l-ascorbic acid

Vitamin C is a mix between class boffin and most popular student, functioning as an antioxidant to protect the skin against environmental damage such as pollution and UV rays from the sun, stimulating collagen to keep the skin in shape, helping to brighten ashy skin, and fading discolouration.

Many Black women make the mistake of thinking vitamin C alone can clear up dark marks. Sadly, it can't, because its primary function is that of an antioxidant to prevent premature ageing. Any skin clarity benefits are a secondary effect. The cynic in me says because most vitamin C products are advertised using yellow and orange colours, it tricks the brain into associating it with brightening and clarity.

FACT 'Lipophilic' refers to substances that like and are able to dissolve in oil and fats. They are also great at water-proofing your skin.

Like retinoids, vitamin C also stirs up a lot of nervousness, but it is a very safe ingredient to use in concentrations up to 20 per cent – anything more irritates the skin. Likewise, it can safely be used in conjunction with your retinoid and other antioxidants: include vitamin C in your morning skincare routine and vitamin A in your night-time routine.

It is well known that vitamin C can go off very quickly when exposed to sunlight and air, so select one that is in a dark bottle with a pump. Better yet, more and more brands (such as Beauty Pie and No. 7) are bringing out single-use capsules, which I think is a leap forward that will save you binning half-used products.

Apart from l-ascorbic acid, vitamin C also goes by other names including ascorbyl palmitate, magnesium ascorbyl palmitate and magnesium ascorbyl phosphate. Let's just say these are watered-down versions that work at a slower pace. The trick is to look out for anything that starts with 'ascorb' on the ingredients list.

(hydroxy) acids

Alpha hydroxy acids, beta hydroxy acids and poly hydroxy acids are, hands down, some of the most hardworking ingredients in any skin health regime. Acids are like henchmen and mercenaries that come from fruits, plants and milk sugars. They don't sound pleasant but they make shit happen, and that's all we're interested in really; they can whip your skin into shape before you can say Jack Robinson.

Their main role is to exfoliate by breaking the glue that keeps old skin cells attached to the skin. In doing so, the skin is prompted to produce newer and fresher skin cells that are smoother and clearer.

Before I go further, it's important to clarify a point: skincare acids of any description are suitable for Black skin. There's a lot of drivel and unfounded claims circulating on the internet, and the best thing you can do is to ignore the noise and listen to your skincare pro! It's all about choosing the right acid and using it in the right way for your particular concern.

You may have to experiment with acids a little bit to find your sweet spot when it comes to exfoliation, because there is such a thing as over-exfoliation that can really damage your skin. If you're also using active ingredients like retinoids, remember that they too are also exfoliating the skin, so your skincare routine should be properly organised.

My approach to acids is to use a little every day and I mainly prefer them in wash-off products like cleansers. What doesn't come off today will come off tomorrow. No stress! Using an acid like a sledgehammer a couple of times a week is a recipe for irritation and hyperpigmentation, so go low and go slow in your use.

Alpha hydroxy acids (AHAs)

These are super common, your star performers and the easiest-available type of acid. This category will include glycolic, lactic, mandelic, citric, malic and tartaric acids. Their function is to exfoliate the skin and stimulate collagen and hyaluronic acid to give the skin volume. They call the top layer of skin to attention, re-arranging the cells into a well-behaved smooth formation, and regulating the rate of cell turnover.

If you're worried about ageing, superficial discolouration or rough texture use *glycolic acid* (my favourite acid). It comes from sugar cane and is famous for being the fastest-acting acid because of its small molecule size.

If your skin is dull, dry and rough, choose *lactic acid*. Not only will it exfoliate gently and smooth your skin, it will also help to hydrate and encourage the skin to hold on to moisture. Lactic acid is a by-product of soured milk but, thank heavens, we now have technology that give us a much more pleasant-smelling synthetic version. A good option if you're nervous about glycolic acid.

Oily and blemish-prone skin types can opt for *mandelic acid*, which is a derivative of bitter almonds. It is a mild lipophilic acid that also exfoliates and reduces the surface oil that makes the skin greasy.

Citric acid is a supportive acid from citrus fruits, used to beef up the popular acids to help tackle signs of sun damage and brighten the skin. I like to call *tartaric* and *malic acid* a fruit cocktail for your skin because their main sources are apples, grapes, pears and cherries. They don't tend to feature in any big skincare starring roles as they are very mild and gentle, but they are good antioxidants.

If for any reason you're dead set against using acids but still want to exfoliate your skin, then consider *enzyme exfoliation*. The main ones in circulation are bromelian, which comes from pineapple, and papain, which comes from papaya. Pumpkin and pomegranate are also quite popular.

Psst...When salicylic acid fails

If salicylic acid doesn't agree with you for any reason, check out benzoyl peroxide instead, which also has an antibacterial action. Start on a low concentration to bypass the usual dryness.

In the same way as acids, they will loosen the bonds that hold old skin cells together at the surface of the skin. They do this at a much slower pace than AHAs and this limits any potential irritation to the skin. It's akin to driving a reliable Fiat as opposed to a super-fast Ferrari. You do eventually arrive, just a little later.

Beta hydroxy acids (BHA)

Salicylic acid ticks all the boxes for blemish-prone, oily, spot- and acne-prone skin. We only use one type of BHA within skincare and it does a fabulous job. Salicylic acid is a very popular ingredient that comes from acetylsalicylic acid or is extracted from the bark of willow trees, so you will sometimes see it mentioned as 'willow bark extract'. It is also lipophilic and a key ingredient in the arsenal for oily/acne-prone skin types, as it can penetrate deep into your pores to help break down the sticky bonds of old skin cells that would otherwise clog the pores, leading to whiteheads and blackheads.

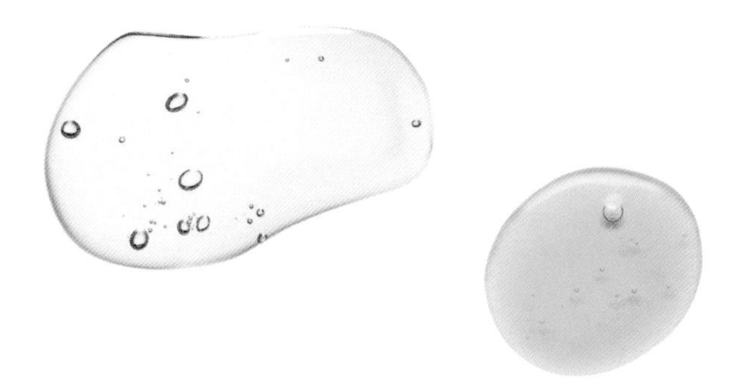

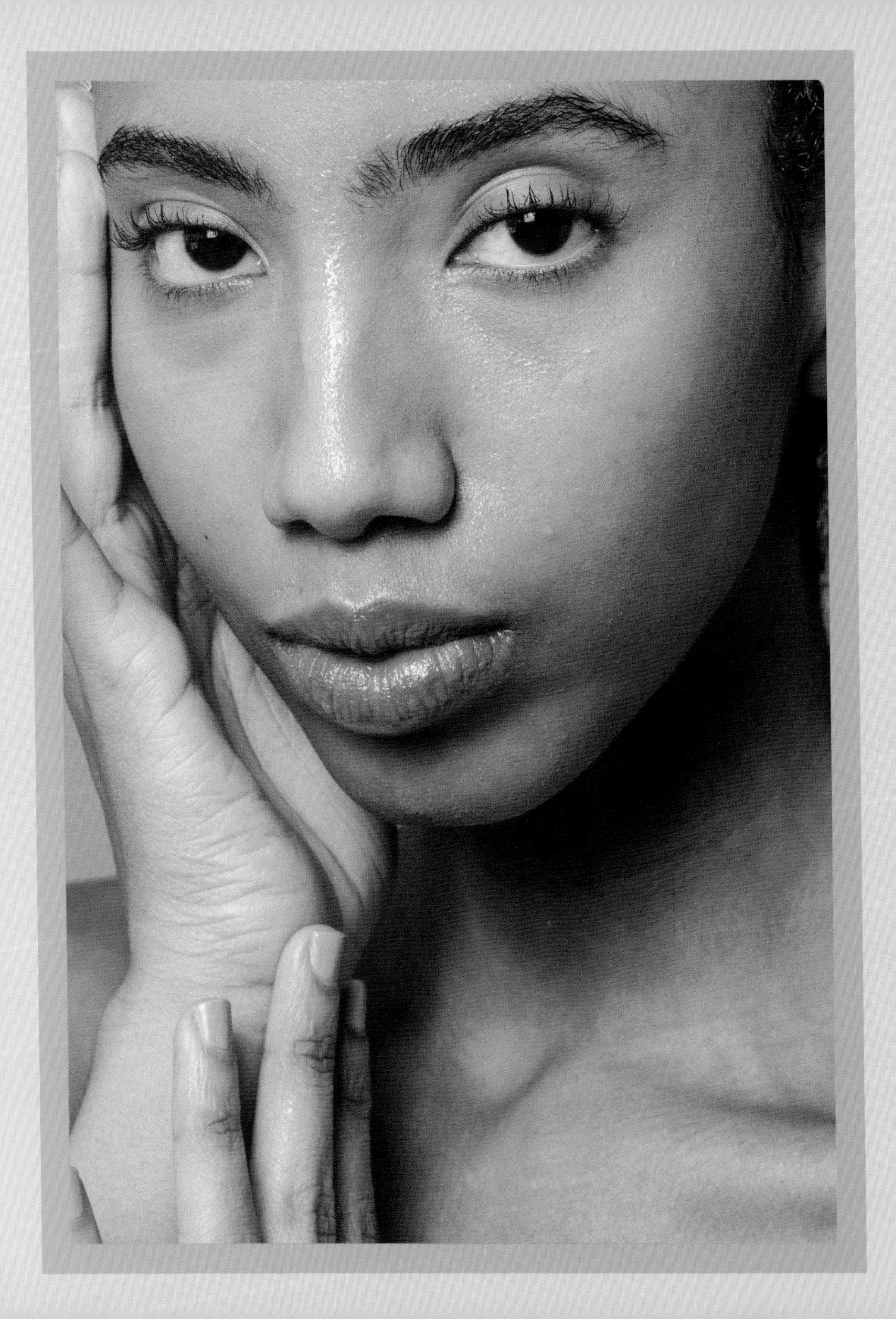

Poly hydroxy acids (PHAs)

Reach for these if your skin is feeling sore/irritated/compromised but you still want some exfoliating acid action. In clinic, I lavish PHAs on the skin after any resurfacing treatments because they help the skin to heal quickly. They are the kindest acids.

PHAs are the newest acids on the block and are known for being extremely gentle because they are full of water, making them hydrating whilst packing a punch, so they are great for supporting sensitive skin and post-treatment skin, and for building up skin strength. Their rate of exfoliation is much slower than other acids, and at first glance they may not seem very powerful. But they are silent multitaskers, supporting and stimulating collagen and hyaluronic acid to minimise lines and wrinkles and protect your skin barrier. I love that PHAs also triple up as humectants and will draw moisture from the air to your skin, which makes them excellent for dry/dehydrated skin conditions like eczema too.

FACT Lactobionic acid is a major part of preservative solutions used to preserve human transplant organs during transfer.

Lactobionic acid comes from milk sugar, and it is a strong antioxidant that's also able to strengthen and deeply moisturise skin. *Maltobionic acid* is similar but is extracted from malt sugar, and is *even more* hydrating and is able to help ease the effects of sun damage. Annoyingly, very few brands have maltobionic acid in the formula because it is hella expensive to use, but it is well worth it in my opinion. *Gluconolactone* is a very effective antioxidant and extremely moisturising. An absolute superstar for sensitive skin, including those with rosacea, and has no irritable elements whatsoever!

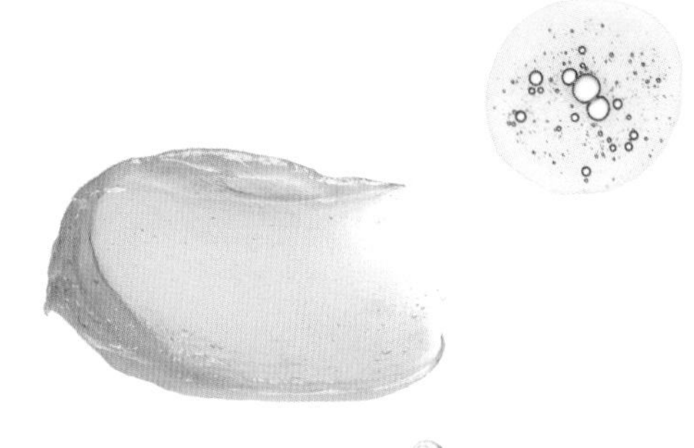

Other acids I think are worth knowing about:

Phenolic acids

Phenolic acids come from plants and have anti-ageing, antioxidant, anti-inflammatory and anti-microbial properties. They reduce DNA damage and encourage effective cell renewal.

Gallic acid is great for treating discolouration and minimising inflammation, so it is handy for acne and breakout-prone skin. *Ellagic acid* is a skin-brightening antioxidant that helps to protect the skin from sun damage. *Azelaic acid* comes from grains such as wheat, barley and rye and is very effective in treating acne because it is antibacterial. It can also be used as a lightening agent for skin to treat hyperpigmentation, and is also prominent in the management of rosacea. *Caffeic* and *ferulic acid* stimulate and regulate skin cell renewal and have anti-acne properties, as well as promoting an even skin tone, making these two all-round good choices for oily skin types.

Hyaluronic acid

Hyaluronic acid is now ubiquitous in skincare and yet I still remember its early days as a topical skincare product. It is a large sugar molecule that is produced naturally in large quantities by the body. Ageing naturally depletes the body's reserves of hyaluronic acid leading to dry skin, wrinkles and loss of shape and volume underneath the skin.

It is a humectant, enabling the skin to retain water and stay hydrated. Unlike all the other acids, hyaluronic acid has no exfoliating qualities. When Black skin is dry and dehydrated, it has a tendency to appear dull and grey, so hyaluronic acid is a great supporting ingredient for radiant-looking skin. It can be applied to the skin in a serum, gel or cream, but bear in mind that not all hyaluronic acid is created equally, so it's important to ensure you select a 'low molecular'-weight hyaluronic acid for optimum beneficial effect.

Hyaluronic acid can also be injected into the skin as a dermal filler to soften lines and wrinkles, tighten skin and encourage improved hydration.

The non-acid you should know about is *N-acetyl-glucosamine* (thankfully called NAG for short!). It's a gentle exfoliator to smooth the skin and brighten and reduce the intensity of dark spots. It's actually a building block of hyaluronic acid, so it also helps to keep the skin hydrated.

tyrosinase inhibitors

A mouthful, I know. But all you need to know is that these are the main ingredients in the skincare world that tackle discolouration. Tyrosinase is one of the main components in melanin production, so if you can reduce or stop it all together, hyperpigmentation can be controlled. This is all you need to appreciate about these wonderful ingredients. That is it, the whole long and short of our science lesson.

For Black women wanting to either maintain or achieve an even complexion, tyrosinase inhibitors is where the magic is at. You will find them doing the most in your pigmentation serums and you must apply straight after cleansing for maximum effect. They are the difference between skin clarity and uneven skin tone, but if you don't know, you don't know. If I could, I would stand at the corner of Oxford Street and hand these out like sweets to every Black woman. I feel they are that important in your skincare.

After retinoids and glycolic acid, the tyrosinase inhibitors listed below are my favourite ingredients because they break down existing hyperpigmentation, reducing the appearance of melanated patches and cleverly supporting your skin to avoid discolouration developing in the first place.

Liquorice extract contains an active ingredient called glabridin and has the ability to treat hyperpigmentation resulting from sun damage and trauma to the skin. It is often seen as a natural skin-brightening alternative to hydroquinone.

Kojic acid comes from several different species of mushrooms that have the ability to limit the production of melanin in the skin. It is often found in skin-brightening products to combat hyperpigmentation, dark marks and scarring.

Transexamic acid is a manufactured version of the protein lysine that is widely used in medicine to prevent excess blood loss. In skincare, some studies have shown that it has beneficial skin-lightening effects, especially with conditions like melasma.

Alpha arburtin is an enhanced biosynthetic form of arbutin, which is naturally derived from bearberry plants. Its main function in skincare is to brighten and even skin tone by interfering with the production of melanin.

Hydroquinone is a high-level, prescription-only skin-lightening ingredient that is used medically to brighten and even the skin tone. Its main function is to control and suppress melanin to lighten darkened patches of skin or to prepare skin for further treatments. Due to its misuse for skin bleaching, this perfectly safe and medically approved ingredient has developed a poor reputation in Black and Asian communities. When used as prescribed with careful monitoring, it is one of the safest ingredients for evening discolouration.

Over-use of hydroquinone can cause exogenous ochronosis, a noticeable condition in which the skin thickens and becomes a patchy blue/purple dark colour. It is not pretty and it's very challenging to treat that sort of discolouration, costing a lot of money and time.

I have seen hydroquinone-laced products being sold under the counter at Afro hair shops. This is not only illegal, but there is no way you can be assured of their safety. Always consult a professional.

Soy is a plant protein that helps to even the skin tone by inhibiting the transfer of melanin pigment from your melanocytes to the surrounding skin cells.

Hexylresorcinol is found in the bran of rye and other cereals and has long been used in the food industry as an anti-browning agent for fresh produce like fruit and shrimps. Makes sense that it should also work in the skincare realm to prevent staining and browning of the skin. Some studies have shown its effects to be comparable to 2 per cent hydroquinone,[18] which is very good.

Cysteamine has its origins in cysteine, which is a natural substance found in our bodies. It is actually an antioxidant that is also able to lighten discoloured skin. I love using it for really stubborn discolouration like melasma and long-term hyperpigmentation, which can be quite distressing. It really does make a difference, not only fading the pigmentation but also improving quality of life and self-esteem. People with a history of vitiligo in their family, or if they are pregnant/breastfeeding, cannot use it though.

Glutathione is actually a peptide comprised of cysteine, glycine and glutamic acid, which is found naturally in the body but decreases with age. It functions as an antioxidant as well as a pigment reducer because it interrupts the enzyme that causes melanin overproduction. This makes it fantastic for targeting hyperpigmentation and dark marks.

Psst… Together is better

Whilst all these ingredients are great, they are better when used together, so look for formulas that contain a clutch of them as that will give the best results. This is because they all attack hyperpigmentation from different angles and using a mix covers all bases.

Other ingredients which also double up as tyrosinaise inhibitors are vitamin C, niacinamide and azelaic acid.

I believe tyrosinase-inhibiting ingredients are a big deal for Black skin, especially in the management of hyperpigmentation and skin discolouration. However, they are not the be all and end all. You can't just slot a tyrosinase-inhibiting serum into your routine and expect to wake up flawless. You have to pay close attention to the rest of your skincare routine, ensuring you are consistent in your approach – especially with the use of sunscreen. Your lifestyle habits will also play a big role in your skin quality, so it pays to have a 360-degree approach and not just rely on one unicorn ingredient, no matter how good I say it is.

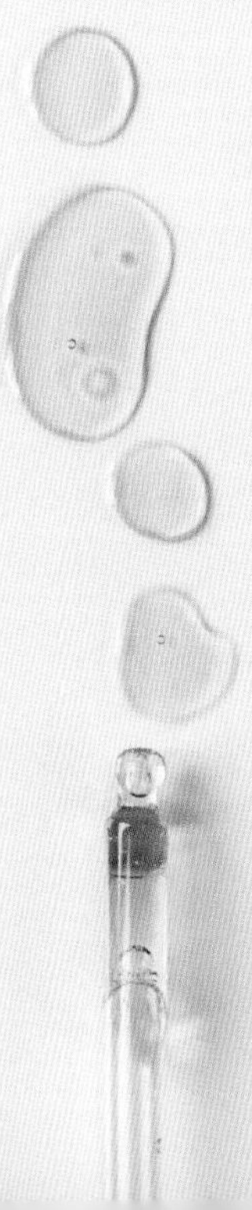

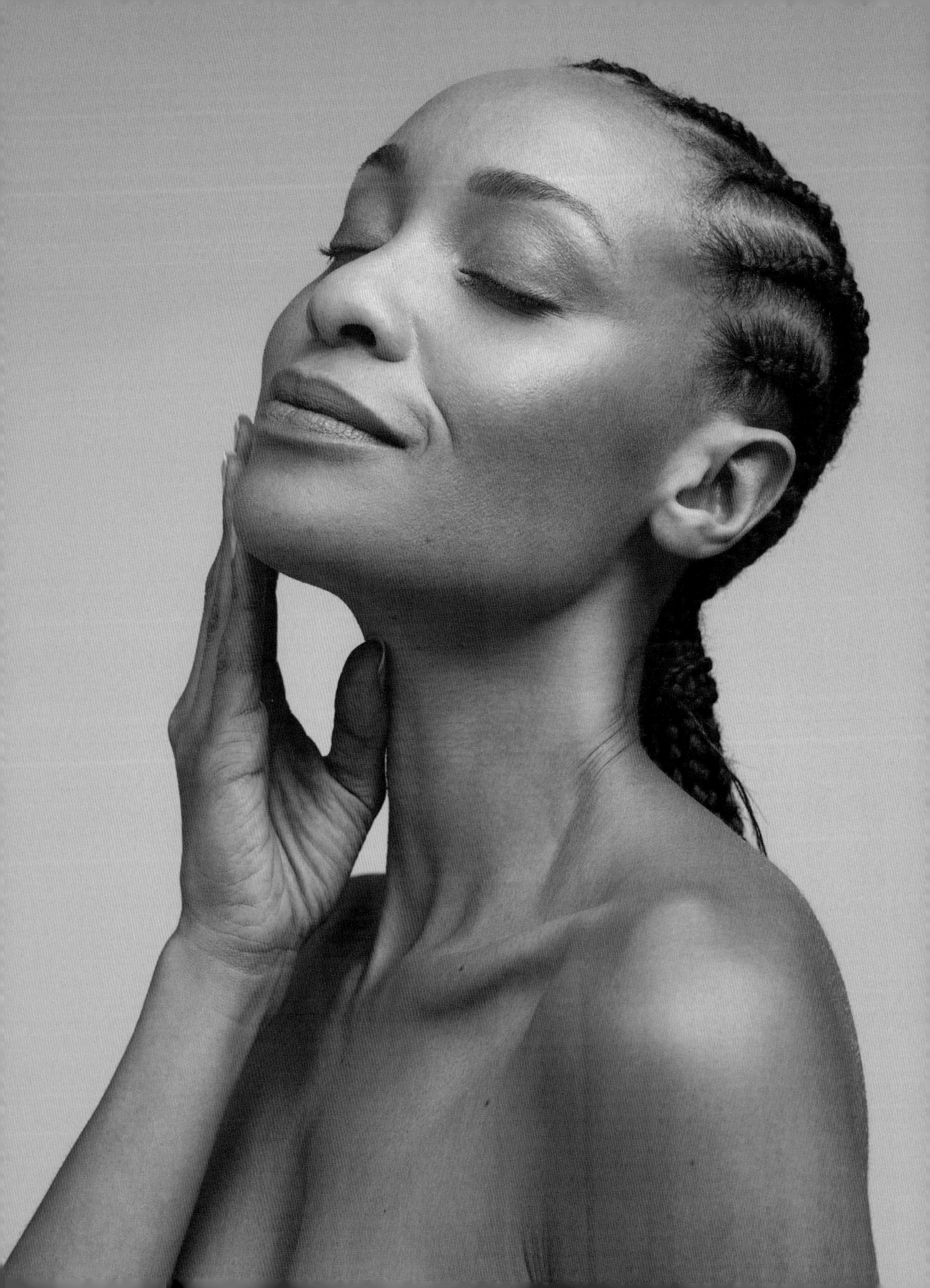

12.

building your skincare regime

building your skincare regime

FOR me, skincare regimes have to be simple and easy to follow. You will never find me giving a client a 10-step routine. I don't hate anyone that much, plus if I don't follow a laborious routine myself, why should I expect anyone else to? Not only is it tedious, it's expensive, and from experience I know that very few people will follow it day in, day out.

And once you fall out of love with using the products because it's a tiresome process, I know you will not see any results and you will resent how much money you spent to have all these products perched on the shelf looking at you whilst you brush your teeth. I do have the T-shirt, self-judgement and bank statements to show for this type of folly.

So nowadays I prefer to keep things simple and limit the steps to only what is essential to maintain skin health. Breaking news – usually this is only 3 or 4 steps, and the routine doesn't have to be complicated or time consuming. On average, it takes me just under 4 minutes to complete my skincare routine, and it's even shorter in the evening.

My favourite words are: Consistency, Commitment and Patience: #CCP. There's no two ways around it. To achieve great skin health you have to be dedicated to the routine as planned, morning and night. It's just like a marriage and you're in it for the long haul.

This is the point at which I get accused of sucking the romance out of skincare, that I have removed the ritual element of self-care, that it's all a bit bish-bash-bosh. What can I say? I'm a functionalist! Jest aside, yes, the routines I design err on the side of simple practicality, but I know they work (and they work fast!), and so many women have been conditioned to think they need an elaborate routine of layering different lotions and potions. Believe me, you don't.

The only caveat that I always add is that if you like using many different products and you enjoy the ritual of skincare, and your skin doesn't mind all the shenanigans, then crack on and continue enjoying yourself.

My philosophy is to use products and ingredients that have been proven by clinical trials and consumer experience to be effective, and that target a number of skin concerns simultaneously. This way you cut down on products and the steps and avoid confusing your skin. I'm here to help you 'reclaim your time', as US congresswoman Maxine Waters famously demanded when her time was being needlessly wasted. Life is for living, with as little time as possible spent in front of the bathroom mirror!

> To achieve great skin health you have to be dedicated to the routine as planned, morning and night.

I do believe you should have a morning skincare routine and an evening routine too, as they serve different functions. In the morning you want to set the scene, revive and protect the skin, whilst in the evening you want to treat and repair. Your routine is the bedrock of your skin health.

When it comes to skincare, I've noticed that we are very impatient and want our products to erase our past dalliances as quickly as yesterday. So when we don't wake up flawless within a couple of weeks, we either cheat on the product by bringing in something new to add to the routine, or kick the product to the kerb like a useless boyfriend, replace it and pin our hopes on a completely new product.

I've done both, and I've seen both being done, and take my word for it when I say: 'Girl, you need to stop and extend some grace to your product and patience to your skin cells. It don't work like that!' I find the impatience is more pronounced when we've spent a pretty penny, too. It's as if all our hopes, dreams and future success get pinned on the one product.

FACT Remember that the skin is an excretory organ, constantly getting rid of waste materials. This doesn't stop whilst you are asleep. Overnight oils, toxins, old skin cells are on the move, being shed with every twist and turn you make in slumber. This is why you have to wash your face in the morning, otherwise you are slowly building up the perfect environment for breakouts and acne.

Also, do you change your pillowcase every evening? I think not. The surface of our pillowcase is littered with hair products, skin cells, dust, oil, mites – things that shouldn't make you think twice whether or not to wash your face in the morning.

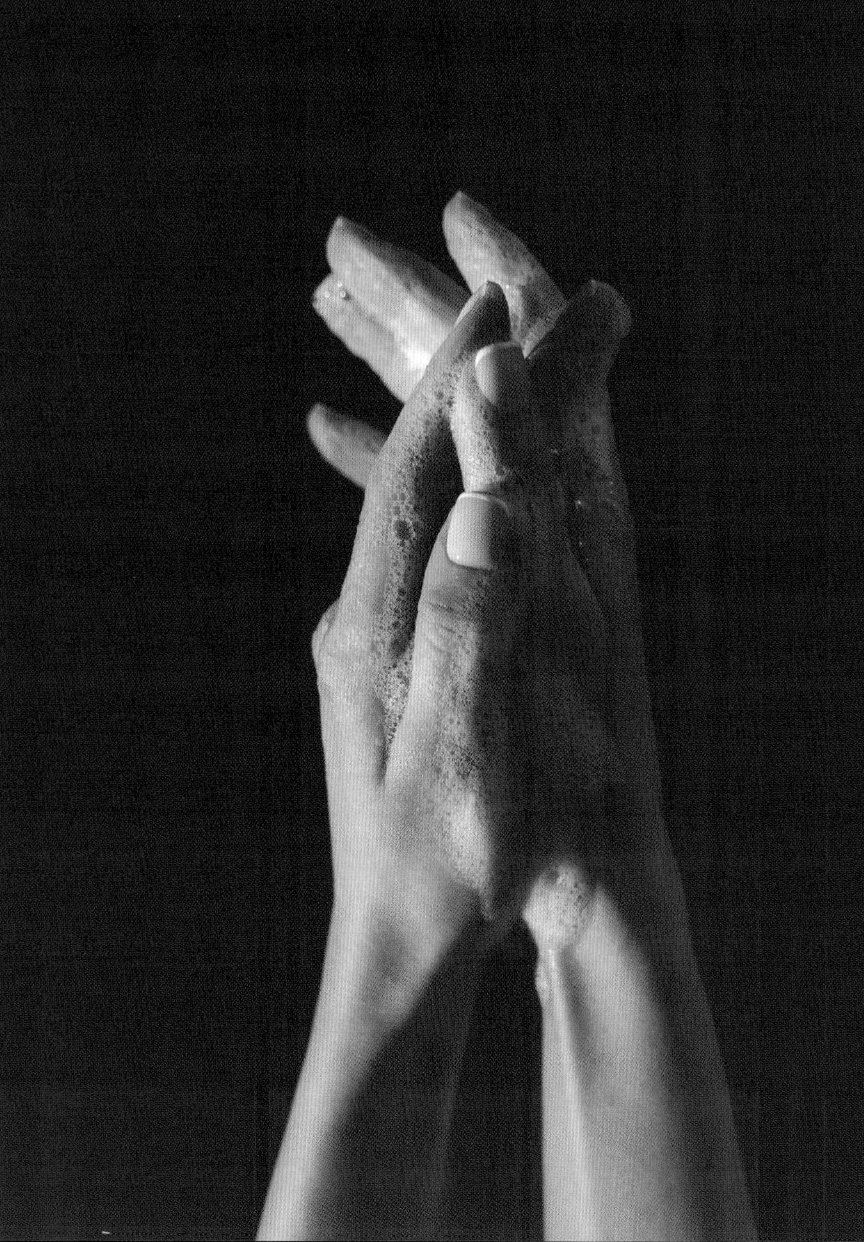

A typical skincare routine will look like this:

morning routine

1. Gentle exfoliating cleanser

An exfoliating cleanser will wake up the skin and get it prepared for the other products that will follow in your routine. Your choice of cleanser will be based on your skin type but, if you can afford it, rotating between two or three cleansers is a good idea so that you can select the best one for the job, depending on what's going on with your skin at that particular time. It's typical to find your skin slightly greasier or oilier as you approach your period, so a more decongesting cleanser, with salicylic acid to remove excess oil and old skin cells deep within the pores, is a good shout. Anything between £20 and £40 will get you a serious cleanser that does the business.

For the people who like to tell me they just rinse their face with water in the morning, the fact box across the page is for you.

> You have to wash your face in the morning, otherwise you are slowly building up the perfect environment for acne.

Types of cleansers:

Cleansers come in different forms and textures, so your choice will be down to a combination of skin type and personal preference.

- **Cleansing Milk –** a very gentle cleanser usually designed for sensitive skin types to help build and restore a damaged skin barrier.
- **Cleansing Gel –** tends to be for oilier skin needing more deep-cleansing action to remove excess oil.
- **Cleansing Cream –** targeted at dry skin to preserve and restore moisture.
- **Cleansing Wipes –** emergencies only, not for daily use.
- **Cleansing Powders** – what's the point, imho? You only have to mix with water to create a paste to then wash your face. Too much faff!

FACT Many cleansers are advertised as 'soap free', but what does this actually mean? Traditional soap is a combination of natural fats and oils, mixed with a strong alkali solution like sodium hydroxide. It works by enveloping oil and dirt on the surface of the skin and allowing water to wash them away. This combination of ingredients can be drying and irritating to the skin. Soap-free cleansers, on the other hand, are alkali free so the potential to dry or irritate the skin has been removed. Instead, they are created with emulsifying ingredients which mimic the same enveloping action.

2. Serum

Serums are full of active ingredients such as vitamin C, alpha arbutin, hyaluronic acid and niacinamide and are the workhorse of your regime to address your core skin concerns, be it dullness, discolouration, dryness, oiliness, fine lines and wrinkles, or just general poor skin quality. Almost everyone needs a serum of one kind or another, and for most Black women, the concern we're guarding against is discolouration. I never devise a routine without a serum to address pigmentation. Serums can also be used to improve hydration, improve skin quality by boosting radiance and brightness, stimulate collagen to smooth fine lines, and clarify the skin by controlling oil. They are most effective when applied straight to damp skin immediately after cleansing. Texture-wise they can range from watery liquids to creams but they will always have a thin and lightweight consistency.

Serums are always where I advise you to spend as much as you can afford, because then your purchase will be your most superior, sophisticated and technically advanced product that penetrates the skin deeply to deliver the results you are after. A serious performance serum will have something called *liposomal encapsulation* and will cost anything between £60 and £150. Above that, I expect the serum to also be able to do housework and cook dinner.

If you feel you have no particular skin concern (lucky you...I'm not jealous...) I would still suggest that at the very least you include an antioxidant serum in your routine. By far the easiest to get hold of would be one containing vitamin C. Antioxidants are the unsung heroes for many Black women, because antioxidants don't always make a visible difference to your skin straight away and good ones tend to cost. In my book they are well worth the money and hype because they protect the skin from environmental and lifestyle damage – such as from UV rays, pollution, poor diet and lack of sleep – that cause premature ageing.

FACT 'Active ingredients' are the chosen ingredients within the products that have a specific benefit for your skin condition. In essence, they make the product work.

Your antioxidant serum does need to be looked after well because if it's exposed to light and air, it will quickly start to break down. Look for one in an opaque or darkly coloured bottle with a pump dispenser – preferably one that retracts so that the opening is covered. It's a waste of time and money to buy anything in clear glass or with a pipette. And whatever you do, don't leave your antioxidant on the dresser or windowsill!

Before we move on, we must talk about the trend I've noticed of using a pipette to apply your product directly to your skin. Pipettes are for dispensing product onto your hands and fingers, not directly to your face. When doing the latter, the pipette invariably ends up touching the skin, which contaminates it with facial oils, dirt, bacteria and old skin cells. This can make your product go off and become less efficient for your needs. Please do jump off that bandwagon.

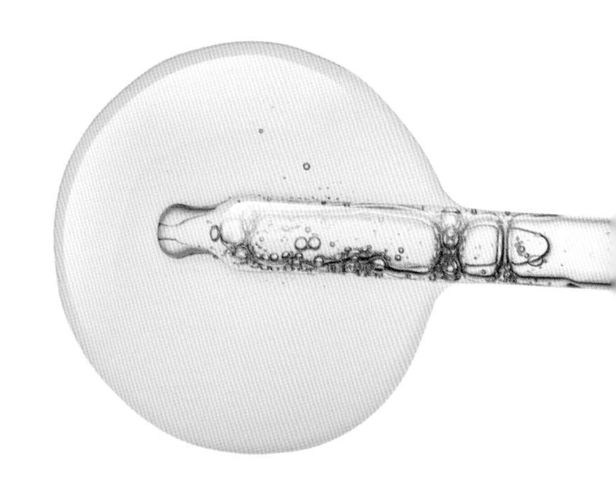

FACT Liposomal encapsulation is a clever way of transporting active ingredients into the deeper layers of your skin. The ingredient is placed within a bubble coated in oil which gives it the ability to penetrate the skin more easily, where it bursts to release the active ingredient at the point where your skin cells can benefit the most. This process is a big deal and an expensive one, so brands will brag about it big time in their marketing. It will be reflected in the product price, too. However, if the brand hasn't beaten you round the head with this information, you can look for the following words on the packaging: phospholipids, phosphatidylethanolamine, phosphatidylinositol or lecithin.

3. Moisturiser

Moisturisers are the overcoat for your skin, and they can either be a lightweight cream or an emollient to seal in your serums and form a soothing protective barrier on top of your skin. Look for moisturisers high in amino acids, ceramides, peptides and glycerine (aka the comeback kid) and that are low in oil, or oil-free if you have particularly oily skin. Not everyone, especially those with oilier skin types, needs or wants to use a moisturiser, and that is fine if your serum or subsequent sunscreen is moisturising enough, but please don't think that because you are an oily skin type you automatically shouldn't use moisturiser.

Moisturiser spend varies anything from £20 to £200 depending on your particular skin concern and budget. You can get some lovely ones from the high street for a little bit less but I find that, as skin matures, you need to spend a little bit more to replace what it loses in the ageing process. Most people won't need a moisturiser above £50, but a treatment moisturiser for deeper hydration – say, for example, for dry menopausal skin – has to be engineered and that will *cost*.

There are three main categories of moisturiser:

Emollients These are oil based and their function is to keep skin soft, smooth, hydrated and balanced. They also help to rebuild skin by replacing lost lipid content on the surface of the skin. Day-to-day moisturisers fall into this category: gels, lotions, creams and ointments.

Humectants These keep your skin hydrated by feeding it moisture from the environment, so they are great if your skincare includes drying agents such as alcohol. Humectants tend to consist of ingredients such as glycerol, amino acids, lactic and hyaluronic acids.

Occlusives These form a barrier on the surface of the skin to prevent water loss and usually come in the form of silicones, oils or waxes. Shea, cocoa and mango butters are all forms of occlusives with lots of beneficial fatty acids for the skin. Their downside is that once on, the skin cannot attract water/moisture from the environment. They are very thick and highly recommended for very dry skin and conditions such as eczema.

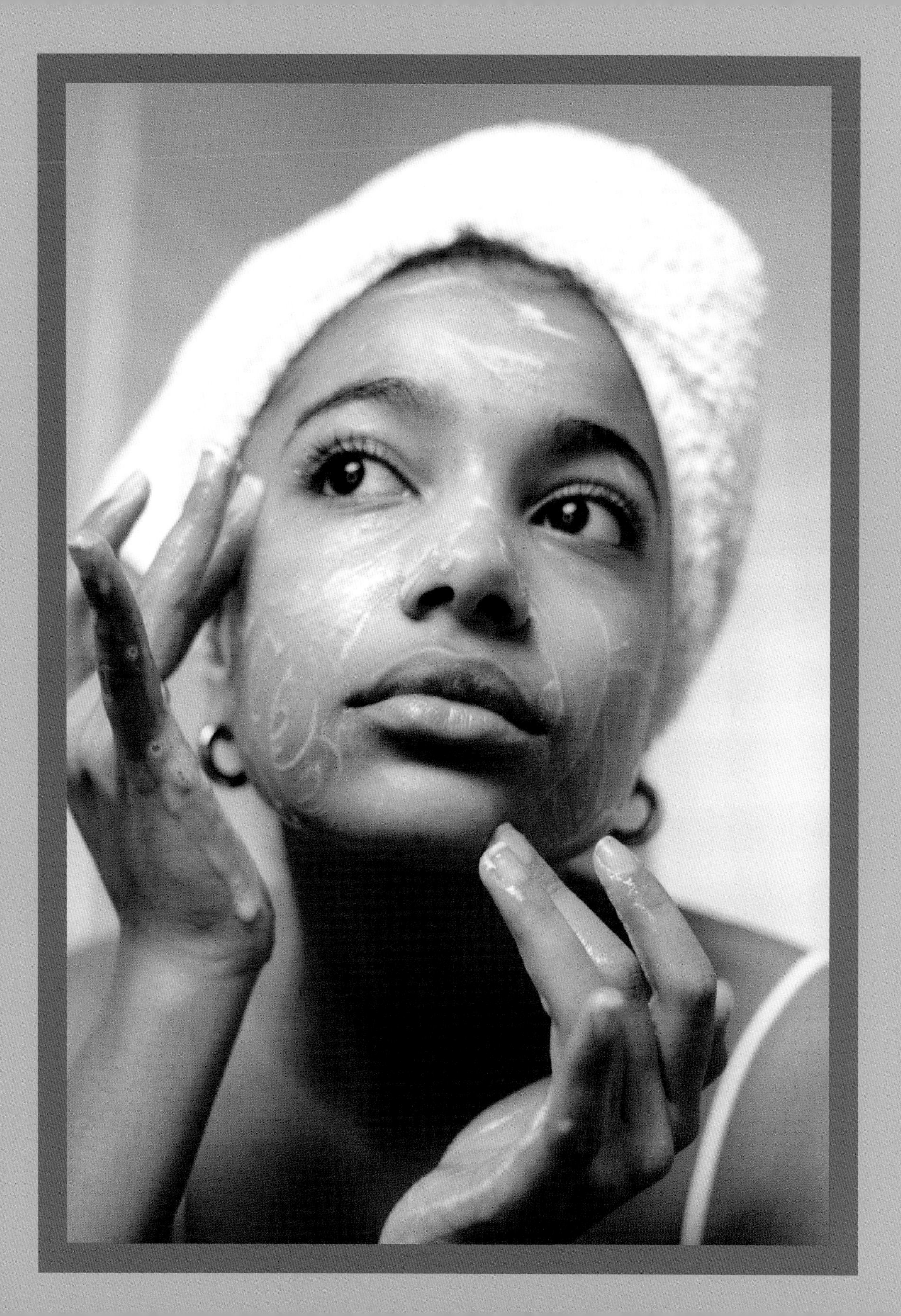

4. Sunscreen

Sunscreen is the ultimate anti-ageing product that will protect your skin against collagen depletion, fine lines and wrinkles, and any worsening of discolouration and hyperpigmentation. I cannot emphasise enough that being Black and having melanin does *not* give you a free pass to leave out sunscreen. Your pigmentation concerns will worsen. Not to mention that sunscreen also protects your skin from burning, which is what leads to sun damage and the potential of skin cancer – which yes, Black people can get too. You should apply two finger-lengths' worth of sunscreen to your face for adequate protection.

Sunscreen doesn't have to cost a packet and for that I am pleased, because I would hate for cost to be the barrier that stops anyone from using it. A good sunscreen should be anywhere between £15 and £30. Expect to pay a little bit more if there are some treatment benefits to the formula.

Whether you use a physical or chemical sunscreen is down to personal preference. A physical sunscreen (sometimes also called a mineral sunscreen) acts a bit like a mirror and reflects some of the sun's rays away from your skin and turns some of them to heat. A chemical sunscreen absorbs the sun's rays, converts them to heat and expels it from the body. Physical sunscreens used to get a bad rap for leaving a white, ashy cast on Black skin. Some still do, but many brands have now invested heavily in technology to stop this happening.

In my opinion, the best sunscreen is the one you like and use every day; so g'on girl, you have no excuse! It can take a while to find the formula that you like, but once you do, applying sunscreen as part of your daily skincare routine will be second nature.

Psst… A word about SPF for the 'I have SPF in my moisturiser or my foundation brigade'

Sunscreen should always be a separate product to ensure you apply enough or even near enough. Research shows most people only apply 20–60 per cent of the required amount, so stop shortchanging yourself.

Caveat: I have been known to recommend a moisturiser/sunscreen combo in order to get a client moving from no sunscreen to some sunscreen, before moving them on to separate sunscreen. Sometimes the reason for this is cost, other times it's mindset. Either way, sometimes we have to take baby steps, so long as we get to the end goal.

evening routine

One of the best pieces of advice I can ever give you is to do your evening cleansing as soon as you get home. The way you whip off your bra for the freedom and comfort when you get home, use that same spirit and do the same for your skin. 'Free the boobs, free the face.'

I know we are busy and tired people, occasionally I have found myself muttering 'Siri, wash my face!' So trust me, I get it, but more often than not I find that people who do their skincare as the last thing before they fall into bed either sometimes forget altogether because they are so tired, or they do a half-hearted, cack-handed job which, over time, leads to clogged, dull skin and breakouts.

1. Pre-cleanse

The purpose of this step is to remove the outside from your skin. By that I mean pollution, dirt, grime, sunscreen and make-up. Use an oil or balm cleanser and really work it into your skin, massaging it into all the nooks and crannies like the corners of your nose and your eyebrows. This is a good time to indulge in a little firm facial massage; spending a few minutes doing this will bring more oxygen to your face and your skin will thank you with increased brightness. Always use a clean, warm, dampened flannel to remove the product from your skin, and use a fresh flannel every evening. Some pre-cleansers turn milky when you apply water, which makes the removal a much easier and pleasant process.

Types of pre-cleansers:

Oil/Balm Cleanser First cleanse in your evening routine to remove make-up and sunscreen. I don't recommend using this in the morning because it may leave a residue on the skin, which can fuel breakouts over time.

Micellar Water A gentle, alcohol-free oil and water combination for removing light make-up as a first cleanse as part of your evening routine. Not always great at removing eye make-up though, so you may need a separate dedicated eye make-up remover.

My inner cheapskate is a massive fan of the pre-cleanse step as it means you use less of your pricier cleanser, which is best used closer to your skin for actual cleaning and exfoliating to have the most beneficial effect.

> My favourite words are consistency, commitment and patience. there's no two ways around it. To achieve great skin health you have to be dedicated to the routine, morning and night.

Psst… A word about flannels

These don't have to be anything expensive. I have a bunch from Tesco that I bought for 50p each and they do an excellent job. Don't get white ones, as they look grubby quickly, and don't use fabric softener when you wash them as it leaves a residue that could irritate your skin.

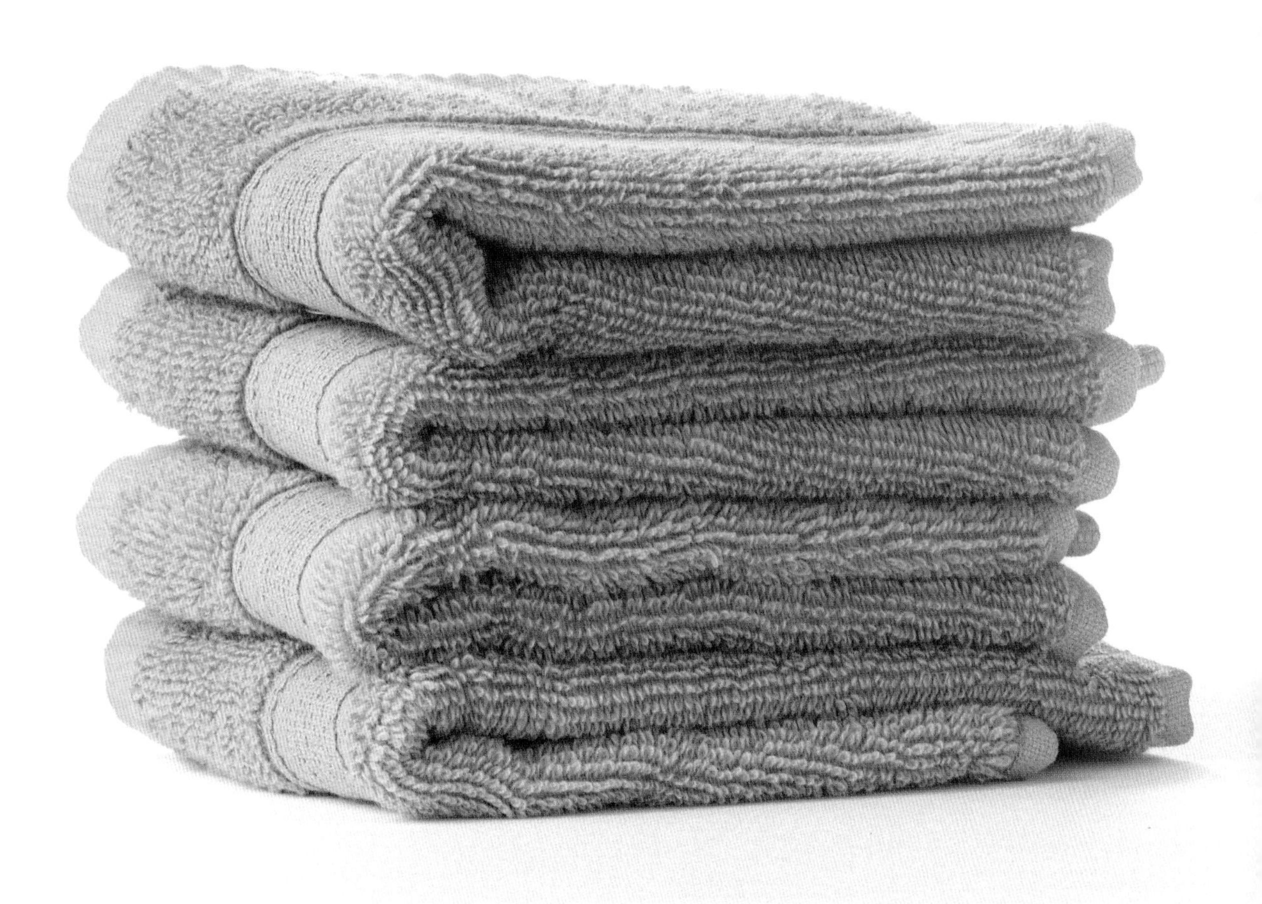

2. Cleanse

Now you actually clean your skin, and you should do this for up to 2 minutes. Yes, 2 minutes! See the list of cleanser types on page 224. Take the time to massage the cleanser into your skin, giving it a chance to get into those pores for a deep clean and loosen old skin cells for increased smoothness. It's fine to just use your hands for this; they are more than sufficient, so no need to use a sonic cleaner or any of those facial bristle-brush cleaners. Typically, we apply extra pressure when we use them and this can be quite harsh on the skin, causing micro tears and wounds. The areas that usually get missed are the hairline, forehead, under the chin and the neck, so pay close attention.

'What sort of evening cleanser should I use? Do I need a different one to my morning cleanser?' This is a popular question and, in an ideal world, I would prefer you to have a morning cleanser and an evening cleanser as they would do slightly different jobs. The evening cleanser has to be much more hardworking, so I prefer a high-potency one with more active ingredients, whereas the morning cleanser isn't doing so much heavy lifting and it's mainly to refresh the skin.

Your choice of cleanser will depend on your skin type, but typically there would be an element of exfoliation to smooth and brighten the skin. Your cleanser should include an alpha hydroxy acid (AHA) such as glycolic, lactic or mandelic acid as the main ingredient, or an enzyme-enriched cleanser with pineapple, pumpkin, pomegranate or papaya as the active ingredient. The former has a faster action on the skin and the latter is slower, but both will deliver results when used consistently.

If your skin is more dry and/or sensitive, then opt for a polyhydroxy-based cleanser with ingredients like gluconolactone, lactobionic and maltobionic acids. They will still exfoliate and brighten the skin, but very slowly and without irritation as these ingredients are padded out with extra water that prevents fast penetration into the skin.

Oily skin types should opt for a cleanser that includes salicylic acid or benzoyl peroxide to decongest your pores and clear away oil and old skin cells that fester and lead to spots and breakouts.

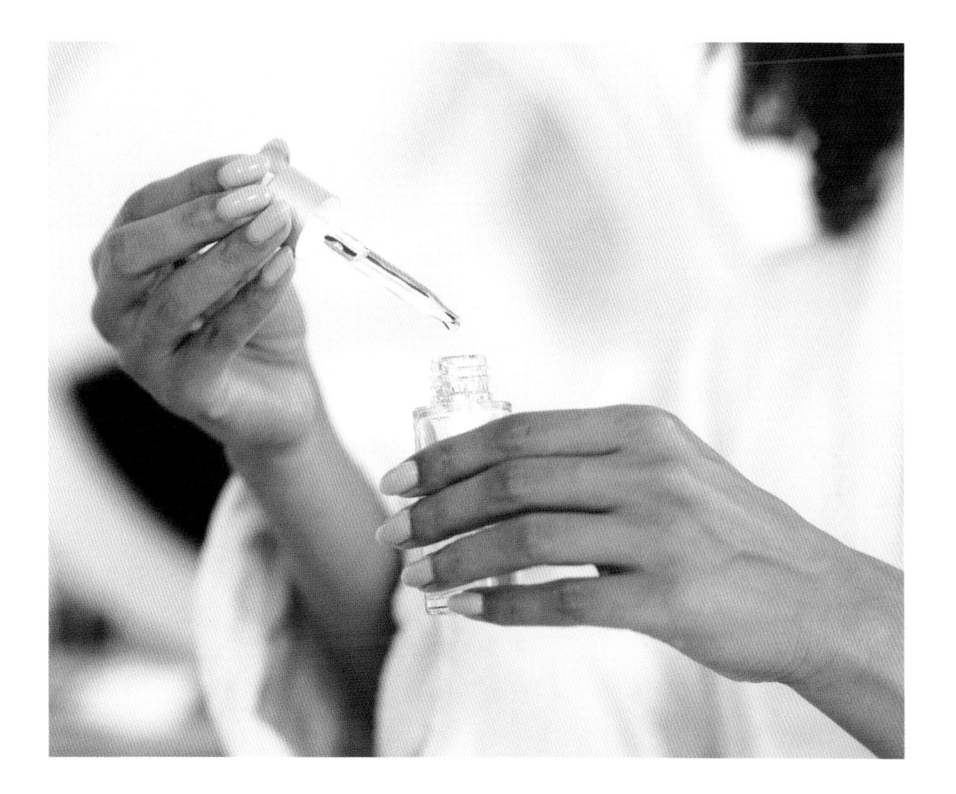

3. Treat

Time to help skin with its regeneration process. Don't get me wrong, skin is always regenerating, it's not a stop–start process, it's continuous. But at night there's less pressure on the skin as you're not fussing with it because you're asleep. My one key product for night-time is vitamin A, aka retinoids. Vitamin A is a gold standard, jack-of-all-trades ingredient that is excellent for stimulating collagen to keep skin plump and firm, improving moisture in the skin by boosting hyaluronic acid, encouraging exfoliation and speeding up cell turnover, fading discolouration and evening out the skin tone, and strengthening the all-important skin barrier.

It's possible to get vitamin A for all skin types; even those with sensitive skin can use vitamin A successfully as it helps to fortify the skin to stave off irritations. But if for any reason you can't/don't want to use vitamin A, make sure you select skin-loving replenishing ingredients that deliver bags of moisture and hydration. The sorts of ingredients that your skin will thank you for are hyaluronic acid, ceramides, glycerol, growth factors and peptides.

Psst... A word about vitamin A

Unless you have acne and your doctor or a dermatologist has prescribed vitamin A after a full and proper consultation, you do not need to be using a prescription vitamin A like Tretinoin. Over-the-counter vitamin A can be just fine.

OVER THE COUNTER	PRESCRIPTION ONLY
Retinol	Tretinoin
Retinaldehyde	Isotretinoin
Adapalene	Tazarotene

There are many more types of prescription vitamin A products, some in combination with antibiotics and/or steroids. They are very strong and can have some severe side effects – which is why they are prescription only. For most people, over-the-counter formulations at different strengths are more than capable of doing the job of keeping your skin in good health, and preventing premature ageing, fine lines and wrinkles. The key is to start using vitamin A early, from age 25 or so, and not wait until you actually see fine lines and wrinkles.

'What about masks, essences, snail juice, scrubs and toners?' I hear you ask.

Masks fall into the 'nice to have' category; they are not essential to basic skin health, but there are some highly effective and results-driven masks that brighten and smooth the skin. My problem with masks is that they encourage some people to ignore their skin day to day, thinking that if they use a big-guns mask once a week, their skin will be fine. Healthy skin is born out of diligence and consistency, not the type of grand gestures an absentee parent would make on their return from being awol!

With toners, it's not uncommon for me to get a follow-up email after a skin health consultation saying: 'Dija, I've just realised you didn't include an exfoliating toner.' The ingredients that these types of toners use have largely been absorbed by advanced cleansers with AHAs and BHAs, serums and vitamin

A and, given the dangers of over-exfoliation – weakened skin barrier, hyper-pigmentation – I largely prefer to stay away from them.

As much as I love Clinique and all it's done since the 1960s to put skincare on the map, I blame them for a clever marketing campaign back in the day that burned the three-step Cleanse, Tone, Moisturise routine into our psyches. I fell for it hook, line and sinker when I was 18 after a consultant used their party trick (the tape test) to show me the amount of dead skin cells I would have without using their Clarifying Toner. It was such a powerful tactic and, for me and a lot of women, I think this is the origin of the reliance on toners.

If you're using toners to re-hydrate your skin post cleansing, I would urge you to make sure your cleanser isn't overly stripping your skin and opt for something a bit more conditioning. If you're spritzing refreshing toners such as mists to keep your skin moist as you work through your routine, go faster so your skin doesn't dry out in between steps.

However, lest I be accused of sucking the fun out of your skincare routine, if it's the case that you simply like a dramatic spritz here and there, keep at it as you're doing no harm. Just choose a spritz that has some beneficial ingredients like glycerine, allantoin or zinc that also add healing value to your skin.

The biggest myth we have about toners is that they are used to remove residual make-up from your skin after cleansing. I'm afraid you've been had if you believe this, because if there is make-up on your cotton pad after swiping with a toner, I'm sorry to say your skin is still dirty and the only solution is to wash your face again.

I feel the same about essences imported from Japanese and Korean beauty regimes. You don't need them, unless you like using them. Snail juice – just stop. Sperm juice – walk away.

As for scrubs with nut kernels for exfoliating the skin, they have been superseded by hydroxy acids in products at other steps in your routine. However, if you are still using grainy scrubs of the St Ives ilk, you need to stop now – but feel free to finish the tube on rough knees and heels. You'll be doing the skin on your face a big favour and saving it from a lifetime of micro-tears and hyperpigmentation.

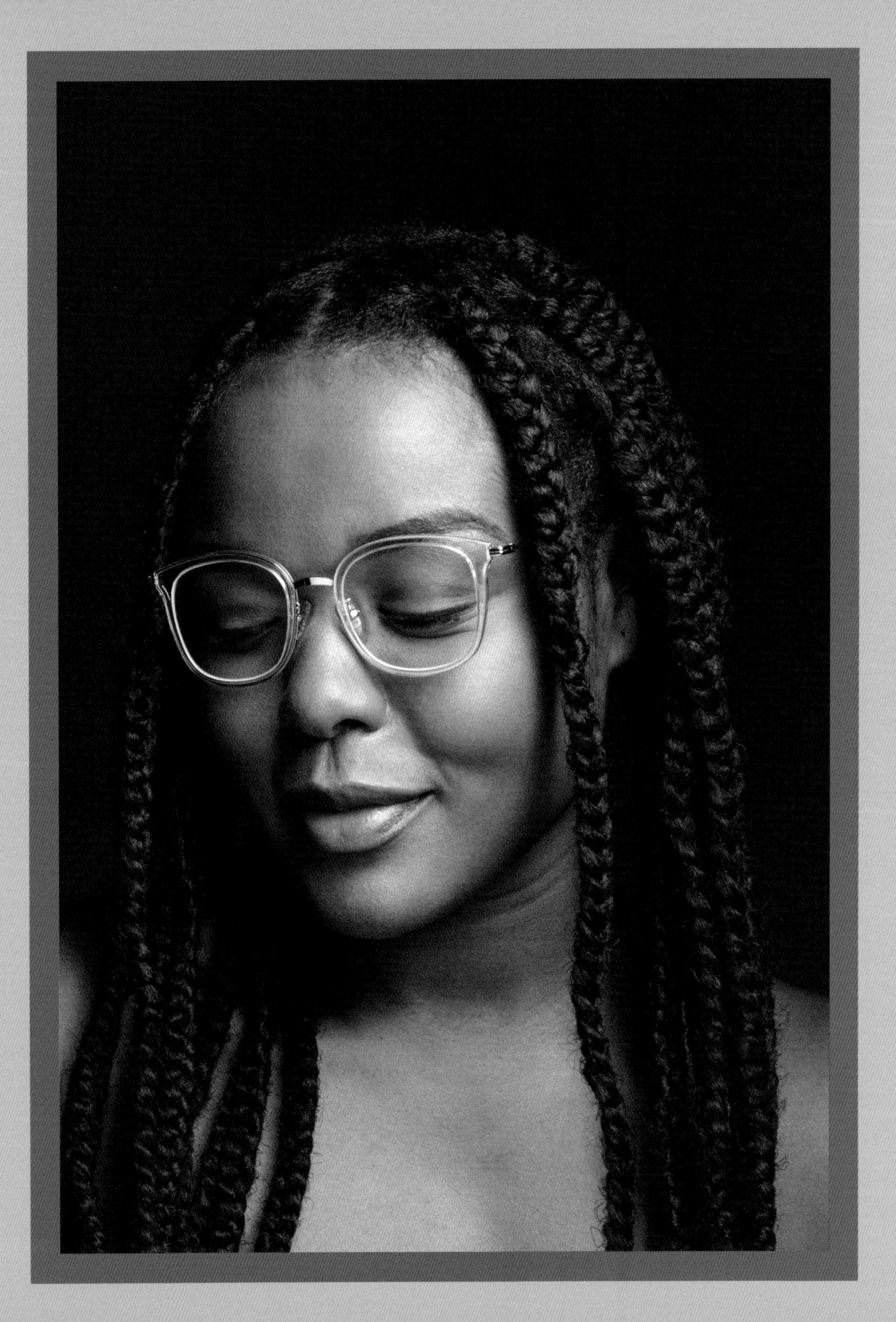

Microbead scrubs are dangerous for the environment and kill fish and wildlife. We are skincare lovers, not fighters.

Whilst I'm here I'll take this opportunity to mention my favourite words again – Consistency, Commitment and Patience: #CCP. Remember, to achieve great skin health you have to be dedicated to the routine as planned, morning and night.

During the course of my career, I've sat in many a consultation listening to clients reel off their product adventures for me to end with only one thought running through my head: How do you have any skin left? Thank God for our detailed consultation forms where you list all your products, otherwise I'd lose track because it can get hella confusing! If I'm confused, think about the effect on your skin.

Chopping and changing your products leads to nowhere but frustration, and routines take a while to bed down and start showing results – sometimes up to four months and longer. If it's any comfort, consumer skincare trials are often run over periods of 12, 16 or 20 weeks, sometimes even longer, so I think it's prudent to always take the same long-term approach when looking at and assessing your skincare products and their effects on your skin. Yes, sometimes you will see some initial results quickly and that is very encouraging, but to see long-term results you need to knuckle down, and patience is key.

There will also be times when a product doesn't work or personally agree with you and that can be for any number of reasons. It doesn't mean that the product is bad; it just means that it wasn't effective for your concerns and we need to move you on to something more suited for your skin, or tweak how you use this product, maybe from every day to three times a week. There's a lot of flexibility in how products can be used, which is why I always recommend you have a skincare professional on your side so they can guide you.

Routines take a while to bed down and start showing results – sometimes up to four months and longer.

Purging and allergic reactions

Sometimes you will start a new routine and find yourself a bit spotty, especially if you're using more potent ingredients. This is fine because the products will initially speed up changes in your skin. Cell turnover will increase, bringing forth with it congestion lurking in the deeper layers of your skin. With patience it does pass, but if the level and amount of spots is getting you down we can make changes to your routine that ease symptoms.

This purging is a process the skin has to go through to build strength and resiliency. It may temporarily increase dark marks and hyperpigmentation, but these will fade quite quickly. Purging is different to experiencing an allergic reaction to a product, which is a sudden reaction, with your skin and body telling you they really don't like what you've just applied.

How to avoid allergic reactions

Some people have skin that easily flares. If that's you then you can keep a lid on things by:

- Patch-testing products first, either in the crook of your elbow or behind your ear. Do this for products that have active ingredients like vitamin A or alpha hydroxy acids, although bear in mind that sometimes they aren't the cause of your reaction – it could be a totally seemingly benign ingredient in the product.
- Keeping a skincare diary. This will help you track any sensations/reactions and how your skin copes with the introduction of new products.
- Not introducing too many products at once. Take it slowly over a number of weeks building up one product at a time, so you're able to spot any potential problems and identify the offending product.
- Keeping a fast-acting emergency skincare kit handy. Mine contains a gentle, sensitive-skin face wash, soothing moisturiser, intense hyaluronic acid and gentle, non-essential oil face oil. I also have OTC antihistamines.

FACT The difference between purging and allergic reaction.

A purge will happen over the course of 4 to 6 weeks (a bit longer for mature skin) as your skin goes through its normal cell-renewal cycle. It will look like an increase in spots, blemishes and bumps on the skin. The only way to solve a purge is to stay the course and push through it, understanding that it will pass.

An allergic reaction will happen almost immediately, within the first 24 hours of applying the product. Depending on your skin tone your skin will look either flushed or red all over, be hot and burning, itchy and rashy. You may even experience swelling and blistering. If this is the case, you need to stop using the product immediately, remove it from your skin and apply a soothing basic moisturiser without any active ingredients. (My go-to is La Roche-Posay Cicaplast Balm B5 Multi-Purpose Repairing Cream.) You may have to seek medical advice if the symptoms don't ease after a couple of days.

A basic skincare routine re-cap

MORNING	EVENING
Cleanser	Make-up Remover
Serum(s)	Cleanser
Moisturiser (if necessary)	Vitamin A/Night Moisturiser
Sunscreen	

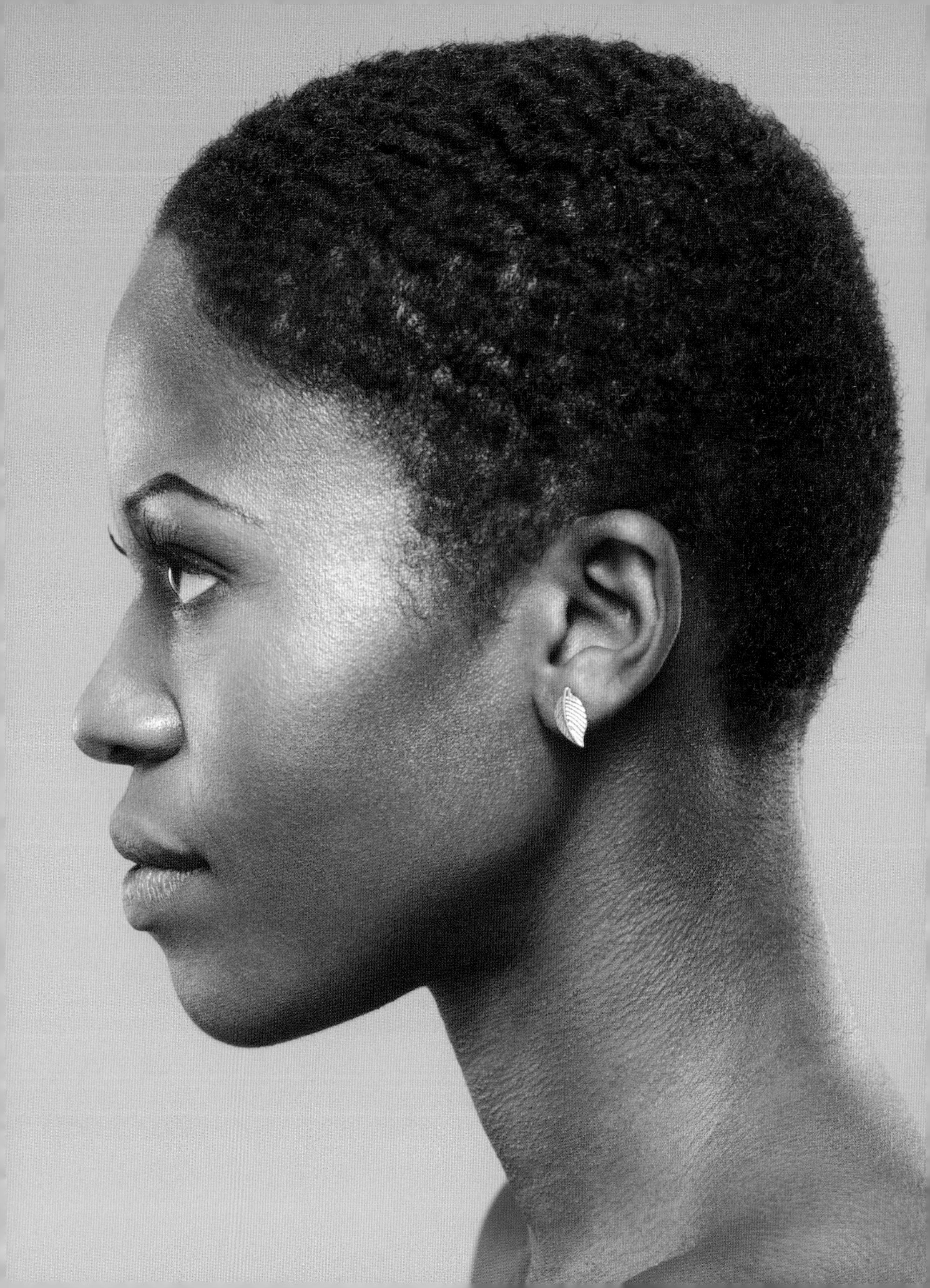

13.

product hall of fame

product hall of fame

I KNOW everyone has different budgets, so I've always tended to base my advice on ingredients as this allows you to find the products at your own pace and that suit your pocket.

However, is there anything better than having a good natter with your gang about new skincare discoveries? One of my most-favourite parts of any skin health consultation is when we discuss your skincare products and how you use them, so it only makes sense that I too give a nod to my favourite products that either feature in my routine day in, day out, year after year, or, at some point, have done such a great job they've stayed in my heart and the back of my cabinet ever since.

cleansers

Everything in skin health starts with cleansing, it is one of your cornerstones. If you leave this step out, or don't do it properly, forget every hope you have for healthy skin.

Make-up removers

- **DHC Deep Cleansing Oil.** Does what it says on the bottle and removes all of your make-up, including mascara, with no fuss.

- **The Body Shop Camomile Sumptuous Cleansing Butter.** A luxe-feeling cleansing balm with a very reasonable price tag. Total thumbs up!

Face washes

- **CeraVe Hydrating Cleanser.** Fantastic for grumpy and dry skin that needs a reset, chockablock with ceramides and glycerine to hydrate.
- **Cosmedix Purity Clean Exfoliating Cleanser.** A treat for combination and oily skin types, with lactic acid to exfoliate without stripping the skin and peppermint essential oil to wake up both your skin and senses.
- **NeoStrata Foaming Glycolic Wash.** Not for the faint hearted, and definitely not for sensitive skin types. With high-strength glycolic acid, I would consider it almost a resetting treatment to smooth and polish the skin. I reach for this if I've neglected my skin and it's looking dull and feeling rough.
- **Sunday Riley Ceramic Slip.** Some cleansers are seasonal and this is one for the summer months when oily skin can become oilier. It's a clay-based cleanser that has magical powers to suck oil and gunk from your pores. Use before a hot and sweaty night out, as oil is instantly tempered. Thank me in the morning.

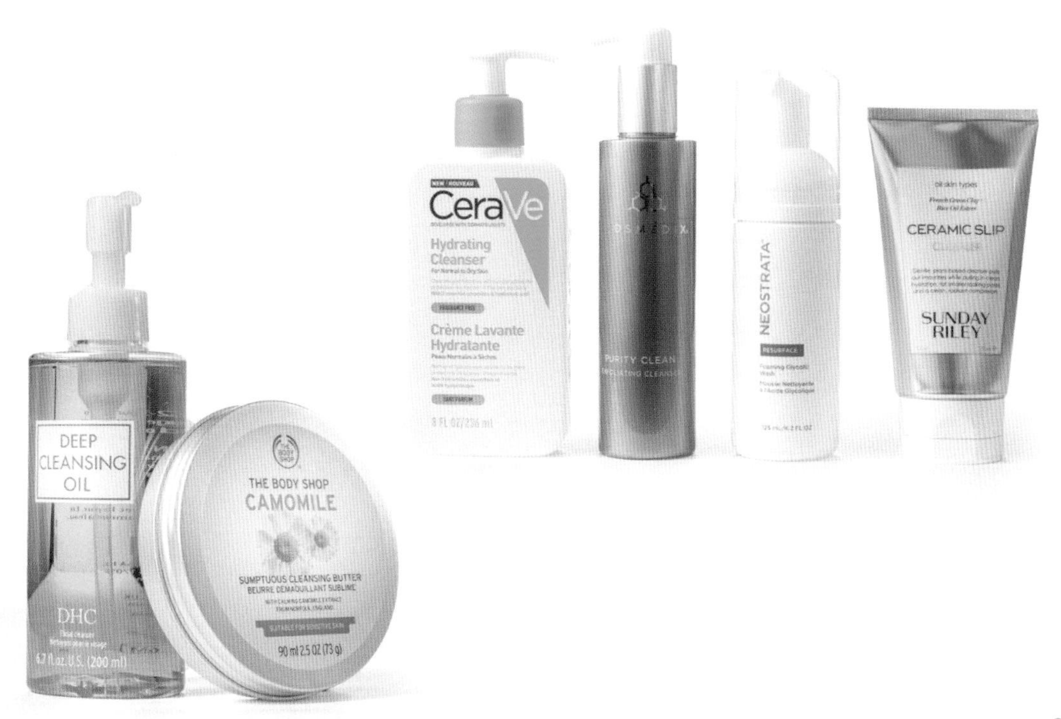

- **The Ordinary Squalane Cleanser.** The easyJet of cleansing: simple, gentle, no-frills for skin that requires no fuss, coming in at under £15.

- **La Roche-Posay Toleriane Dermo-Cleanser Wipe-Off Milk.** For when you've overdone it. Insert your reason but whatever you've done, or even reacted to, and it has left your skin sore, irritated and sensitive, this cleanser restores your skin's peace with glycerine and LRP's soft magical spring water. You apply with fingers and remove with damp cotton pads. Better yet, cotton pads that have been soaked in cool bottled water as hard water can up the levels of irritation.

- **Dermalogica Skin Resurfacing Cleanser.** Lactic acid is the star ingredient to exfoliate deeply but gently remove dead and dull skin cells. Skin is visibly brighter after one use, and it is gentle enough for most people to use easily.

- **Youth to the People Superfood Cleanser.** I've got through bottles of this deliciously fresh cleanser. If you could have a healthy green smoothie for your face, it would be this. It's chockablock with antioxidants – kale, spinach and green tea – to cleanse and refresh your skin without stripping it. Great for all skin types too!

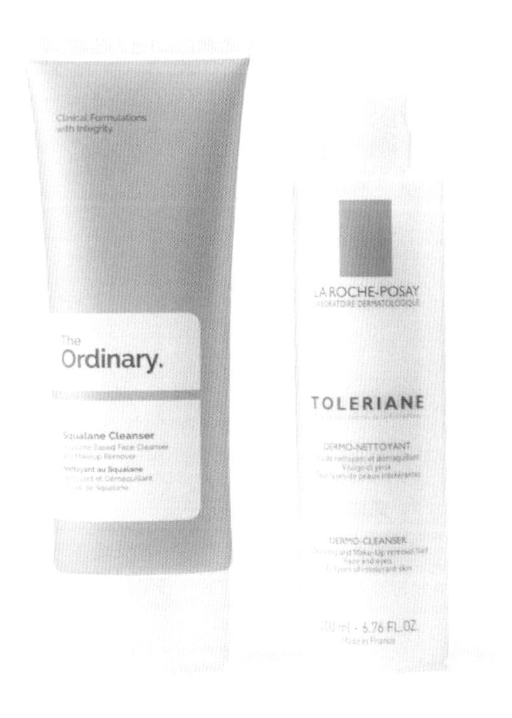

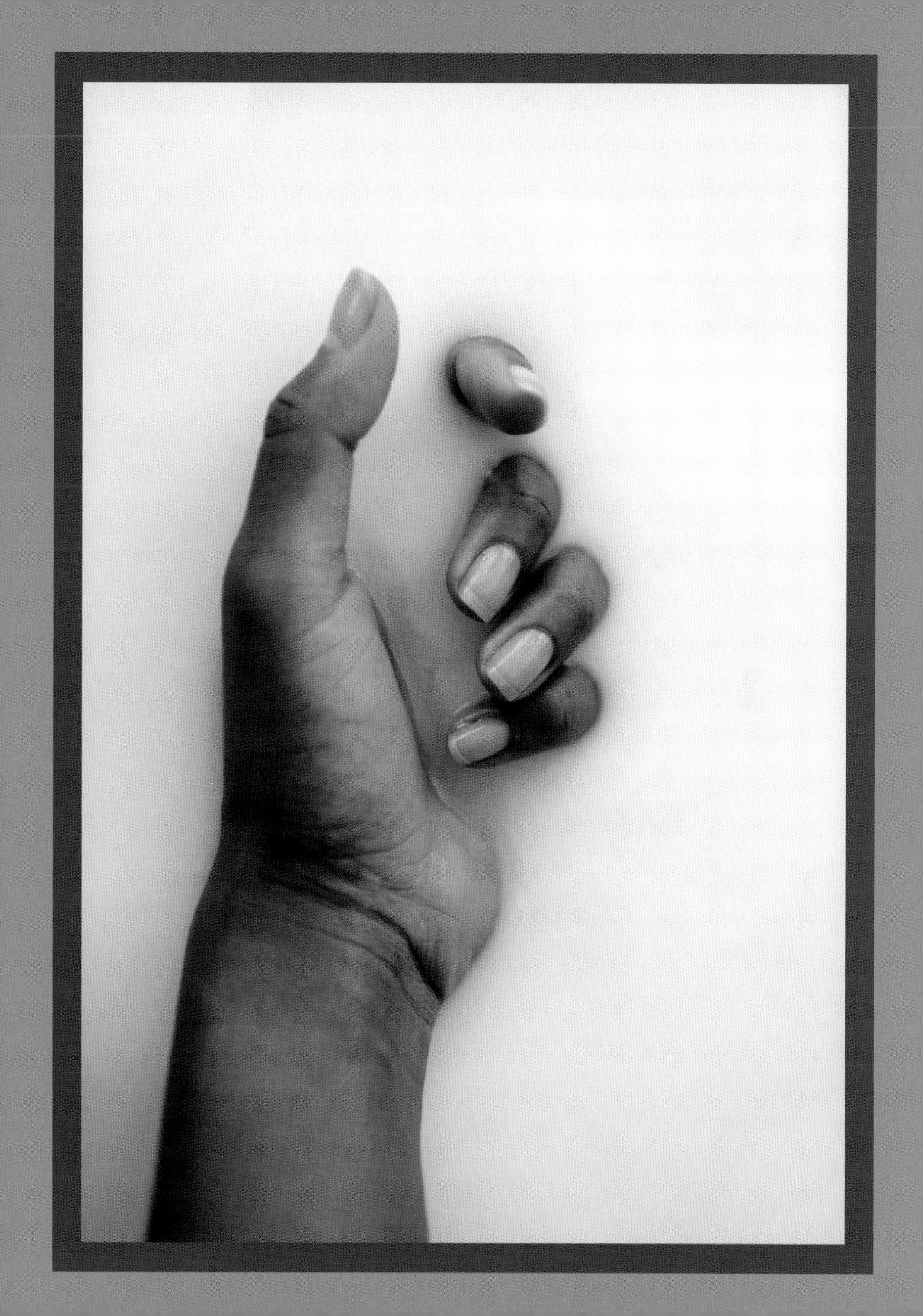

Exfoliating Pads

If you're salty about taking toners out of your skincare routine, exfoliating pads used two to three times a week are an excellent replacement if you need an oil-control boost, and also to brighten the skin and make it pop.

- **Dr Dennis Gross Alpha Beta Universal Daily Peel Pads.** A lauded combination of 5 skin-friendly acids, including glycolic and salicylic, plus vitamin A and antioxidants in a two-step regime.
- **SkinBetter Science AlphaRet Exfoliating Peel Pads.** With salicylic acid and vitamin A to improve exfoliation. I've found them really helpful in minimising milia. Great for travel as they are packaged individually.

FACT Milia look like tiny cysts, usually under the eyes, and they are filled with compacted old skin cells that have become trapped under the skin.

- **Strivectin Advanced Resurfacing Daily Reveal Exfoliating Pads.** These micro-peel fibre pads will resurface and polish your skin using a potent concoction of gylcolic acid, tranexamic acid, salicylic acid, azelaic acid and gluconolacctone. Your pores, texture, glow and clarity will be refined.

antioxidants

- **SkinBetter Science Alto Defense Serum.** The biggest and baddest antioxidant to date, with 19 different types of antioxidants to protect the skin and improve its quality. We're talking vitamin C, grapeseed extract, ubiquinone, turmeric, coffee, liquorice root extract, ginger...

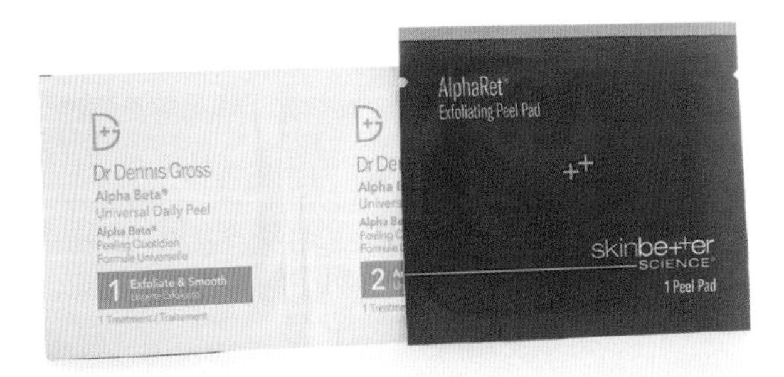

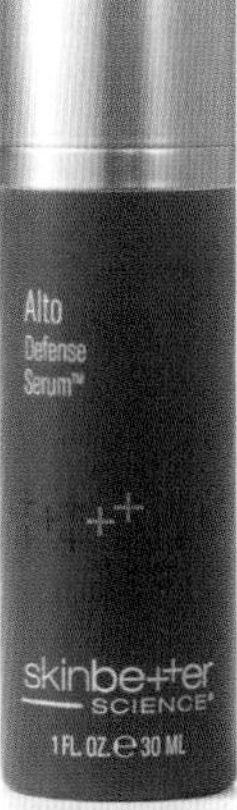

pigmentation serums

When it comes to skin discolouration, I like serums that get to work fast. The best ones fade the visible dark marks on the surface of the skin, but they also work within the skin to prevent dark marks from developing in the first place.

- **Cosmedix Simply Brilliant 24/7 Brightening Serum.** This is the 'aha' serum that turns most people on to the power of pigmentation serums. Obscure ingredients such as whitonly and waltheria give you a glow from within and it's still jam packed with the usual faders: niacinamide, vitamin C, liquorice root extract, lactic and salicylic acid.

- **SkinSense Advanced Anti-Pigmentation Perfecting Serum.** My favourite ingredient, hexylresorcinol, as well as niaciniamide are responsible for the clarity this serum delivers. It's good for all skin types and with continued twice-daily use the complexion is brighter and more even.

- **NeoStrata Enlighten Illuminating Serum.** The first-ever product that showed me the true power of cocktail ingredients: vitamin C, liquorice extract, niacinamide, all in a cooling gel that fades pigmentation and brightens the skin too.

- **SkinBetter Science Even Tone Correcting Serum.** The queen of pigmentation serums that cleverly tackles red, yellow and brown pigmentation stains but also gives your skin a supersized radiance kick. It's fast acting, with encouraging results in as little as 4 weeks. I recommend it for all my impatient clients.

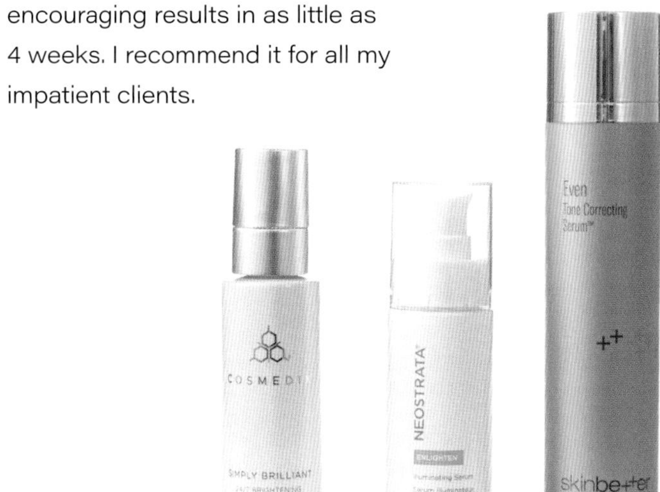

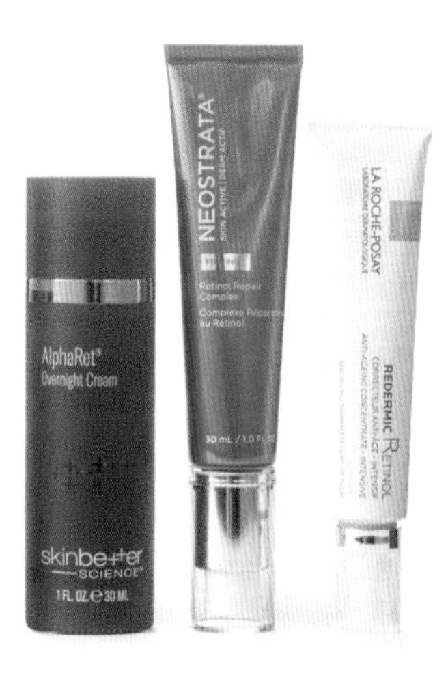

retinoids (vitamin a)

These are the jack-of-all-trade marathon runners of your skincare. They are for the long haul to rejuvenate, prevent lines and wrinkles, encourage clarity, boost hydration, and keep your skin in good all-round condition.

- **CeraVe Resurfacing Retinol Serum.** I love that this is specifically for blemish-prone skin that experiences dark marks. The retinol will help to tackle and fade them, while still being gentle, and has supportive barrier ingredients like ceramides and niacinamides. If you're caught out, it also doubles up as a fast-acting spot treatment.

- **SkinBetter Science AlphaRet Overnight Cream.** This is a special advanced retinoid combined with lactic and glycolic acid. I reserve it for experienced users of retinoids, or mature skin types who need rejuvenation quickly.

- **NeoStrata Retinol Repair Complex.** This was my first go on the retinoid rodeo over 10 years ago, and it's a goody for all skin types bar sensitive. If you're after skin clarity, improving hydration, firming and plumping your skin, this does the business.

- **La Roche-Posay Redermic Retinol.** This is my first choice high-street retinoid. It has a very gentle action on early lines and patchy skin tone with consistent use. A good option for the 20–30 age bracket.

- **Skin Rocks Retinoid 1.** If you're new to retinoids or want to dip your toe back in, this is your option. This will clear up dark marks, soften fine lines and visibly reduce breakouts. Use Retinoid 2 to step it up a gear.

parched skin

Thirsty skin needs water, and it needs to be able to hold on to the water you give it. That is where these products come in. Hyaluronic acid is like a tall drink of H_2O for your skin and is famed for its ability to refresh, revitalise and restore your skin so that it can function better.

- **Indeed Labs Hydraluron Moisture Serum.** The original product that brought the powers of hyaluronic acid to the mainstream.
- **Vichy Minéral 89 Hyaluronic Acid Booster.** Moisture!
- **Medik8 Hydr8 B5 Intense.** Even more moisture!
- **NeoStrata Tri-Therapy Lifting Serum.** Moisture but with added amino acids and poly hydroxy acids to gently exfoliate too. You're getting moisture, smoothness and clearer skin. It's the class prefect of hyaluronic acids and perfect for mature skin types.
- **Shiseido Treatment Softener Enriched.** My first thoughts were 'unnecessary expensive face water!', but in reality it's an excellent hydrator that's the texture of glycerine. Not a hyaluronic acid like the others in this category, it's got Japanese yuzu seed extract going for it, which improves your skin's ability to hold in moisture. If you don't mind the spend and you don't get on with hyaluronic acid, this may be the one for you.

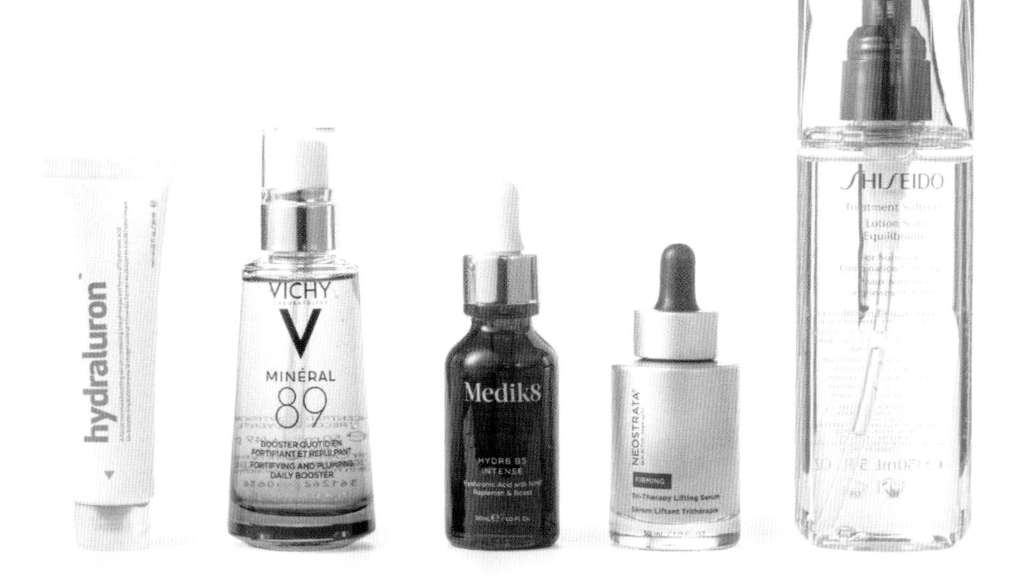

emergency fixers

Sometimes you just need to insert a short-term product into your routine that quickly puts out the fire.

- **Cosmedix Clarity Skin-Clarifying Serum.** A fully loaded retinol and salicylic acid firecracker for acne breakouts and spots that are more frequent than at that time of the month.

- **Medik8 Blemish SOS Rapid Action Target Gel.** For the odd spot that pops up from time to time. Just dab this after cleansing and it will show itself out. And quickly too!

- **NeoStrata Glycolic Renewal Smoothing Cream.** For skin that's dry, rough, and dull textured on the face or body, this is a creeping introduction to the smoothing powers of glycolic acid. Also, my secret weapon for getting skin ready for advanced in-clinic treatments.

- **Osmosis Rescue Epidermal Repair Serum.** Time out but for tantrum-like skin that's inflamed, flushed, hot and congested: one or two cycles of Rescue resets your skin. The key ingredient is trioxolane, prized for its ability to soothe and repair cellular damage.

- **No7 Radiance + 15 per cent Vitamin C Serum.** For when your skin needs a brightening pick-me-up. My trick is to use this morning and night at least 10 days prior to a big event. I can only describe the resulting glow as like a 'lightbulb under your skin.'

- **Clinisoothe+ Skin Purifier.** If you're into popping spots (which you shouldn't be), then this keeps your skin sanitised without stripping it.

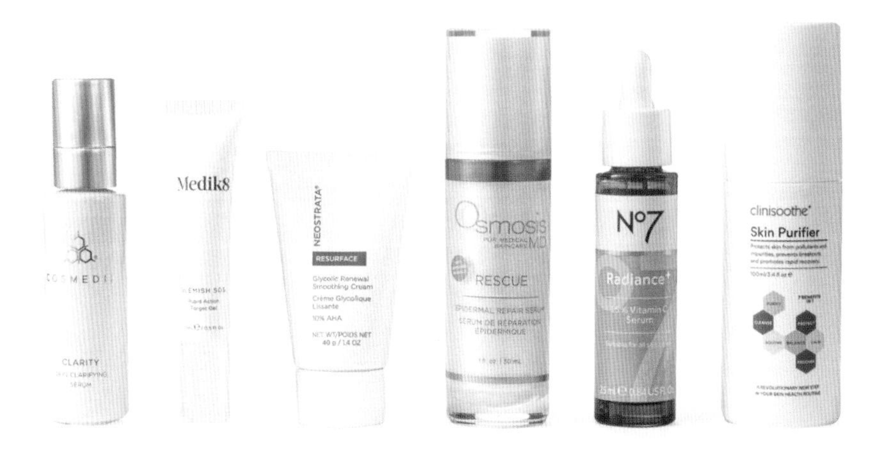

face falling off – over-processed, dry, tight, irritated

One of the main after-effects when skin is over-processed is extreme dryness, because your skin is losing moisture really fast. This is accompanied by intense itchiness and sometimes flaking. It's just a mess! These are my go-tos: they are high-emollient moisturisers that soothe extremely dry skin. And fast too!

- **La Roche-Posay Cicaplast Baume B5.** Panthenol, glycerin and shea butter balm; basically a plaster that prevents dehydration and keeps moisture inside the skin, exactly where it should be! Also good for hands and babies' bottoms.

- **Weleda Skin Food.** There are times when I find the scent a little overpowering, but there's a reason it's been around for nearly 100 years and still flies off the shelf every 16 seconds. It's a fixer for all manner of dry skin.

- **Cosmedix CPR Skin Recovery Serum.** It's called CPR. Need I say more other than it brings your skin back to life?

- **Dr Jart+ Ceramidin Cream.** Most ceramide-boasting moisturisers have 3 at the most. This has 5 different types of ceramides (a fatty wax substance that is already naturally produced by the skin) to coat the skin and prevent moisture loss.

- **NeoStrata Restore Bionic Face Cream.** With a thick and balm-like texture, this is really a puffer jacket for your face. No chance of moisture escaping. My favourite in-clinic point-treatment moisturiser, as well as for rosacea skin.

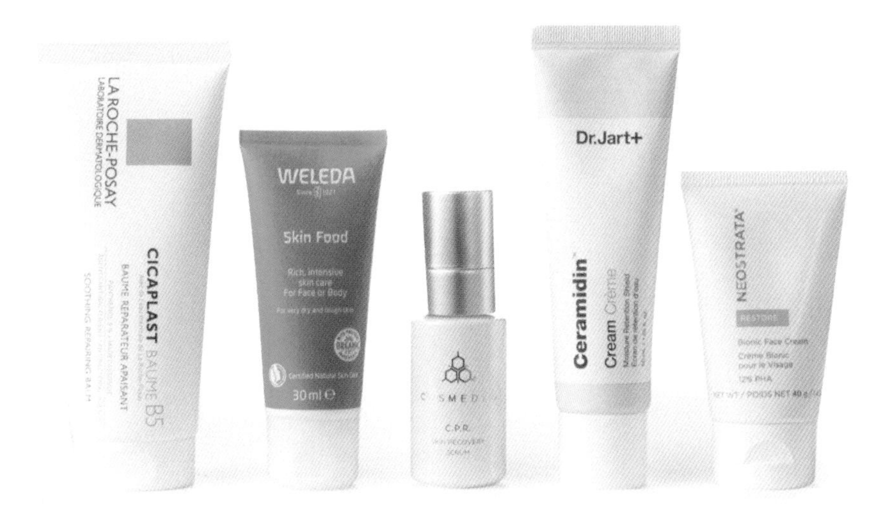

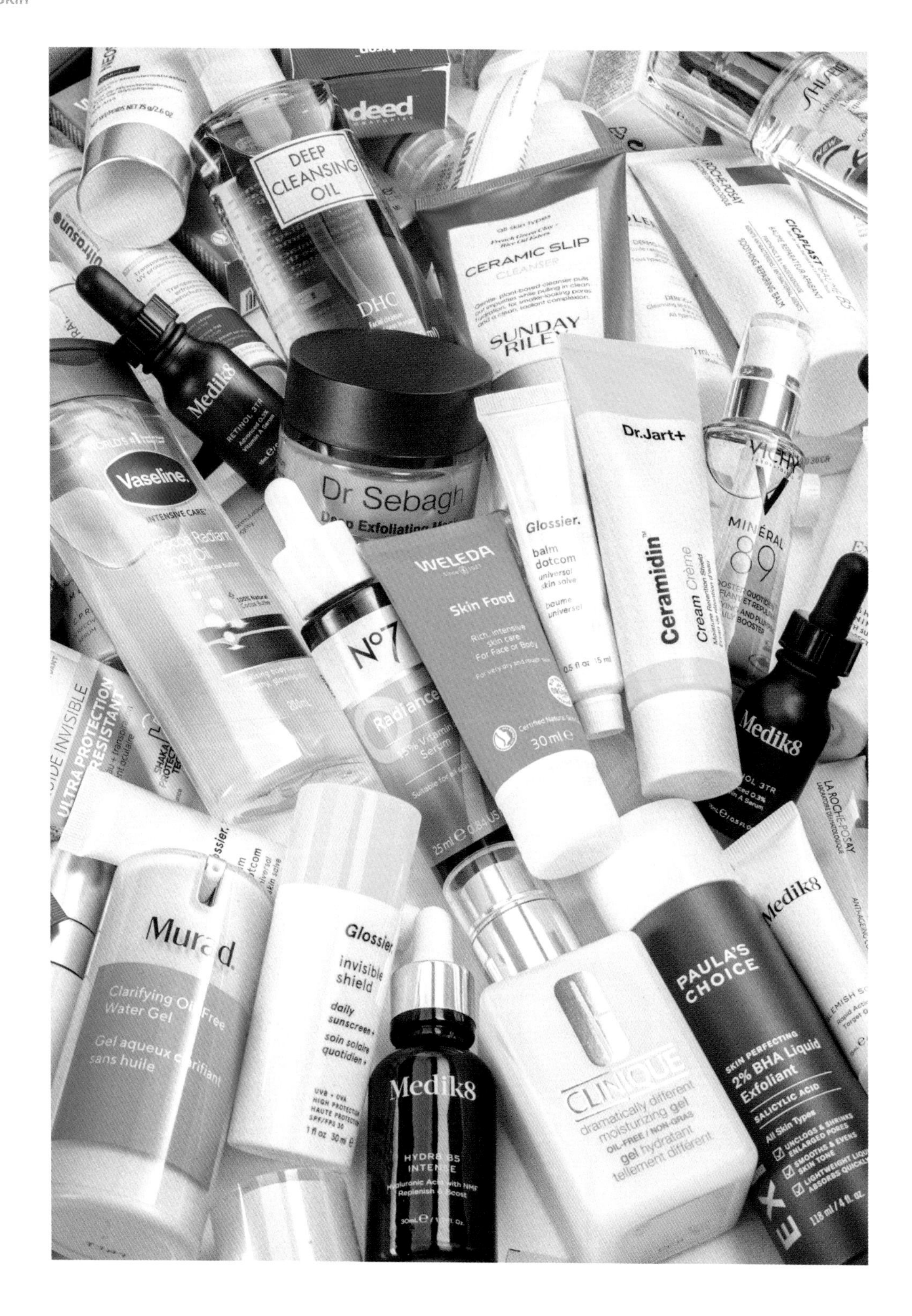
DEEP
CLEANSING
OIL
DHC
CERAMIC SLIP
CLEANSER
SUNDAY
RILEY
CICAPLAST BAUME B5
SOOTHING REPAIRING BALM
Medik8
RETINOL 3TR
Vaseline
INTENSIVE CARE
Dr Sebagh
Dr.Jart+
Ceramidin
Cream Crème
Glossier.
balm
dotcom
universal
skin salve
baume
universel
0.5 fl oz 15 ml
WELEDA
Skin Food
Rich, intensive
skin care
For Face or Body
30ml
No7
Radiance
VICHY
MINÉRAL
89
ULTRA PROTECTION
RESISTANT
LA ROCHE-POSAY
Murad.
Clarifying Oil-Free
Water Gel
Gel aqueux clarifiant
sans huile
Glossier.
invisible
shield
daily
sunscreen+
soin solaire
quotidien+
1 fl oz 30 ml
Medik8
HYDR8 B5
INTENSE
CLINIQUE
dramatically different
moisturizing gel
OIL-FREE / NON-GRAS
gel hydratant
tellement différent
PAULA'S
CHOICE
SKIN PERFECTING
2% BHA Liquid
Exfoliant
SALICYLIC ACID
All Skin Types
118 ml / 4 fl. oz.

moisturisers

- **Murad Clarifying Oil Free Water Gel.** Lightweight moisture without greasiness. Oily skin types often skip moisturiser for fear of turning into an oil slick and developing more spots. This is the perfect antidote, with salicylic acid to control oil and Korean red pine extract that disrupts bacteria to prevent spots.

- **SkinBetter Science Trio Rebalancing Moisturising Treatment.** This has all the big guns to settle the driest of skin, especially mature or menopausal skin that tends to be naturally dry, hence why this is more a treatment and not a regular schmegular moisturiser. It has the same elements that make up the skin's natural moisture system, but super-amped.

- **The Ordinary Natural Moisturising Factors + HA.** Basically, everything that makes up and keeps the surface of our skin healthy: amino acids, fatty acids, triglycerides, urea, ceramides, glycerine, hyaluronic acid, and more, in one tube. I like this for the teens just starting out on their skincare journey.

- **Clinique Dramatically Different Moisturising Lotion+.** An icon in the skincare world and a steadying hand that you can always depend on to moisturise and balance the skin. Does what it says it will do and, with the addition of the gel option, even oilier skin types get a look-in.

- **Tatcha Silk Cream.** A desert island moisturiser. It has a lush lightweight gel texture and is made with liquid silk proteins similar to the protein structures of our skin. I have been through countless pots and if it came to it I would shamelessly fight for the last one!

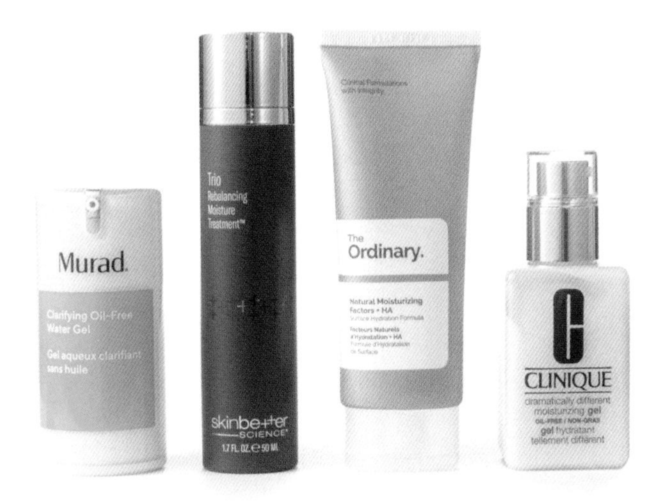

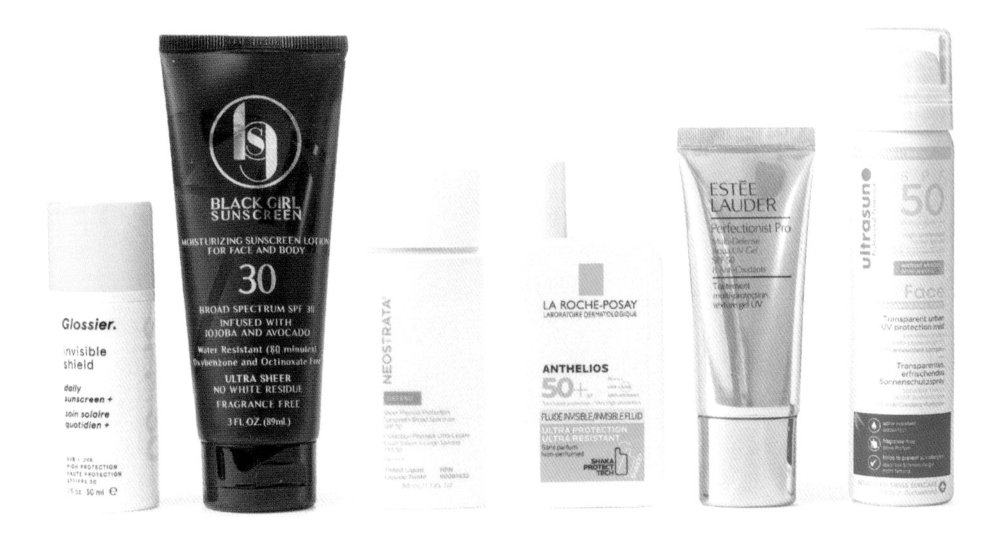

sun protection

- **Glossier Invisible Shield Daily Sunscreen SPF30.** My only complaint is that this doesn't come in a bigger bottle, but there is nothing to not like here. It's light, it's colour- and streak-free, and plays well with make-up.

- **Black Girl Sunscreen SPF30.** For us, by us, and infused with nourishing ingredients such as avocado, jojoba and sunflower oils and vitamin C. The finish is flawless – and Black women did that!

- **Ultra Violette Supreme Screen SPF50.** No white cast, superior protection (it's an Australian brand and we know how stringent they are with sun protection), very moisturising, easy to apply. Ticks all boxes from combination skin to normal skin. Also a good primer underneath make-up. Still yet to meet anyone who's not a fan.

- **NeoStrata Defend Sheer Physical Protection SPF50.** This is a physical sunscreen that does leave a subtle white chalk-like cast on the skin, which is easily covered up with make-up. But boy, does it act as a primer, and literally cements your look into place! I love it for that alone, and if I want budge-proof make-up, this is my go-to.

- **La Roche-Posay Anthelios Ultra-Light Invisible Fluid SPF50.** Accessible on every high street and well formulated. I actually prefer the tinted version, which is a sheer peach but the colour perks up Black skin and isn't noticeable under make-up.

- **Estée Lauder Perfectionist Pro Multi-Defence Aqua UV Gel SPF50.** I actually look forward to using this; I can only describe it as lightweight, lush, and easily layered with other items in your routine. It's so lovely to use that the sunscreen element is simply a bonus.

- **Ultrasun UV Face & Scalp Mist SPF50.** It's so hard to find a decent sunscreen to top up with during the day; no one likes the faff of re-applying, so Ultrasun has rescued us with an easy-to-use hygienic mist that you can also use on your centre parting. Stick it in your handbag and go.

facial oils

In the main, I very rarely use facial oils, neither do I recommend them freely. But for the odd Sunday skincare session or to protect your skin in extreme cold weather, they are handy. My top picks are:

- **Soho Skin Facial Oil.** This is lightweight and non-oily, meaning it is absorbed effortlessly into your skin. It's also full of antioxidants from the pomegranate and raspberry seed oils. A few drops is all you need to feel totally grounded.

- **Decléor Green Mandarin Aromessence Glow Serum.** Glow becomes me is how I like to think of this oil. My skin and mind feel like I've had a good therapy session. I do my signature facial massage, apply a mask and sit in a hot bath. Bliss.

Side note: all the Decléor oils are expertly formulated and are indulgent treats for your skin. Not to be sniffed at at all.

masks

For someone who famously declared 'I don't do masks' I sure do have a few favourites. In my defence, these are performance masks, not the lie-back-in-the-bathtub types.

- **The Ordinary Salicylic Acid 2 per cent Masque.** This clay-based mask is great for congested and spotty skin, especially younger skin. It can also be used as an overnight spot treatment.
- **Cosmedix Pure Enzymes Cranberry Exfoliating Mask.** If acids aren't for you, then you may want to try this instead. You still get exfoliation but more slowly and without the stress. Add a squirt to your face wash a couple of times a week and leave it on for a few extra seconds for an intensive clean.
- **Beauty Pie Super Pore Detox Mask.** This is super for a reason. The ingredients are comprehensive – glycolic, salicylic and lactic acids, Kaolin Clay, micro-buffing bamboo and natural liquorice and eucalyptus. I use this ahead of any big event to smooth my skin, control oil and shine, and create a flawless base for make-up. Definitely not suitable for sensitive skin types!
- **Dr Sebagh Deep Exfoliating Mask.** One day, almost 10 years ago, my husband woke up with an acute acne breakout that had no rhyme or reason. We used this to coax his skin back to form, and every time I get a slew of spots I use it, too. Azelaic acid and lactic acid are what makes it tick.

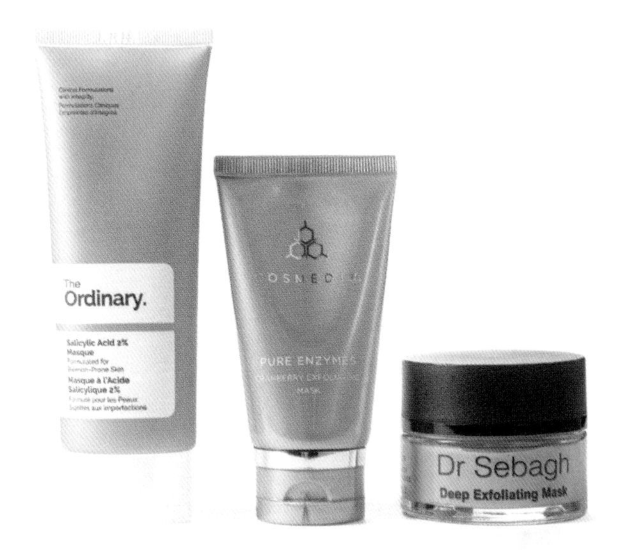

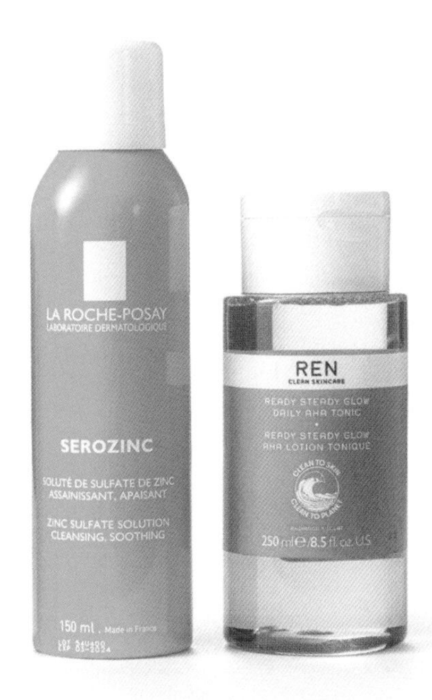

toners

Most times I regard toners as a defunct category, when a lot of their usefulness has been absorbed by other products in your routine. However, these ones actually do something.

- **La Roche-Posay Serozinc Face Toner Mist.** Zinc is highly regarded as a healing mineral, so this is handy for spotty and acne-prone skin. Also backne!
- **REN Ready Steady Glow Daily AHA Tonic.** Is there anyone who hasn't tried this yet? If you don't have many concerns about your skin but want to maintain brightness and glow, this cult classic is it.
- **Paula's Choice Skin Perfecting 2 per cent BHA Liquid Exfoliant.** Great as an extra mattifier for oily skin during periods where you find your skin even oilier, e.g. before or during your period or in the summer months.

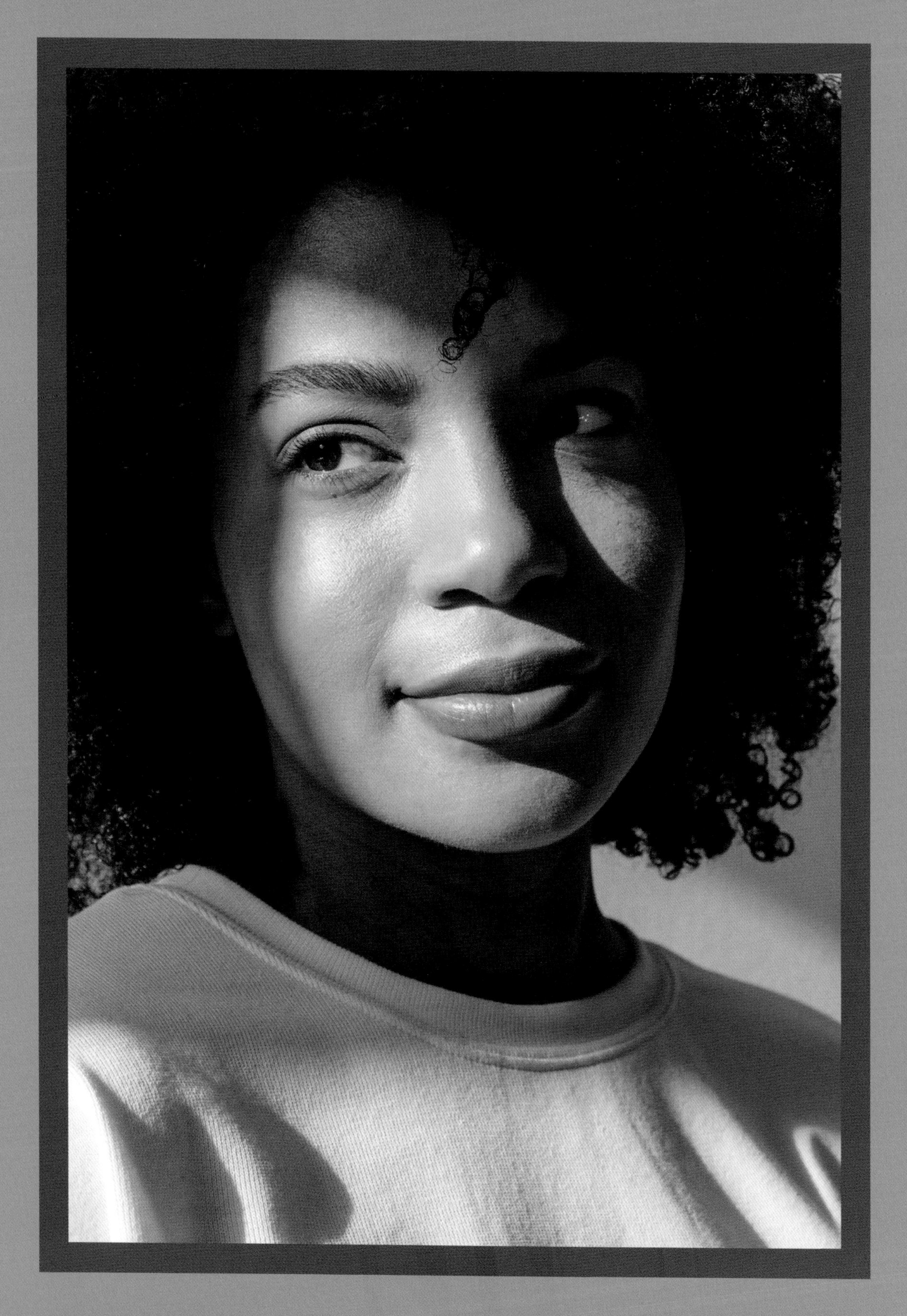

eyes

It's well documented that I'm not the biggest eye cream fan. The skin around the eyes is so tricky, and as many of the concerns have multiple sources it's impossible for one product to provide a total solution.

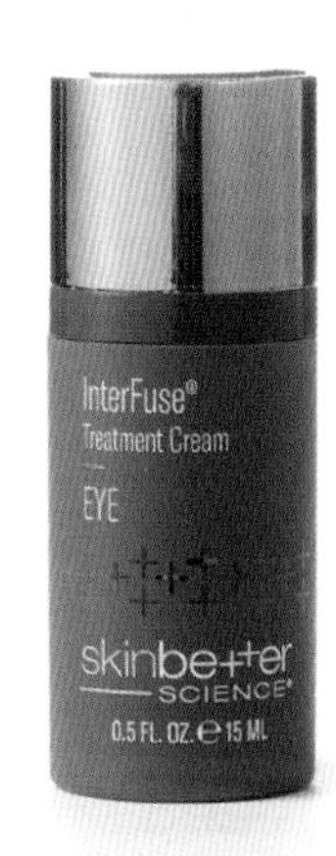

- **SkinBetter Science Interfuse Treatment Cream EYE.** This is the only eye cream I take a bet on. It's an all-rounder, easing the outward signs of crows' feet, reducing puffiness and bags, moisturising and brightening with vitamin C. It's what you call comp-re-hen-sive.
- **EyeMax AlphaRet Overnight Cream.** If you want some retinol firepower in your eye cream, then EyeMax AlphaRet Overnight Cream (also from Skin Better Science) is your best bet.

lips

- **Glossier Balm Dotcom.** A modern classic in tons of flavours, using heavyweight hydrators such as castor oil, beeswax and lanolin for severely dry and chapped lips.
- **Alpha H Absolute Lip Perfector.** This lives on my bedside table and I use it every night to keep my lips smooth, soft and moisturised. Peppermint oil and wild mint also stimulate to plump the lips.
- **Rhode Lip Peptide Treatment.** Everyone is mad for Rhode lip treatments and so am I. I have one in my bathroom, my handbag and my nightstand. The combination of shea butter, cupuaçu, peptides and babassu is a recipe for perfectly long-lasting moisturised lips akin to a soft, plump glazed doughnut.

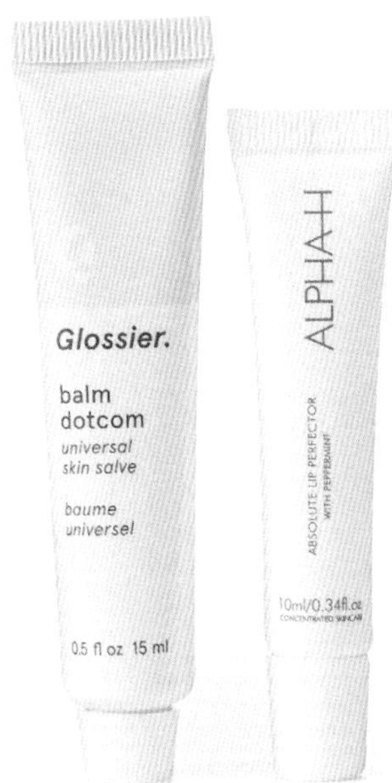

body

- **NeoStrata Problem Dry Skin Cream.** High-strength 20 per cent glycolic acid that quickly solves dry and chapped heels (especially!), elbows and knees. Once tights season is over, I use this for a few weeks and my feet are ready for summer sandals.

- **CeraVe SA Smoothing Cream.** If you have bumpy skin on the back of your arms or thighs, that's keratosis pilaris: a build-up of old skin cells that need exfoliation with salicylic acid. This is your answer. Partner with CeraVe SA Smoothing Cleanser wash for maximum effect.

- **Vaseline Intensive Care Cocoa Radiant Body Gel Oil.** A perfectly textured lightweight gloss for your skin without any of the downsides of a slippery oil. It's best to remember that less is more with this.

- **Dove Body Love Intense Care Body Lotion.** We forget that skin barrier damage can happen all over the body. This everyday lotion goes the extra mile to keeping it intact, focusing on restorative and repairing agents to nourish dry skin. I love that it's easily accessible and purse-friendly too.

- **Cantu Skin Therapy Coconut Oil Hydrating Body Lotion.** All of my best sunny beach holidays delivered in each pump, leaving my skin smelling glorious and moisturised. Shea butter, aloe vera, cocoa butter, jojoba oil – everything good you want in a moisturiser.

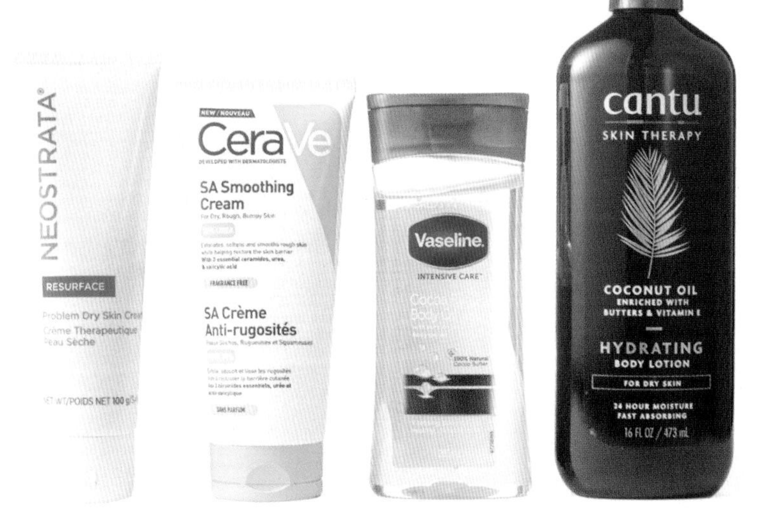

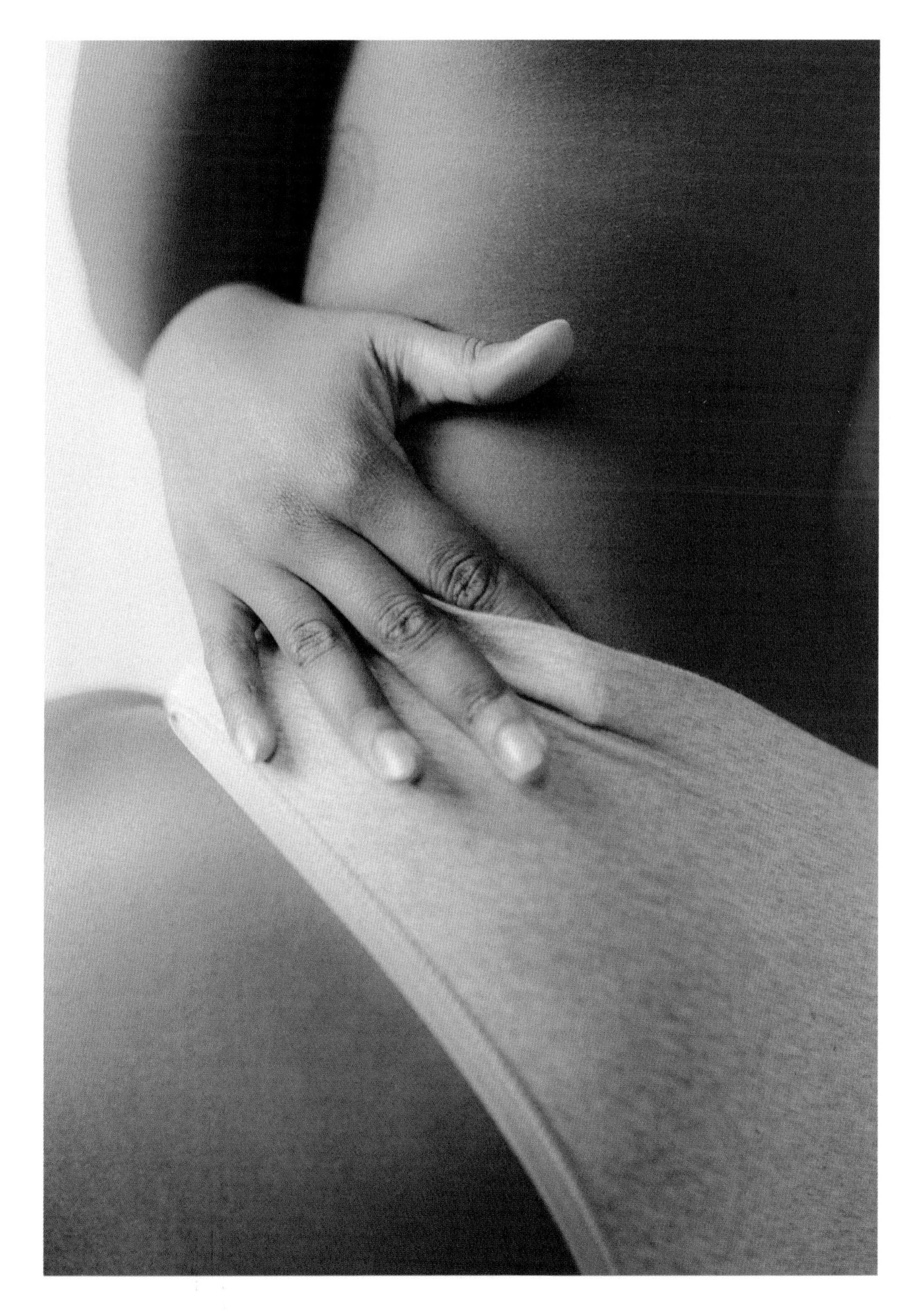

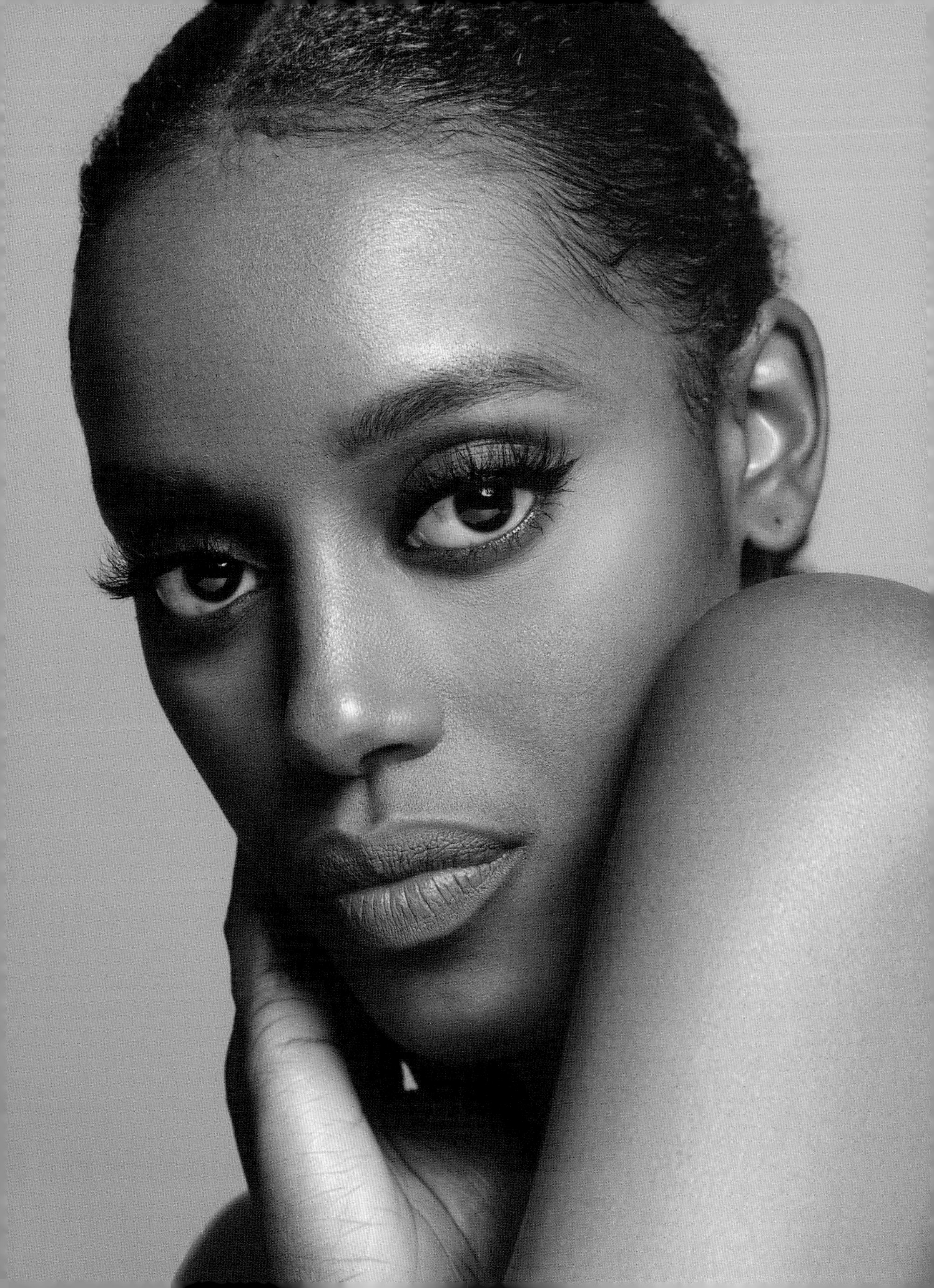

14.

go pro or stay home?

go pro or stay home?

THERE'S no denying that skincare treatments can cost a pretty penny, so naturally you want to make sure you make the right choice about where your hard-earned money should go. On products? On treatments? Or both?

If you're looking for the best results and to have your skin in its best health, then you want to be having both: high-quality in-clinic treatments on a regular basis, as well as using expertly formulated products high in active ingredients at home. There isn't a short cut I'm afraid.

Over the years I have learned that with consistent and diligent use skincare products will get you 80 per cent on the way to achieving skin health, but to get to 100 per cent you must also invest in non-invasive professional skin treatments, such as chemical peeling, micro-needling, light therapy and laser treatment every 4 to 6 weeks. These will do major heavy lifting that home skincare products cannot and will act like a turbo-booster for the skin. The effects and results of injectable treatments last a while longer, so those are only needed quarterly, biannually, or sometimes only yearly.

Seeing a skincare pro will also help keep on top of any issues, trouble-shooting any problems before they occur, especially if you have concerns about hyperpigmentation or the natural ageing process of the face. Whenever I see my aesthetic doctor, we always talk about the tweaks and support my face and skin need now to prevent more major work in the future, and I appreciate her for that. It's about fine tuning as you go along.

Also, as a pro, I can ensure you get more bang for your buck with your products, because each time you attend the clinic our conversation is naturally a mini review. We go through how you're using your products, what you find enjoyable, and what is bothersome, and again we fine tune things to make sure you are getting the most out of your skincare shelf.

The question of affordability comes up frequently because, let's face it, some treatments and products can be pricey. If long-term affordability is a concern, the first thing you should do is book yourself a skin health consultation so you can get the best advice possible. Most practitioners will have their preferred products they stock in their clinics, but they are also familiar with products that suit a variety of budgets. So if you're upfront about your spending power, they will design a plan for you that stays within your budget. I love when clients say, 'I can afford *x* amount every month.' It saves us a lot of time and makes planning so much easier.

In my opinion it is better to have affordable daily-use skincare products than to spend big money on one-off treatments only to then use sub-par products at home, especially if your skin has already started showing signs of ageing. That is a false economy.

'What about at-home professional treatments?' you ask. To be honest, unless you bootleg an actual in-clinic treatment to use at home, there is no such thing as a professional at-home product because, quite simply, the strength and potency will be missing. It's just marketing-speak to get you to hand your card over. The active ingredient(s) would have been buffered to temper their potency as no brand wants any mishaps that could land them in court. When a brand says their product gives you professional results at home it's important to dig a little deeper to find out what that really means, because legally (and morally) unless they've sighted your skin health qualifications, professional kits should not be sold to consumers.

You can tell by now that I don't advocate professional treatments at home, especially when you're doing it as a means of bypassing seeing a professional in clinic. I know there are websites where you can buy professional-strength products containing all manner of concocted ingredients with promises of glowing and flawless skin. I take a dim view of these sites, and the questions I always urge you to bear in mind are: 'Do I know what to do if I experience a reaction to this product?' 'Who can I turn to if I accidentally burn or injure myself?' If you cannot answer these questions, then you shouldn't be buying products aimed at professionals.

One of the chief reasons why professional treatments should be left to the pros is that we are trained to manage complications if you suffer an unexpected reaction. We have the knowledge and training (and remedial products at hand) to know what to do quickly, and how to reassure and advise you on what to do when you get home. Plus, we stay in close contact with you until the issue is resolved.

The bonus on top is that we are also insured, so if you need to sue us (and I pray it never comes to that!), you know we're good for the payout.

choosing a skincare professional

From facialists to dermatologists, there is a skincare professional for every need, but I appreciate that it can get confusing trying to understand and select who you should see. Regardless of who you choose, the bottom line is that they must understand and have experience in treating Black skin and empathise with your concerns. I'd go as far as to say, they must also have some sort of cultural awareness so they can place your concern in the context of your daily life and environment.

Dermatologists

Dermatology is the branch of medicine concerned with the diagnosis and treatment of the three thousand possible diseases affecting the skin, scalp, hair and nails.

Dermatologists are qualified medical doctors who have completed an additional 8 years of post-graduate training to specialise in this field, earning themselves the grand title of Consultant Dermatologist. That's 14 years' worth of training and education, so they sit at the top of the skin-health pyramid. They are qualified to work with a whole range of patients, from new-born babies to the elderly, and are usually based in hospitals or their own private practices. They provide skin consultations and can treat a range of conditions including skin cancer (big, big part of their job!), moles, eczema, psoriasis, rosacea and acne.

Speaking to my hospital-based dermatologist friends and colleagues I realise that a big focus of their role is cancer care and prevention. This really impacts on their time and it unfortunately means that cosmetic skincare concerns fall down the priority list. Lately, though, there is a new crop of dermatologists coming through who have an interest in cosmetic skincare and who practise non-medical aesthetics too, performing an extensive range of cosmetic treatments such as peels, laser therapy, intense light therapy (IPL), Botox and dermal fillers.

FACT Dermatologists and aesthetic doctors must be registered on the General Medical Council (GMC) register. Nurses must be registered on the Nursing and Midwifery Council (NMC) register. Both these registers are in the public record and it's good practice to check your pro's professional record.

Beauty therapists

Qualified to do it all – waxing, nails and facials, eyebrows, tanning – they are your beauty generalists that you will find in your local high street salons and spas.

Aesthetic practitioners – doctors and nurses

Aesthetic medicine is an umbrella term to describe practices that focus on improving cosmetic appearance. Qualified medical doctors and dentists are able to enter this field immediately post medical degree. Nurses must have a minimum of three years' general adult nursing experience and hold a prescribing qualification. Some practitioners may also have a post-graduate qualification in aesthetic medicine.

Aesthetic practitioners perform a variety of minimally invasive and non-invasive treatments, including injectables like Botox and dermal fillers. The patient base is mainly adults, and they would usually refer complex or sinister skin-health cases to a dermatologist.

Most aesthetic practitioners have their own private practice or work within a medi-spa environment.

Aestheticians (in some circles referred to as facialists)

Aestheticians like me are skin specialists who are trained to address skin disorders holistically. We undergo extensive training focused only on skin health, usually in the form of a Level 4 diploma, after completing basic broad beauty therapy qualifications.

This additional training can take up to 2 years to complete and provides in-depth knowledge about the skin's anatomy, physiology and microbiology, alongside skincare ingredients and how medical conditions, nutrition and lifestyle contribute to overall skin health. We work privately in our own clinics or in salons and medical practices alongside dermatologists to help you look after your skin on a daily basis, develop an effective skincare routine, and choose the right skincare products. We also perform a variety of treatments from chemical peels to laser, and we point you in the right direction if you need more intervention.

I'm biased, but a good aesthetician is worth their weight in gold and can keep you and your skin happy and healthy for a long time. We are the lynchpins that connect you to other aspects and people within the beauty industry, because a good aesthetician will have an extensive list of other professionals in their network.

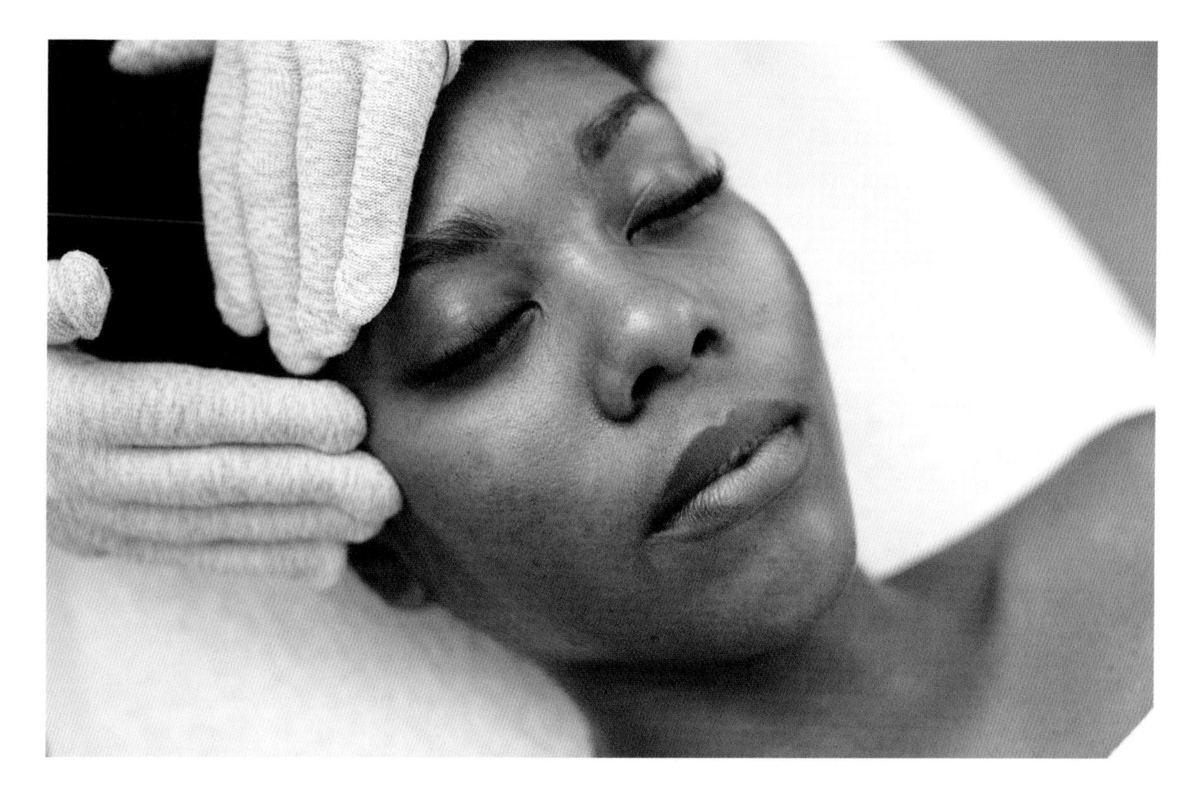

There's always some level of overlap, but if you're trying to decide who you should book in with:

- For a quick pick-me-up for an instant fresh-faced glow, your best bet is a beauty therapist, who will also do lots of blissful massage.
- To address skin conditions like acne, rosacea, pigmentation and scarring, start with your aesthetician, who can give you a comprehensive view of what's happening to your skin and/or refer you to a dermatologist for more intensive treatment if needed.
- If you want to make structural cosmetic changes to your face and body, e.g. more definition in your lips, reshaping your nose, smoothing out wrinkles, go to an aesthetic practitioner.
- If you have a mole or scar that is constantly weeping or crusting, difficult to treat or heal, then heading straight to a dermatologist for further investigation is the best action you can take. The same goes for any chronic and acute skin conditions that you can't seem to resolve: see a derm.

Price points will always vary amongst professionals depending on where they are located: London will cost more than Sheffield; Harley Street will cost more than Tottenham – simple economics. Professional standing, level of expertise and experience will also make a difference. This is why it's good to have a consultation with a number of practitioners before committing to anything. With professional skincare you tend to get what you pay for – and cutting corners just to save a few pounds usually backfires and costs you more in the long run to put right.

WORD OF WARNING

Shockingly, there are no rules preventing Ronke from down the road from attending a one-day injectable course and then setting up shop to fill lips and whatever else she feels like. Trust me when I say she has no idea of the blood and nerve network of the face, and also – seeing as some injectables are only available on prescription – God only knows the back of which truck they came from.

Please only use reputable and registered practitioners (check the registers) for your injectables treatments. Whilst I sometimes gripe that they may not always have the highest and most in-depth skincare knowledge, I know for certain they have the physiological and anatomical knowledge to be able to treat you successfully – i.e., without the potential of disfiguring you or, worse, killing you, and they know what to do if things don't go as planned and you experience a complication.

Put your smarts on when considering injectables; it can be the difference between blindness, disfigurement, life and death.

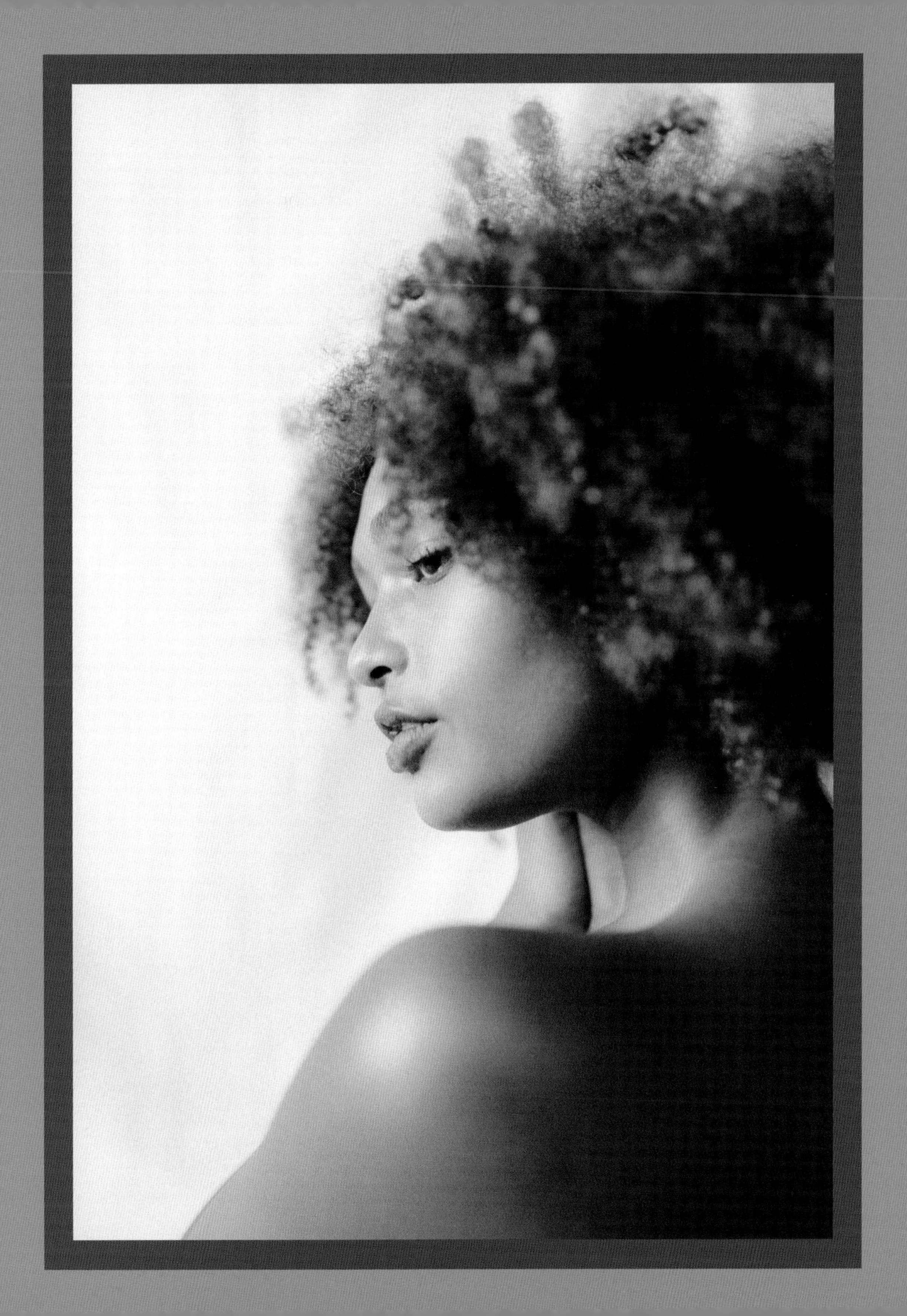

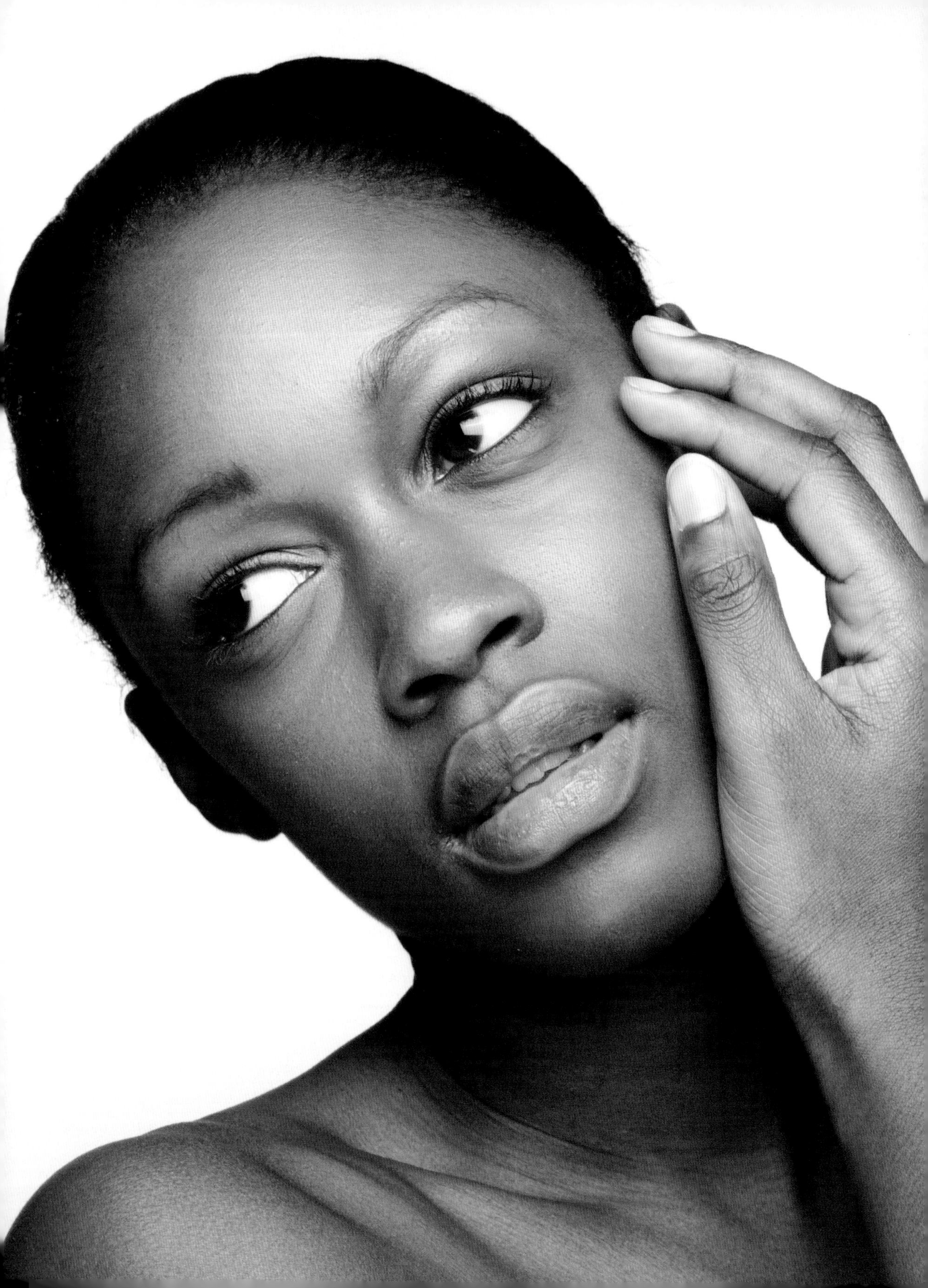

treatments

15.

treatments

IN my experience, most Black women are wary of treatments. This is completely understandable and there are lots of reasons for this, including that treatments have never really been specifically advertised or marketed to Black women, so we have been left out of the conversation and lack the necessary knowledge to make a decision on the suitability of treatments. People tend to be apprehensive of the unknown, so this wariness makes sense. On top of this, many clinics can be reluctant to treat darker skin tones and turn clients away because they themselves lack the appropriate knowledge, practical hands-on experience and confidence to treat Black skin safely. There is a general unfounded fear that dark skin is problematic to treat with advanced procedures, which creates a vicious circle that only results in one thing: Black women are unable to access treatments in the same capacity as white women.

There is a general unfounded fear that dark skin is problematic to treat with advanced procedures.

We also have the issue of brands that don't clinically trial or consumer trial their products, ingredients and treatments on darker skin tones. They either infer that the treatment would be suitable based on results they've seen on lighter skin tones, or they say the treatment isn't suitable (without having even tried because, at the end of the day, no one wants a lawsuit on their hands). We know that there is a small number of treatments that would be unsafe and unsuccessful for Black skin, so there is very little need to trial these, but that is no excuse not to include Black skin in the majority of trials. I make it a point at my clinic – West Room Aesthetics – to only partner with brands that have evidence of their product or treatment performance on Black skin. I also set up Black Skin Directory to highlight clinics and practitioners who support this ethos and are experienced and confident in treating Black skin.

The amount of leg work and anxiety that Black women face as consumers in the beauty world is considerably higher than white consumers because we have been subjected to so many myths, we just don't know what and who to believe. This is something I can personally testify to, so I know it helps massively if you have some idea of the different types of treatments out there. This takes away some of the fear and uncertainty and you can play a more confident and active role in the management of your skin concerns.

It's great that new treatments are introduced all the time, but the standard repertoire also delivers outstanding results on Black skin and I hope this final chapter will give you more faith and confidence to explore advanced skincare treatments.

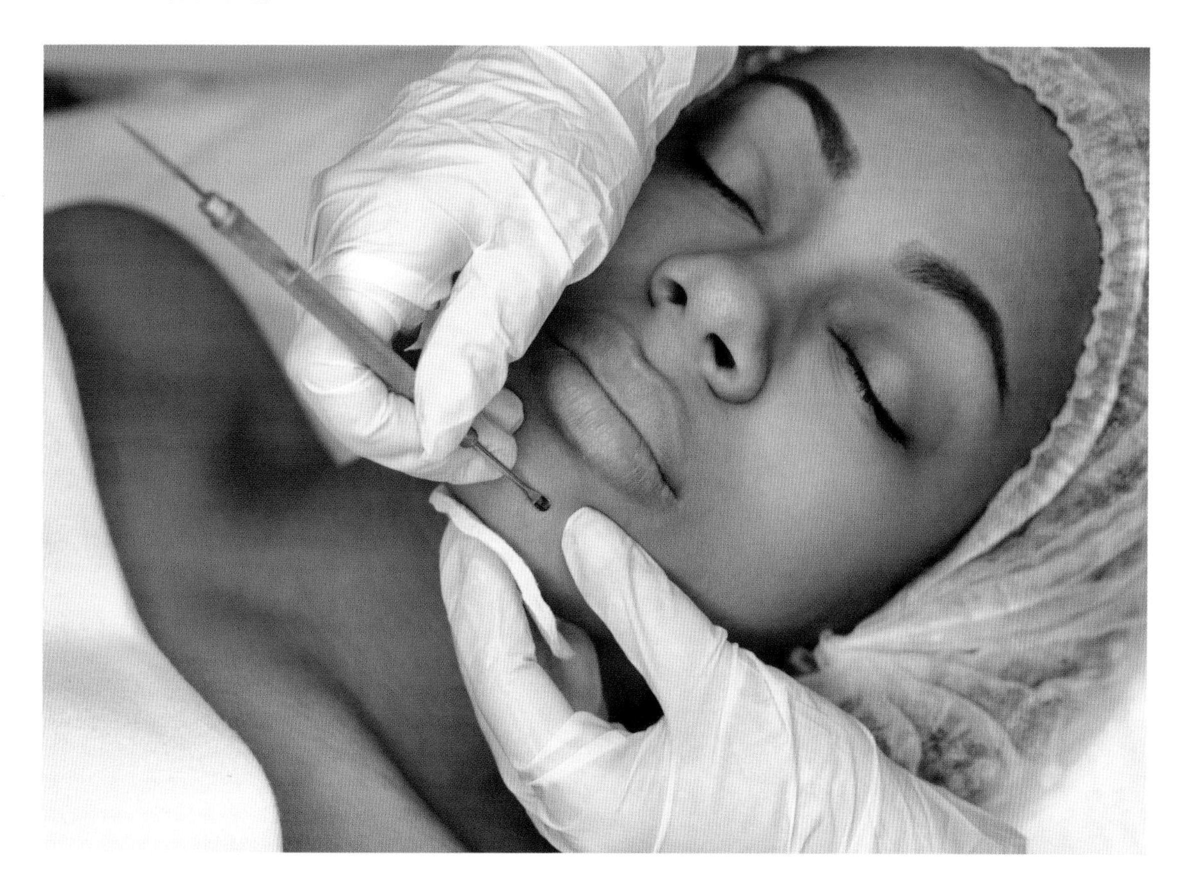

chemical peels

These are the workhorses of the skincare industry because they are so versatile and can be tailored to suit every skin tone and skin type easily. It is hands-down my favourite treatment to give and receive, as the results are visible anything from immediately to just a few days later. Although we use much more advanced ingredients now, chemical peels have been going for millennia: Cleopatra used to bathe in asses' milk to smooth and brighten her skin, milk being a source of lactic acid and therefore an exfoliant.

I find that once clients get over their initial fear and apprehension, they are always impressed by the instant improvement in their skin. Everyone seems to remember the *Sex and the City* storyline when Samantha Jones had a chemical peel and ended up looking red raw.

Chemical peels are suitable for all types of skin conditions, from acne and hyperpigmentation to scarring and even rosacea. Their function is to improve your overall skin condition. They also decongest and remove oil from your pores, so not only is pore size minimised but you have improved oil control. Peels stimulate collagen and hydration too, so your skin is plumper and firmer, and help to fade hyperpigmentation and dark marks so your overall skin tone is evened out.

Chemical peels are really a jack-of-all-trades treatment and it is easy to see why they are a favourite as they tick so many boxes. The normal pH value of the skin is 5.5, which is slightly acidic, and for a chemical peel to be effective it must have an even lower pH. In clinic for professional treatments this can be anything from pH 0.6 to 1.6. This is what powers the peel to loosen the bonds that hold old skin cells together so they can be shed from the surface of the skin, revealing new, fresher and healthier skin underneath.

The main acids used for chemical peels are glycolic, lactic, mandelic and azelaic acid. Citric acid is sometimes included to boost the strength of the peel; salicylic acid also features if the peel is designed for an oily skin type. Retinoids are also used for chemical peels and can be used successfully on darker skin tones. They give a slightly deeper peel with visible skin shedding, but when done properly the results are outstanding.

Chemical peels come in three main categories: superficial, medium and deep.

Superficial peels sometimes also called light peels or lunchtime peels, are the gentlest. They work on the upper layers of the epidermis and they are ideal for brightening the skin, boosting radiance, improving clarity, controlling oil and breakouts, and shrinking pore size.

Medium peels are a bit more intensive and they penetrate a bit deeper into the skin, but they are great for stimulating collagen for firmer skin, treating mild to moderate acne, and softening lines and wrinkles. You may require a few days of downtime to recover in peace and privacy.

Both superficial and medium peels are fine for Black skin and can be used safely for skin health and rejuvenation.

Deep peels are intense, delivering very dramatic improvements and changes to the skin. Due to the intensity and the depths that deep peels can go to, you only need one treatment. Deep peels are notable because they use phenol and croton oil (which, by the way, can be poisonous in inexperienced hands) to instigate the burning and peeling in the skin to literally erase wrinkles, dark marks and other signs of ageing. They are definitely unsuitable for Black skin and can lead to all manner of hyperpigmentation and hypopigmentation problems.

We tend to have an image in our heads that a chemical peel will initiate some sort of snake-like shedding of the skin, and that couldn't be further from the truth. It's nothing that dramatic – mostly you get tightness, dryness and localised 'skin dandruff' perhaps around the nose or chin. Deeper peels will cause more visible flaking of the skin.

On Black skin my preference is for 4–6-weekly superficial or medium peels that keep the skin in good nick across the year, rather than the sledgehammer approach of one-off deep peels. It is also important to prepare the skin before a chemical peel and you won't catch me doing a chemical peel on your first visit. A prep time of 3–4 weeks using similar ingredients and acids to the peels will acclimatise your skin so that it tolerates the treatment, saving you potential issues of irritation and hyperpigmentation.

After a peel your skin can take anything between 5 and 10 days to fully heal. Moisturiser is your friend and now is the time to slather your skin, keeping it juicy and well hydrated. It is crucial to apply sunscreen liberally too to protect your skin as it will be more vulnerable and delicate. Wide-brimmed hats and sunnies are also good investments to protect your skin from unnecessary sun, especially in the summer. The more consistent you are with your peels, the shorter the healing time as your skin develops strength and resilience. Sounds like a lot but the results are well worth it!

Enzyme peels

These are a gentler alternative to acid-based chemical peels that will give some results, but nothing as dramatic or as quick. The main agent is usually a fruit enzyme such as papaya, pumpkin, pomegranate or pineapple, and through enzymatic action the bonds that hold old skin cells together are dissolved so that exfoliation can occur. If you cannot tolerate acids, they are a good option.

> **Both superficial and medium peels are fine for Black skin and can be used safely for skin health and rejuvenation.**

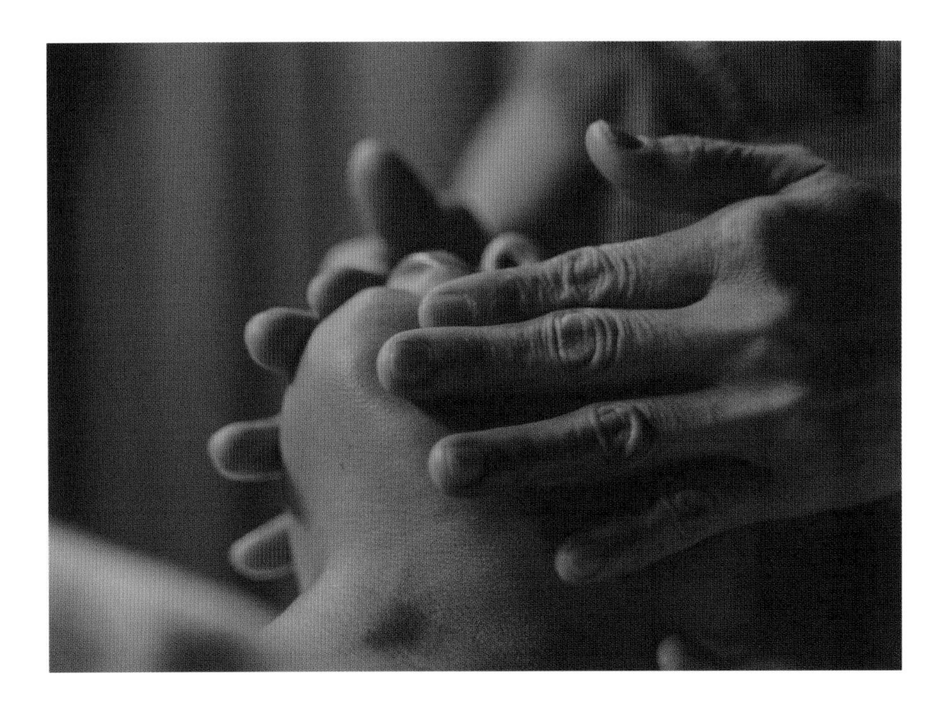

laser and intense pulse light (IPL)

Laser treatments are also often viewed with scepticism. Everyone knows someone who's been told that lasers are not suitable for Black skin, that they will cause burns and result in hyperpigmentation. Yes, that is true (and can happen to any skin colour, to be honest, not just Black skin), but it's not true that lasers are not suitable for Black skin; it simply all depends on the type of laser and the practitioner wielding the wand.

Lasers work on the principle of wavelengths and using concentrated beams of light, aka energy, on the skin to address specific concerns. Up until about 20 years ago, lasers had a really bad reputation because they just weren't suitable for Black skin – they didn't have the wavelength range or sophistication to treat dark skin. They primarily worked on the principle of the light beam being attracted to a dark spot (or hair) on a light surface, so they were literally unable to distinguish between a dark spot on Black skin, or a Black hair on Black skin. Also, melanin itself proved to be a hindrance as it would absorb the light and convert it into heat, leading to blisters, burns, scarring and discolouration. Additionally, melanin would also reduce the intensity of the light beam, reducing the efficacy of the treatment and making it time consuming and expensive. Easy to see and understand why Black women tread carefully around talk of laser treatments!

Over the last 10 years, lasers have come on in leaps and bounds and are much more versatile and advanced, so Black women and other darker skin tones can now get a look-in. They have longer wavelengths, longer pulse durations and more efficient cooling devices that prevent heat accumulation. The light beam is more controlled and more slowly deposited in the skin, all in all reducing the likelihood of injury. Some laser beams will see black/brown pigment, which will address hyperpigmentation and hair removal; some will see red, which is great for treating thread veins. For some it's more about focusing the energy in particular areas of the skin to stimulate collagen or maybe tackle an overactive sebaceous gland that is producing excess oil.

> Lasers have come on in leaps and bounds and are much more versatile and advanced, so Black women and other darker skin tones can now get a look-in.

Lasers are suitable for treating a variety of skin conditions: overall skin rejuvenation, where they stimulate collagen to keep the skin plump and bouncy; tackling acne by helping to kill bacteria, temporarily shrinking oil glands and tightening pores; easing and soothing rosacea-prone skin; and destroying excess melanin pigment for clearer skin. They help to build the strength and resiliency of the skin whilst slowing down signs of premature ageing such as wrinkles and fine lines.

FACT Laser treatment is not a permanent form of hair removal; it is for hair reduction, and you will need top-up sessions once or twice a year to maintain hair free results.

Facial hair can be annoying for some women (me included) and lasers are a godsend, providing a long-term solution and saving hours of plucking, threading, tweezing and shaving. The laser beam destroys the hair bulb to stunt hair growth.

FACT There are two types of lasers: ablative lasers, such as Fraxel and CO_2, resurface by targeting the top layer of skin and peeling it off. These are not great for Black skin, avoid, avoid, avoid! Non-ablative lasers do deep work targeting specific concerns without peeling or troubling the top layer of skin.

For Black men in particular lasers can bring relief from conditions such as pseudofolliculitis barbae (razor bumps) on the cheeks or lower neck area, and acne keloidalis nuchae, usually on the nape, when hair follicles become infected, leading to hyperpigmented scarring and keloids.

Whilst laser treatment can occasionally be used as a quick fix that gives dramatic results, especially if you have a big event ahead, they are best viewed as a long-term addition to your professional treatments. That is why they are usually sold as a course of anything from 6 to 10 sessions, especially if it's for hair removal. This time allows the practitioner to err on the side of caution, treat the skin without any aggression, and allow for sufficient healing between appointments.

The best laser technology for Black skin is the Nd:YAG. When you ask a clinic what laser they use and they don't mention the Nd:YAG, it is OK to run for the hills. Jest aside, remember that even when using the Nd:YAG, which has a high tolerability for Black skin, you must have a patch test at least 48 hours before the actual treatment.

Intense pulse light

Or IPL for short. This is quite different to a laser but very often the two things are mixed up. This treatment is definitely less suited to Black skin because it is based on the principle of using multiple scattered light beams (remember that lasers use only one light). This light scatter creates an extra energy capability that is difficult to control and target in Black skin, ultimately damaging the skin by causing burning and discolouration.

Psst… A bit more on patch tests

Also ask for a new patch test if you've been on holiday, because a simple thing like a tan will change your skin colour, albeit temporarily, but the device settings must be adjusted to prevent injury.

micro-needling/dermal rolling

I've yet to meet the client who doesn't pull a face when I suggest micro-needling as a treatment option, and I can totally understand why – it's needles! On your face! Most of us are barely tolerant of one needle going into our arm, let alone hundreds of needles in the most public-facing part of the body. I also find that Black women tend to be apprehensive, squirming in fear when I pick up the micro-needling device. But, honestly, there is nothing to fear. Micro-needling (sometimes called collagen induction treatment) is a brilliant skin-rejuvenating treatment and very safe for Black skin when done by a competent practitioner.

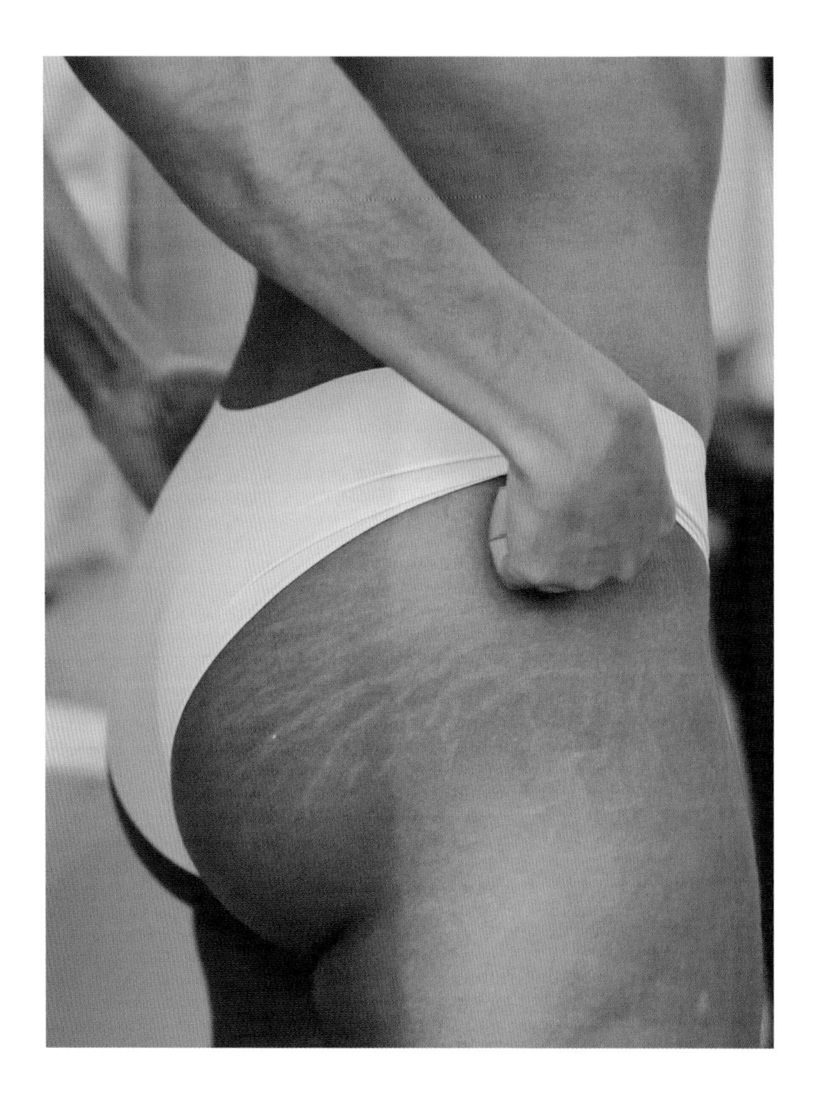

Micro-needling involves using very short and extremely thin but densely packed needles, arranged in a neat pattern, to pierce the skin and create shallow micro-wounds. The needle lengths can range from anything from 0.25mm to 3mm. The shallower needles are great for improving product absorption into the upper layers of skin so that you have the appearance of healthy, revitalised skin. Longer needles can do anything from reduce scarring (in particular, the type of uneven and bumpy scarring you get from acne) and hyperpigmentation to removing wrinkles and stimulating collagen so that the skin feels plumper, firmer, and more radiant. Micro-needling can also be done on the body to tackle stretch marks, and on the hands to refresh and revive them.

On Black skin the shallower the needle the better. Longer needles can injure the skin, which will cause hyperpigmentation. SkinPen and Dermapen are popular advanced mechanical devices you'll find in clinics, but it's also common to see derma-rollers which are manually operated.

Personally, I don't think micro-needling is painful, but for your comfort a numbing cream can be applied to the skin about 30 minutes before the treatment, just to take the edge off. Like most advanced treatments, you will always need more than one session to really see the benefits and any long-lasting gains for the skin.

WORD OF WARNING

Be wary of home-use micro-needling devices. For starters, the needles are usually either too short to penetrate the skin for any beneficial effect, so you'll unconsciously (or maybe even consciously) press harder into your skin and end up wounding yourself. Likewise, the needles may also be too long and will therefore penetrate too deeply, causing significant injury. Both scenarios will lead to post-inflammatory hyperpigmentation!

These tools can also become breeding grounds for bacteria and viruses. No matter how clean you are, if you are unable to sterilise to clinic standards, each time you use your micro-needle, you're leaving yourself vulnerable to infections.

micro-current

If you think of your facial muscles and skin cells as mini mobile phones that lose power over time, then micro-current treatment is the charger. It brings your skin back to life in the most stunning way, by stimulating your muscles and skin cells using small charges of electrical current that encourage healing and recovery.

There are 43 muscles in the face and, over time, they get weaker as their tone and structure change; micro-current is a great treatment for improving muscle firmness at any age and also for generally improving the vitality of the skin. As we age, the skin cells become sluggish and less active, collagen and elastin production slow down as well. Micro-current gives these processes a kick up the backside. Well-cited studies by Dr. Emil Y. Chi at the University of Washington's department of pathology in 2003 showed that collagen can be boosted by up to 10 per cent, elastin by 45 per cent and blood circulation by 40 per cent.[19]

It's a totally pain-free procedure. How it works is that dual-pronged wands are passed over your skin and they gently send electric waves through the skin to stimulate lazy muscles and energise the cells. The results are visible and immediate: facial muscles are tighter, and the lift to the skin is noticeable. There is more definition to your jawline, the cheeks are inflated, and eyebrows are more pronounced. The best way to describe it is that it feels like your face is higher on your head. Micro-current = mini face lift.

Another effect of the treatment is that it helps your body remove toxins and waste fluid faster, and this really wakes up your face, giving you the ARB effect – alert, radiant and brighter! Additionally, our skin cells are dependent on an energy system called adenosine triphosphate (ATP), which also depletes with age. Micro-current turbo-boosts ATP by 500 per cent,[20] making it work more efficiently to respond to cellular damage quickly.

I like to include micro-current in as many treatments as possible, especially if you have a big event coming up. It's great as a course of weekly treatments or just included in your standard monthly professional visit. Its benefits are endless, it perks up your skin and, long after you've hopped off the treatment couch, you'll find your products are working harder for your skin and delivering better results because micro-current increases their absorption rate so they can penetrate your skin better.

led light therapy

I love Light Emitting Diode (LED) treatments so much that I include it as standard in all our in-clinic treatments to finish off the service, accelerate healing and soothe the skin. After all, it's a Nobel Prize-winning technology.

Advanced treatments tend to aggravate the skin in some way, in order to instigate the healing process that strengthens the skin; LED is a super effective way of helping that healing process along. In addition, it calms inflammation, zaps bacteria, helps to fade pigmentation, temporarily shrinks pore size, improves skin texture, boosts the vitality of the skin and guards against environmental damage. Phew! The benefits are actually endless.

FACT The red light is for stimulating a healing response in the skin and boosting collagen, and the blue light is great for killing bacteria. Lastly, the green light plays a role in reducing melanin production, helping to prevent hyperpigmentation and dark marks forming.

The LED device, such as Dermalux or LightStim, is made of a panel of red and blue bulbs positioned a few inches above your skin during the treatment. It can feel claustrophobic, so if you're scared of being in small spaces, do speak up. The lights are very bright, so protective goggles are needed, but essentially your skin cells absorb the lights' energy to repair damage and improve your skin's healing response. Additionally, there are increased flows of blood and oxygen, which boost your natural glow. A massive bonus is that you can use LED treatment on any part of the body.

Whilst LED has only become popular in facial treatments in the last 10 years or so, the science and the technology have their origins in the nineteenth century. In fact, it was the ancient Greeks who first recorded the healing properties of light, in 1500 BC. We're all familiar with how a few minutes soaking up the sun's rays can improve our mood and heal certain skin conditions. I certainly remember as a child my grandmother saying '*mek san wam am*' (Creole for 'put her under the sun') if I had a rash or some skin complaint. I guess to a certain extent sunlight will always be seen as restorative.

Although small in size, some studies have shown that blue light kills bacteria in oily/blemish-prone skin, so it's great to include LED in the treatment plan for current acne complaints, and to prevent further breakouts.

'Are at-home LED devices safe?' Yes, you can't really overdo LED, and home devices are a great way to boost the skin in between clinic visits; if you can make the investment in an approved home-use unit then go for it. There are many out there, but I like the faceLITE Led Mask, which has a flexible lightweight fit on the face. If you're flush with cash, the Dermalux Flex is a fantastic option because you can use it on the face and body. I've seen it work wonders on sprained ankles and sore backs as much as on the face.

I do stress purchasing from a reputable brand, because if the LED lights have been calibrated poorly, at best there's no effect on your skin but at worst they can exacerbate issues like hyperpigmentation.

high frequency

This is an 'oldie but goodie' treatment for treating acne and breakouts, enlarged pores, fine lines and wrinkles, puffy eyes and, in some cases, thinning hair. There are still quite a few places that include it in their clinic programmes.

A glass electrode (a wand really) is run over the face and, when it is in contact with the skin, a mild electrical current passes through the gas (usually neon or argon) in the electrode. During the treatment, which usually lasts about 20 minutes or so (longer when combined with other procedures), your skin will feel warm, and this creates an antibacterial effect that cleans and purifies whilst also enriching your skin with nutrients and hydration. Blood circulation is improved, collagen is boosted, and the skin looks rejuvenated and softer even after only one treatment.

With the talk of electrical current, glass and gas, it's easy to imagine this is a scary treatment. It's really quite safe and gentle, and the bonus is that there isn't any down time.

mesotherapy

Mesotherapy is the secret to improving dull and tired skin by pushing a rejuvenating concoction of vitamins, minerals and amino acids into the deeper layers of the skin. It's usually done after or alongside micro-needling, because there are already open channels in the skin to allow the concoction to penetrate.

The treatment also has benefits for pigmentation concerns, acne scarring, fine lines and wrinkles, and, interestingly, it can also stimulate hair growth and so is a good option for thinning hair lines. Mesotherapy is suitable for Black skin, but as with any treatments which involve controlled trauma to the skin, it is important to see a competent and experienced practitioner to minimise any potential post-treatment inflammation and hyperpigmentation.

platelet-rich plasma (PRP) therapy

PRP is a well-known treatment popularised by the Kardashian girls as 'the vampire facial' because, without mincing any words, it can be quite bloody. Gore aside, it's a powerful rejuvenating treatment that stimulates the body to go into repair-and-rebuild mode.

It involves taking a small sample of your blood, running it through a machine called a centrifuge that separates the blood into two parts – the red blood cells and the plasma, which is rich in proteins and stimulating growth factors. It's the plasma that is carefully injected into damaged skin to accelerate healing along with increasing collagen production and connective tissue formation, leading to skin tightening and overall rejuvenation.

Sometimes a micro-needling device is used to inject the plasma into your skin. The whole process takes about 45 minutes and has real benefits for skin texture and tone. Results last several months. If you have a few treatments, the results can last up to 18 months.

WORD OF WARNING

PRP therapy can only be carried out by a medical professional such as an aesthetic doctor, nurse, dentist or surgeon with a current registration with the GMC, GDC or NMC.

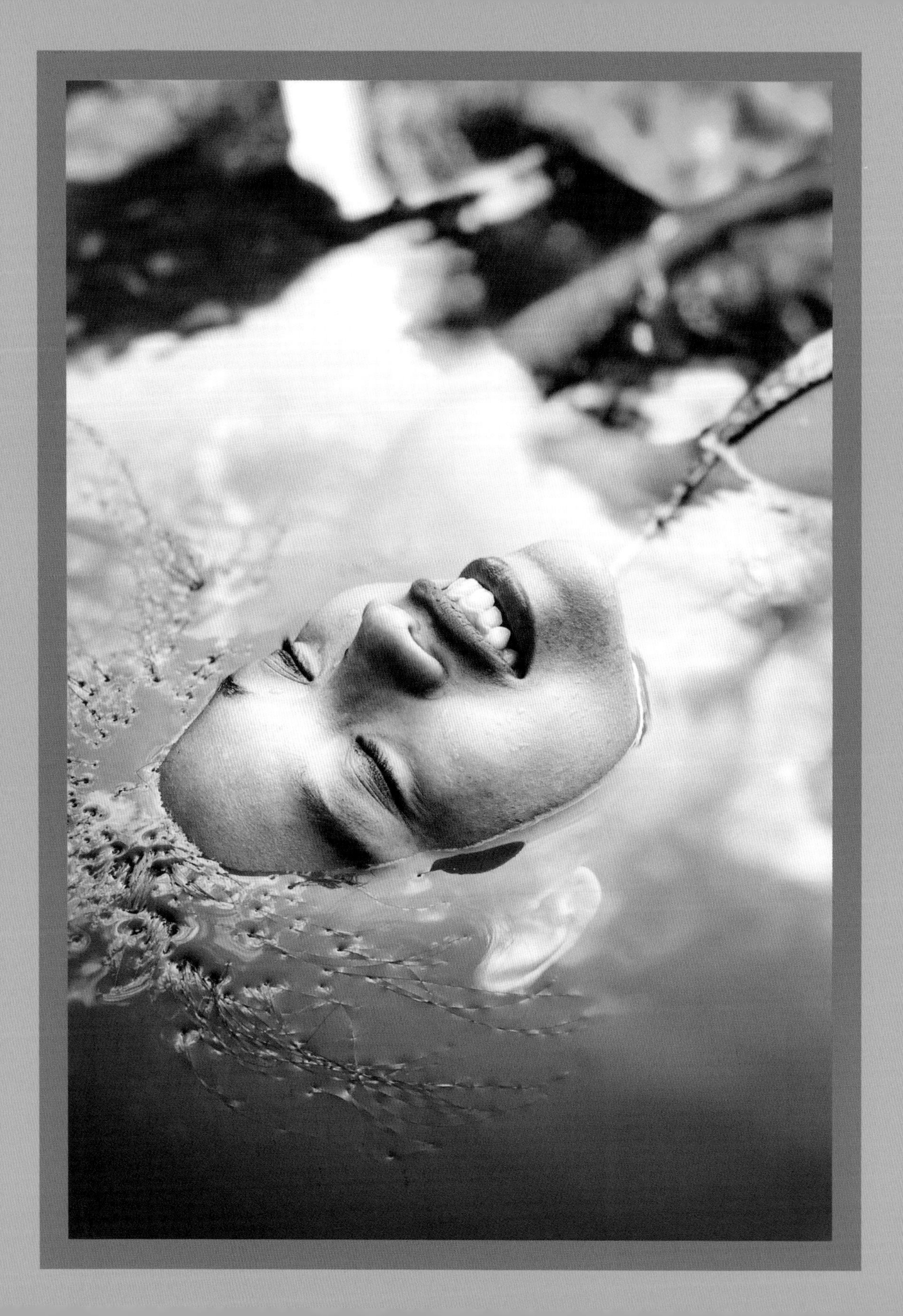

profhilo

If your skin needs deep moisture – if either you have naturally dry skin or hormonal fluxes like the menopause are causing you to feel intense dryness – Profhilo will be a game-changer for you. Even if you are neither of the above, Profhilo will give you an intense radiance boost like no other. It is, literally, the equivalent of injecting moisturiser into your skin. Even though it uses hyaluronic acid, this a next-level, super-stabilised version that is designed to last for longer in the skin and stimulate four different kinds of collagen and elastin. The effects are a marked improvement in skin quality, tightening and lifting underlying muscles, and smoothing wrinkles and lines.

Psst... Not the prettiest treatment

The treatment can look unsightly because you're left with 5 bumps of solution on either side of your face that slowly melt into the skin over 12 hours. Your Profhilo day may not be the day you also want to have public meetings. I have given you fair warning!

A full treatment consists of 2 sessions, a month apart, and an additional session may be recommended after approximately 6 months in order to prolong the effect. In total, there's 10 injection sites and from them the solution slowly spreads underneath the surface of the skin. You have the option to use numbing cream to reduce discomfort from the injections, but don't let that put you off! What I like about Profhilo is that it has no competition and doesn't replace another procedure. It is a well-behaved child that gets on with everyone, but it is not an excuse not to look after your skin using good skincare. You still have to do that!

Results should last for around 6 months. Remember, it is an injection, and only qualified medical professionals can give injections. Ask for proof of qualification if necessary.

Spot Extractions

Extractions are best left to professionals. That will always be my advice, but you and I both know advice is take-it-or-leave-it, especially in the face of a juicy, come-to-mama kind of spot. No matter how much I say do not pop your spots at home, there will always be someone who does and in doing so will leave dark marks on their skin that they sheepishly confess to at their next appointment. Sigh! So I figure if you're going to go at your spots at home, I may as well give you my all-time failsafe tips on how to do it properly and minimise any potential damage.

First things first, it has to be a ripe spot; it cannot be one that is still under the skin without a head. If that's the case forget it, otherwise you will injure your skin trying to force the blockage out and definitely get a black mark for your efforts.

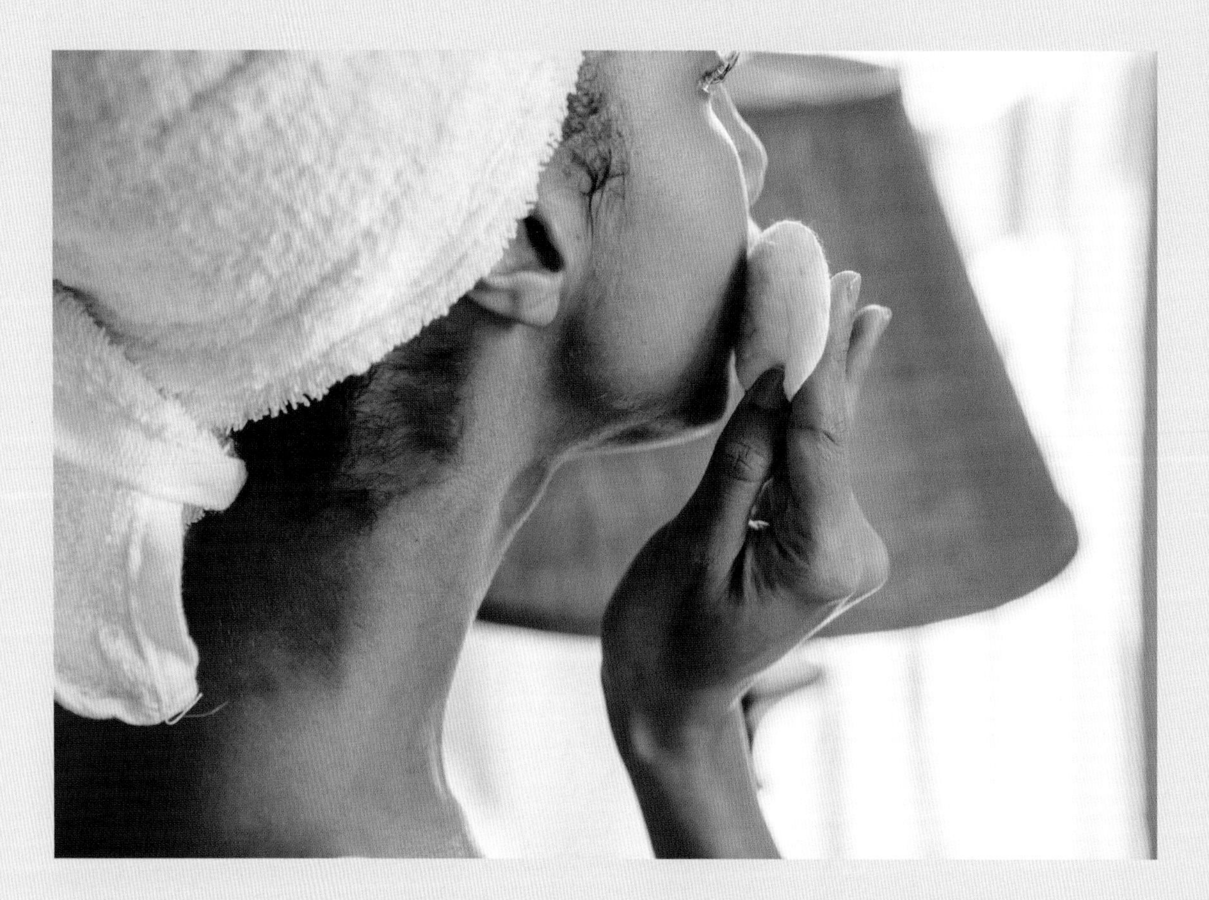

Things you will need:

Clean skin and clean hands so you don't introduce more dirt and bacteria to the area.

A small facial steamer will be handy.

Facial oil.

Clay mask.

Cotton pads or clean tissues. Don't be tempted to play amateur aesthetician by using the metal implements you can find online. Used incorrectly, they can seriously damage your skin, risking post-inflammatory hyperpigmentation, tissue and capillary damage.

Salicylic acid toner or exfoliating pad.

Spot treatment gel.

Micro plaster (optional).

1. Put the steamer on and let it waft in your face whilst you wash your face. This will gently warm and soften your skin to loosen blackheads and congestion in your pores.

2. After this, I like to massage the skin with a light facial oil to encourage the spot to rise to the surface. The aim is to push the congestion as close to the surface of the skin as possible because when you pop the spot, you want to get everything out.

3. Apply some clay mask on top of the spot to further tease out the congestion. Remove after 5 minutes.

4. Using the cotton pads, firmly press down and under the spot. It should literally erupt but you may have to wiggle your fingers to gently ease the congestion out. You should hear a rather satisfying plop as the gunk comes out or, if you're very lucky, you'll get a 'shoot and splatter' against your mirror!

5. Once out, use a clean cotton pad (preferably soaked in a salicylic acid toner, or an exfoliating pad, to cleanse the area. Dot a blob of spot treatment gel on top. The antibacterial properties will disinfect and stop the spread of bacteria.

6. If you are a fiddler and will keep touching the area, put a micro plaster over the top to protect the area from pesky fingers and give it time to heal.

7. The way melanin is set up in Black skin, it's likely that a dark mark will develop when you pop a spot, but by doing it like this, you will lessen the likelihood of this happening. And if you do get a dark spot, you've treated the skin so well it will fade quickly. Apply lashings of your pigmentation serum and massage it into the area to speed up healing and improve skin clarity.

injectable treatments

There are two types of injectable treatments – neurotoxins and fillers. Both are used to make small and usually temporary changes and enhancements to the face, skin and body. Whilst I don't personally administer injectable treatments, this is a topic that comes up quite a lot in consultations, especially as there comes a time when creams and potions won't be able to restore volume or smoothness lost through ageing. Also, sometimes, regardless of age, we can be unhappy with aspects of our appearance and want to be able to make small tweaks here and there. This is where injectables are really handy.

In my experience, Black women have always shied away from injectables, for plenty of understandable reasons: expense, lack of representation and knowledge about procedures, stigma, and fear and mistrust of the aesthetics industry. Up until the last 5 years, many brands didn't even feature Black women in their advertising, so injectables haven't been a procedure intentionally marketed to the Black community.

I know for sure that Black women are curious about tweakments, and I can see light bulbs go off when I talk about procedures that I've had. I love that I'm able to bring Black women into a conversation and a world that many assumed was closed off to them.

Psst... Beware of man-sized prices

Some clinics add a surcharge of between £25 and £50 for men, because they have stronger facial muscles and need bigger doses.

Neurotoxins

Sounds awful, doesn't it? But I assure you it's not. In essence, neurotoxins are made up of proteins that help to relax and temporarily paralyse your facial muscles so that lines and wrinkles are softened. The effects last for anything between 4 and 6 months and the most common places neurotoxins are injected are where muscles get scrunched up – your number 11s, which are the vertical frown lines between the eyebrows, forehead lines, crow's feet and smile lines. Botox is the most popular brand by far, but there are many others such as Dysport, Jeuveau and Xeomin. The costs vary depending on where you are based, but expect to pay anything from £250 upwards.

I have a particularly expressive forehead, which I've made less mobile with a few sprinkles of Botox.

FACT Baby treatments, sprinkles, droplets, micro-dosing, dusting – what are these terms? The lite, or as I like to joke, the low-fat version of a treatment. These are great when you are new and nervous to cosmetic treatments and I always advise my clients to take these sort of baby steps. Just be mindful that the effects won't last as long as the full-fat treatment, and you may not be able to see the full effects. Nevertheless, it's enough to give you an idea of whether you would like the treatment and what it may possibly look like.

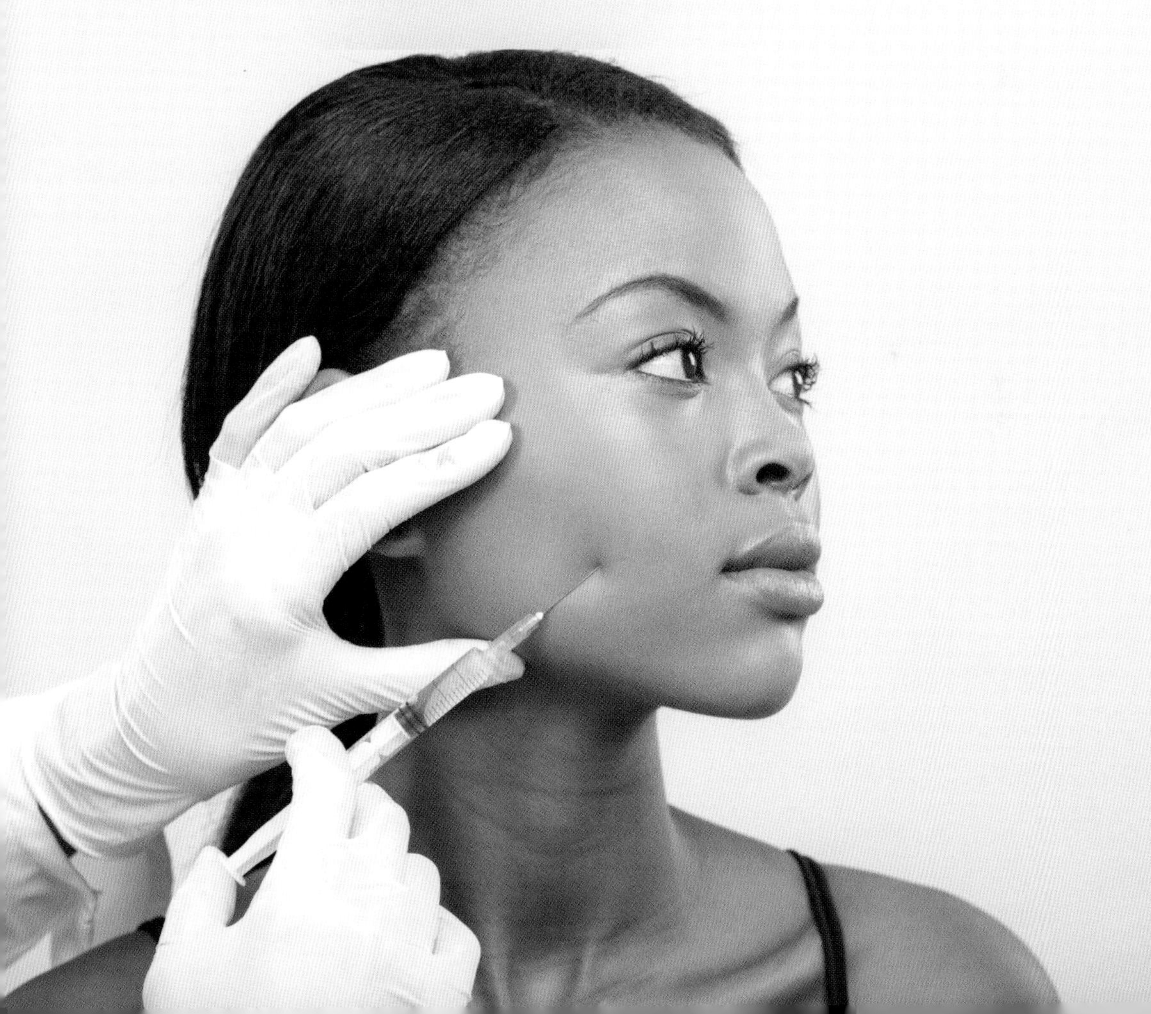

Fillers

I am also partial to a sprinkle of filler here and there and I love the rejuvenating effect they have on my skin, especially now that I'm starting to see the slow decline of collagen.

Fillers are made of gel-type substances that are injected just below the surface of the skin to replace volume, improve the smoothness and tautness, and to plump out lines and wrinkles. You can also use them to shape the face with new contours. Think sharper jawline, straighter nose, higher cheekbones, fuller lips and re-plumping the hollow area under the eyes. It is all temporary, of course, but depending on the filler and the purpose you can go anything from 6 months to 2 years before needing a top-up.

Most fillers are typically made from a variation of hyaluronic acid and, as explained in previous chapters, is a natural substance already found in the body. Popular brands are Juvederm and Restylane, which are reversible so if for any reason you don't like the results they can be removed. Fillers like Sculptra tend to last a little longer and have the added benefit of encouraging your body to produce new collagen. Radiesse is a non-reversible filler that can be used for face and hands.

Once injected, some fillers help your skin produce more of its own natural hyaluronic acid. Talk about buy one, get one free!

Psst... Lip fillers

Black people genetically tend to have fuller lips and shy away from lip fillers, but apart from increasing the size of your lips, fillers do so much more. They smooth lip lines and wrinkles, hydrate and moisturise, give more definition, and can help improve the position of your lips.

It goes without saying that injectables should only be administered by doctors or nurses because, God forbid, if anything goes wrong or there is a complication, they know how to immediately deal with it.

It's always worth finding out how much experience the practitioner has had treating Black skin, because that will make the difference to both how you experience the treatment and your end result.

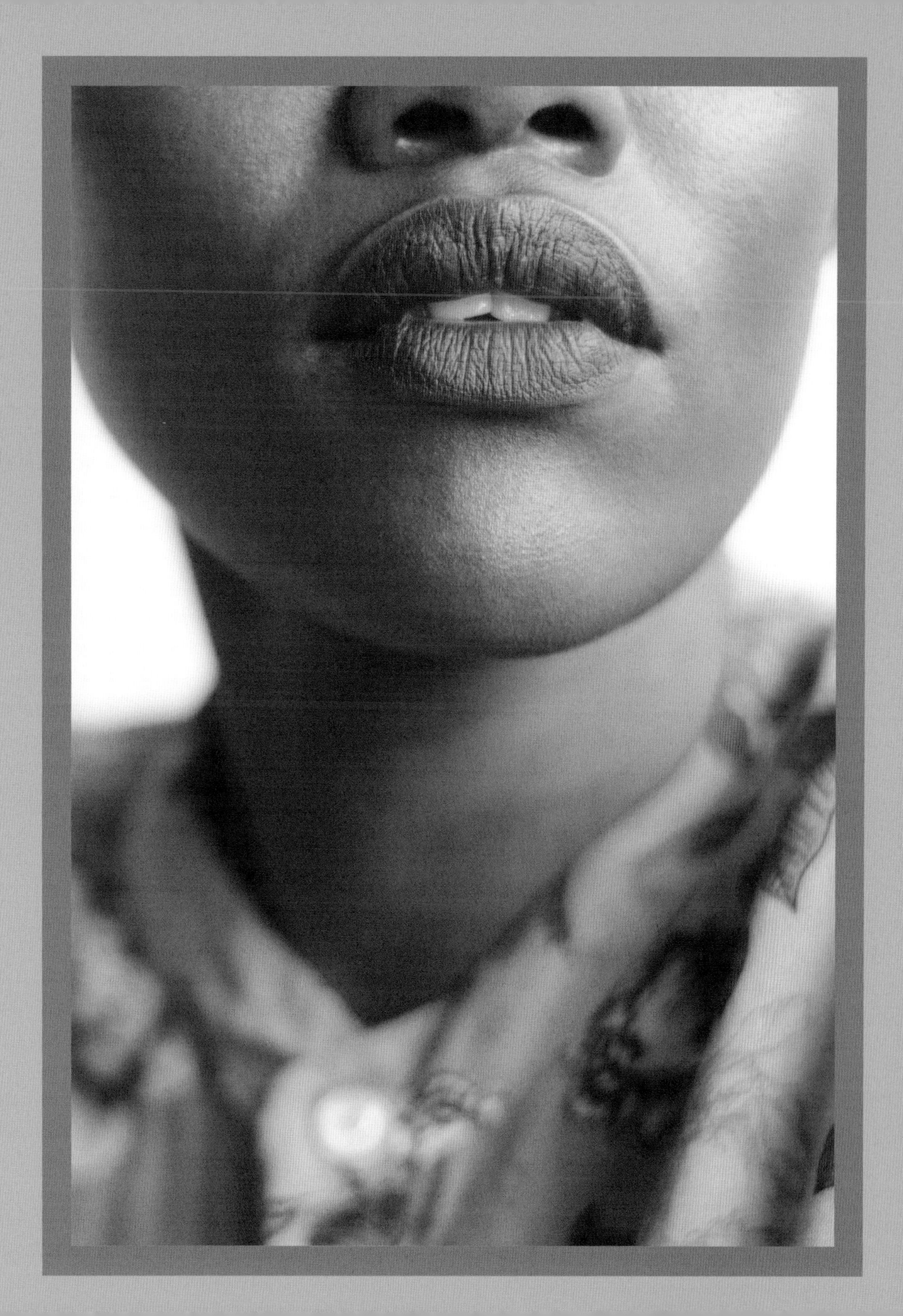

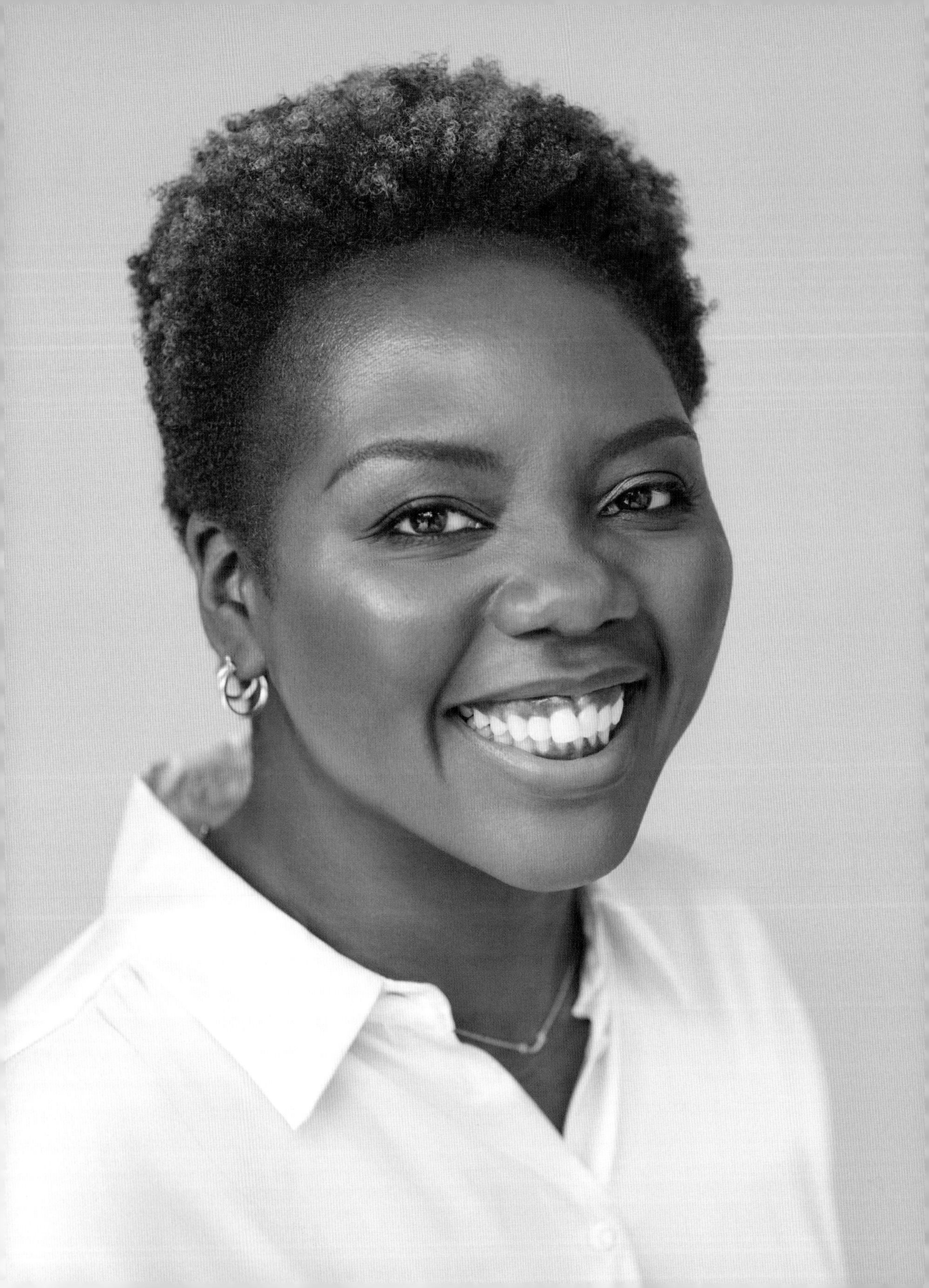

16. final words

final words

WOW! If you didn't appreciate your skin before, I bet you do now! Black skin signifies so much and shows itself to be truly resilient; to you as an individual but also as a collective to the world, Black skin tells a story.

I hope that you have learned some new truths about your skin: what it does, how it protects you and, in turn, how you can look after it by using the right products, ingredients, treatments and techniques to keep it in its healthiest condition. There are plenty of skincare options available for our skin and we have nothing to be afraid of.

Whilst your skin may be strong in more ways than one, it is also sensitive – so be kind to it. Don't for one minute think that melanin gives you a get-out-of-jail-free card if you abuse your skin. In many respects, melanin will make your skin even more sensitive to the daily knocks and tribulations of life.

I hope through the historical look back you have been able to gain a deeper perspective of how you interact with beauty and the beauty industry, and I hope non-Black readers are able to see the vital role they can play in helping Black women to catch up by advocating change on our behalf. I really want girls the same age as my daughter to grow up fully knowing about their skincare options, knowing they are beautiful and valuable, and celebrating their uniqueness alongside their peers. It is up to all of us to see to it that this dream comes true.

All it remains for me to do is to leave you with my own personal skin rules.

For skin that remains in its best possible health all of your days, keeping and protecting all that is within:

Seek bespoke professional advice and treatments where necessary. This is the only way you can ensure you get the best for your skin without potentially causing damage that can result in discolouration and hyperpigmentation.

Be patient with your skin. It is dynamic, changing month to month, season to season. Follow the changes to keep your skin and mental health intact.

Don't treat your skin aggressively. Avoid harsh treatments and products, as 'high strength' or pain doesn't mean benefits for your skin health.

Foster a healthy dose of realism and try to keep expectations in check. Patience, consistency and concealer are good things to have. It can take a few months to see positive changes in your skin health, so hang in there.

Wear sunscreen. It is the cheapest and easiest way to keep your skin healthy and beautiful. Really.

Good luck, and wishing you all the best in your skin health journey!

Dija x

references

[1] [new] B. Barankin and J. DeKoven (2002), 'Psychosocial effect of common skin diseases,' *Canadian Family Physician*, 48, 712–16

[2] Scott Oldenburg (2001), 'The riddle of Blackness in England's national family romance,' *Journal for Early Modern Cultural Studies*, 1 (1), 46–62, www.jstor.org/stable/40339499

[3] David Olusoga, *Black and British: A Forgotten History*. London: Macmillan, 2016

[4] http://banmarchive.org.uk/collections/newformations/03_33.pdf

[5] Textbook of the Madam C. J. Walker Schools of Beauty Culture

[6] https://npg.si.edu/exh/noir/broch3.htm

[7] Neelam A. Vashi et al. (2016), 'Aging differences in ethnic skin,' *Journal of Clinical and Aesthetic Dermatology*, 9 (1), 31-8, https://www.ncbi.nlm.nih.gov/pmc/articles/PMC4756870/#B29

[8] Alpana K. Gupta et al. (2016), 'Skin cancer concerns in people of color: risk factors and prevention,' *Asian Pacific Journal of Cancer Prevention*, 17 (12), 5257–64, https://www.ncbi.nlm.nih.gov/pmc/articles/PMC5454668/

[9] G. La Ruche and J. P. Cesarini (1992), 'Histologie et physiologie de la peau noire [Histology and physiology of black skin],' *Ann. Dermatol. Venereol.*, 119 (8), 567–74, https://pubmed.ncbi.nlm.nih.gov/1485761/

[10] A. V. Rawlings (2006), 'Ethnic skin types: are there differences in skin structure and function?' *Int. J. Cosmet. Sci.*, 28 (2), 79–93, https://pubmed.ncbi.nlm.nih.gov/18492142/.

[11] K. C. Allah et al. (2013), Cicatrices chéloïdes sur peau noire: mythe ou réalité [Keloid scars on black skin: myth or reality],' *Ann. Chir. Plast. Esthet.*, 58 (2), 115–22, https://pubmed.ncbi.nlm.nih.gov/22542368/

[12] Derrick C. Wan et al. (2014), 'Moisturizing different racial skin types,' *Journal of Clinical and Aesthetic Dermatology*, 7 (6), 25–32, https://www.ncbi.nlm.nih.gov/pmc/articles/PMC4086530/

[13] Alexis B. Lyons et al. (2019), 'Circadian rhythm and the skin: a review of the literature,' *Journal of Clinical and Aesthetic Dermatology*, 12 (9), 42–5, https://www.ncbi.nlm.nih.gov/pmc/articles/PMC6777699/

[14] Won Yen-Kim et al. (2014), 'Clinical efficacy and safety of 4-hexyl-1, 3-phenylenediol for improving skin hyperpigmentation,' *Archives of Dermatological Research*, 306 (5), 455–65.

[15] Cordain L, Lindeberg S, Hurtado M, Hill K, Eaton SB, Brand-Miller J. Acne Vulgaris: A Disease of Western Civilization. Arch Dermatol. 2002;138(12):1584–1590 doi:10.1001/archderm.138.12.1584

[16] P. U. Giacomoni, et al. (2009), 'Gender-linked differences in human skin,' *Journal of Dermatological Science*, 55, 144–9

[17] U. Jacobi et al. (2005), 'Gender-related differences in the physiology of the stratum corneum,' *Dermatology*, 211 (4), 312–17

[18] https://www.dermascope.com/treatments/the-physiological-effects-of-microcurrent

[19] A. P. Kelly and S. C. Taylor, *Dermatology for Skin of Color*. New York: McGraw-Hill, 2009

[20] Cheng, et al. (1982) 'The Effects of Electric Current on ATP Generation, Protein Synthesis, and Membrane Transport in Rat Skin' Clinical Orthopaedics and Related Research,(171), 264 - 72

index

U–Z

thank you

My A-Team: Hammed, Amariah and Abraham. Gang-gang, we full ground. One of one special edition, I do it all for you.

The matriarchs: Ya Alimamy, Ms Bangura, Mrs Koroma, Mrs Ayodele Snr, Memuna and Yalamba, I am sharp and switched on because of you. My brother Abdul, all shade and all love. Dad, I was 8 when you told me I had a way with words, I've never forgotten. I wish you were here.

The entire HQ team: Nira Begum, I guess if I'm writing this we got the magical land of 'there'! Lol! Lisa Milton, Lucy Richardson, Vickie Watson, Katrina Smedley, thank you for giving me space. Emily Voller, Haya Junaid and Micallar Walker, you rock! Kate Fox, you will always have my gratitude.

My inner circle: Deborah Johnson, Tom Wright, Etta Martin, thank you for always challenging me to be better. You're doing the Lord's work. Bev James, I love your quiet presence. Thank you. Ruvimbo Kuuzabuwe and Nateisha Scott, you always understand the assignment.

My cheerleaders: Karen Tippett, Tosin Jegede, Toyin Oluwanisola, Halima Bepo, Tomilola Adu, Ronke Oke , Jess Ratcliffe and Dr Ifeoma Ejikeme. My clients who took a vested interest in this book especially Ola, Shakira, Nneoma, Kishan, Aline and Antonia. Marylebone Massive: Joanna and IreAyo, we do big things! Thank you Emiola Oke, I will never forget your help. My therapist, Mr O, thank you for always holding a mirror up.

My beauty industry family who gives me soft spaces to land especially Caroline Hirons, Andy Millward, Alexandra Forbes, Lisa Potter-Dixon, Lesley Blair, Mary Sommerlad, Lorna Bowes, Millie Kendall MBE, Emma Bracey-Wright and Alice Hart-Davis.

My journalist friends who have supported my endeavours tirelessly to advocate for the needs of Black skin. Shout out to Claire Coleman, Sarah Jossel, Deborah Joseph, Donna Dia, Shannon Peters, Sonia Haria, Jacqueline Kilikita, Irene Shelly, Sali Hughes, Joy Joses, Chloe Gronow, Shannon Kilgariff , Twiggy Jalloh and Georgia Seago.

My glam team: Stacy Wodu, Shada Jenkins, Subrina Kidd, Debbie Thomas, Dr Joanna Christou, Sara at VCC Nails, Tinu Bello, Gina Knight, Andrée Marie, Abisoye Odugbesan, Calvin Da-Silva, Elisabeth Hoff, Christopher Oakman and John Godwin for saving me at the last minute!

My Insta-fam, far and wide, your support means the world. I will always be grateful.

Thank you to all the beauty brands I've worked with over the years, your support of me and *Black Skin* is much appreciated.

And finally, to Black women, I thank you for your sisterhood.